Psychotherapy of the Combat Veteran

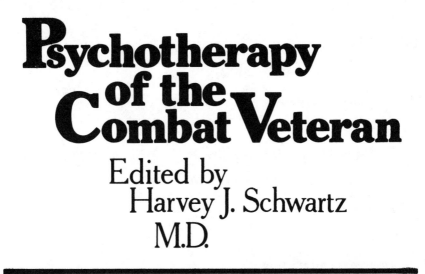

Psychotherapy of the Combat Veteran

Edited by
Harvey J. Schwartz
M.D.

Department of Psychiatry and Human Behavior

Jefferson Medical College

Philadelphia, Pennsylvania

SP

SP MEDICAL & SCIENTIFIC BOOKS
a division of Spectrum Publications, Inc.
New York

SPECTRUM PUBLICATIONS, INC.
175-20 Wexford Terrace
Jamaica, NY 11432

Library of Congress Cataloging in Publication Data
Main entry under title:

Psychotherapy of the combat veteran.

  Bibliography: p.
  Includes index.
  1. War neuroses—Addresses, essays, lectures.
2. Veterans—Mental health services—Addresses, essays,
lectures. 3. Vietnamese Conflict, 1961–1975—Psychological aspects—Addresses, essays, lectures. I. Schwartz,
Harvey J. [DNLM: 1. Military psychiatry. 2. Combat
disorders. 3. Stress disorders, Post-traumatic—Therapy.
4. Psychotherapy—Methods. WM 184 P974]
RC550.P78 1984   616.85'21206   83-23022

ISBN: 0-89335-200-4

Printed in the United States of America

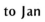

Contributors

D. Wilfred Abse, M.D. • Clinical Professor of Psychiatry, University of Virginia, Charlottesville, Virginia; Director of Psychiatric Education, St. Albans Psychiatric Hospital, Radford, Virginia; Teaching Psychoanalyst, Washington Psychoanalytic Institute

Robert Blitz, Ph.D. • Psychology Technician, Psychiatric Research Section, VA Outpatient Clinic, Boston, Massachusetts

Immanuel Cohen, M.D. • Head, Mental Health Branch, Israel Defense Army, 1976-1980

Richard B. Cornfield, M.D. • Clinical Assistant Professor of Psychiatry, University of Pennsylvania School of Medicine, Philadelphia, Pennsylvania; Attending Psychiatrist, The Institute of Pennsylvania Hospital, Philadelphia, Pennsylvania; Candidate, Philadelphia Association for Psychoanalysis

Victor J. DeFazio, Ph.D. • Associate Professor of Student Personal Services, Director of Veterans Services, Psychotherapy Supervisor, Queensborough Community College, City University of New York; Consultant to the Vietnam Veteran Outreach Centers, New York; Candidate, New York University Postdoctoral Program in Psychotherapy and Psychoanalysis

Ramon Greenberg, M.D. • Professor of Psychiatry, Boston University School of Medicine, Boston, Massachusetts; Faculty Member, Boston Psychoanalytic Institute

John A. McKinnon, M.D. • Assistant Professor, Department of Psychiatry, University of California, San Francisco, California; Chief, Mental Hygiene Clinic, San Francisco VA Medical Center

Rafael Moses, M.D. • Visiting Professor of Psychiatry, Hebrew University, Jerusalem, Israel; Supervising and Training Psychoanalyst, Israel Psychoanalytic Institute

Erwin Randolph Parson, Ph.D. • Assistant Clinical Professor of Psychology, Institute of Advanced Psychological Studies, Adelphi University, New York; Regional Outreach Manager, Northeastern Region, Vietnam Veteran Outreach Centers; Member of Adelphi Society of Psychoanalysis

Harvey J. Schwartz, M.D. • Director of Residency Training, Clinical Assistant Professor of Psychiatry and Human Behavior, Thomas Jefferson University, Philadelphia, Pennsylvania; Attending Psychiatrist, Coatesville-Jefferson VA Outpatient Clinic, Philadelphia, Pennsylvania

Robert B. Shapiro, Ph.D. • Supervisor of Psychotherapy, Columbia University, New York; Visiting Faculty, Postgraduate Center for Mental Health, New York; Supervising Psychoanalyst, Faculty Member, William A. White Psychoanalytic Institute

Contents

Contributors   vii

Introduction: An Overview of the Psychoanalytic Approach
to the War Neuroses   xi
      Harvey J. Schwartz, M.D.

Acknowledgments   xxix

1   Brief Historical Overview of the Concept of War Neurosis
    and of Associated Treatment Methods   1
      D. Wilfred Abse, M.D.

2   Psychoanalytic Psychotherapy and the Vietnam Veteran   23
      Victor J. DeFazio, Ph.D.

3   Unconscious Guilt: Its Origin, Manifestations, and
    Treatment in the Combat Veteran   47
      Harvey J. Schwartz, M.D.

4   Transference, Countertransference, and the
    Vietnam Veteran   85
      Robert B. Shapiro, Ph.D.

5   Nightmares of the Traumatic Neuroses: Implications
    for Theory and Treatment   103
      Robert Blitz, Ph.D. and Ramon Greenberg, M.D.

6   Brief Psychotherapy of the Vietnam Combat Neuroses   125
      John A. McKinnon, M.D.

7   The Role of Psychodynamic Group Therapy in the
    Treatment of the Combat Veteran   153
        Erwin Randolph Parson, Ph.D.

8   Traumatic War Neuroses: Some Pharmacologic and
    Psychophysiologic Observations   221
        Richard B. Cornfield, M.D.

9   Fear of the Dead: The Role of Social Ritual in
    Neutralizing Fantasies from Combat   253
        Harvey J. Schwartz, M.D.

10 Understanding and Treatment of Combat Neurosis:
    The Israeli Experience   269
        Rafael Moses, M.D. and Immanuel Cohen, M.D.

    Index   305

Introduction

AN OVERVIEW OF THE
PSYCHOANALYTIC APPROACH
TO THE WAR NEUROSES

The survivors of traumatic events have long been known to suffer psychological sequelae. Of all possible stressors, combat is one of the most devastating. Wartime exposes its victim to a myriad of stimuli that are far beyond those of civilized life. The impact that remains can affect generations to come.

In recent years there has been a paucity of research on the long-term effects of battle. Particularly after the recent war there was initially an inclination to minimize the psychological impact of combat. It was only after concerted effort by a few dedicated clinicians that formal recognition was granted to the current version of the war neuroses. In the parlance of the day it was called the Post-traumatic Stress Disorder (Figley, 1978).

This phenomenologic diagnosis has been instrumental in bringing the necessary attention to this condition. Its applicability has been tested across a wide range of stressors, from man-made to natural. Few workers in the field now doubt the power of traumatic events to leave a profound impression on the victim. Contrary to previous thought, it has now been found that this imprint often becomes a chronic scar.

Having established the existence of the syndrome, the next step is to investigate its inner workings. This leads us to study the individual psychological make-up of each patient, and ultimately to the unconscious. This journey is of course not new. Freud elaborated the conceptual possibility and the technical means to understand the unique inner-life within each person. He revealed the therapeutic power in metaphoric listening, transference reenactment, and unconscious reconstruction. As has been amply demonstrated by clinicians through the years, these skills are no less essential in treating victims of external trauma. This is due to the fact that the chronically disabled victim of battle has not only been overstimulated by stress he has also had his internal fantasy system altered. This volume is intended to reintroduce these fundamental dynamic notions of psychological functioning to the work with trauma victims.

The contributors to this book have studied the unconscious processes of their stressed patients. As you will see, some of their findings reaffirm the value of the traditional approach to treatment. This is in and of itself a major contribution. For too long these patients have been relegated to supportive counseling when more depth work was actually required. Although full analysis may not be possible or advisable, skillful adherence to the derivative principles of psychoanalytic psychotherapy is generally indicated. For many possible reasons clinicians have not been using tried and true methods of treating these patients. The guidelines offered here should help reinforce the usefulness of our basic concepts.

While remaining grounded in the basic paradigm of transference, countertransference, resistance, and working-through, we have had on occasion to widen our theory and technique. This parallels and draws upon the broader research into "parameters" that has occurred in recent years within psychoanalysis and psychotherapy in general. Insights into early infant development, maternal stimulus regulation, regression, and primitive transference states have been the basic science of our clinical modifications. Being relatively new areas of study, the conclusions drawn in this volume are varied. Many of the ideas presented will be controversial. They are not intended as the final word. They are designed to engage the clinical community in the dialogue of learning that will enrich our understanding of this condition. This will bring us closer to our goal of alleviating the suffering of some of the victims of the terrible man-made trauma that is war.

CASE EXAMPLE

A 30-year-old man was referred for treatment. He found himself in difficult straits and did not know how he got there nor how to get out. He was engaged in an extramarital affair that was not at all satisfying. Yet he felt helpless to break it off and return to his wife from whom he was recently separated. Efforts at marital and supportive counseling were to no avail and he continued his compulsive behavior. He was on a path of self-destruction and could not stop.

The patient's history revealed that his extramarital affair began soon after his younger brother became seriously ill. Additionally, lifelong conflicts with his intermittently depressed mother and distant father were the fertile soil for his reawakened neurosis. Within the marriage, idealization of his wife led to passionless sexual activity and defensive self-blame. The patient was a Marine in Vietnam 12 years earlier, but saw minimal combat and suffered from no post-traumatic symptomology. My impression was of a man suffering from a not atypical neurotic conflict. Clues to latent themes suggested oedipal level pathology.

Treatment was begun. In the initial phase I noted somewhat greater than usual resistances to the free associative process. These took the form of an authoritarian transference and some concreteness. While I expected such a reaction given his obsessive character, we had great difficulty working through it. He evaded the therapeutic regression through many means including a defensive identification with me. Within that phase he ended his affair and returned to his wife. Still, he could not bring in his associations.

From the beginning of treatment, he would often lapse into a bitter state and proclaim his wish not to come to the sessions. His associations suggested a punitive father transference, towards whom he experienced both submissive and competitive urges. However, I was unable to meaningfully work with him around these issues even in their derivative form. At that time all I could do to sustain the treatment was to draw upon his nascent curiosity about himself. I also listened carefully to the details of his protests. Again and again he would complain, "I don't want to be here—I'm only here because you tell me to!" These exclamations were interlaced with long periods of rebellious silence, blank withdrawal and physical discomfort. We were at a standstill.

Ever so gradually the word *Vietnam* entered his verbalizations. A dream here, a memory there. In the piecemeal fashion so characteristic of the associative process, a theme slowly emerged from seemingly desperate images. A passing reference to the hot weather would lead to his remarking on his irritability when it rained. Discomfort with humidity would elaborate jungle imagery. Sensitized by my work with grossly ill combat veterans, the threads of his past coalesced into a meaningful whole.

Again he protested, "I can't stand being here—but you won't let me leave!" I finally asked him if that was how he felt in Vietnam. The door was opened. Not to a floodgate of affects, for this was a functioning obsessive, but to powerful memories from the war. In the transference I was the commander who physically abused him and forced him to stay in Vietnam against his will. I was to learn about his heretofore never spoken of overseas history. This included rage outbursts at officers, terror-filled nights of bombardment, and conflicted feelings of sympathy and sadism toward the war victims. Repeatedly he would relive these states within the transference. As painful as this was for him, it spared him from remembering. It was only with persistent work that we were able to bring to consciousness his warded-off reactions to male authority figures. He was struggling against his passive cravings for love as well as his rage toward me, his Marine commander, and his father. His deep conviction that the transference relationship was infantalizing and humiliating was derived from the perceived sadomasochistic relationship with his father. Aspects of this reality-fantasy amalgam were acted out in his Marine training and wartime experiences.

While our work did inevitably lead to the release of strangulated affects, it was a good deal more complex than that. It involved analysis of intricate drive-defense compromise formations. War was not solely a generic traumatic overload, but was also a stimulus to specific long repressed drive derivatives. The unconscious guilt he suffered, a prominent aspect of his current self-destruction, was partly a result of infantile fantasies being acted out in boot camp and battle. This conflicted past was interweaved with and reawakened by his renewed aggression and guilt toward his sick brother.

I learned a great deal from treating this man. He is not the typical overwhelmed trauma victim. While our work did reveal acute post-stress acting out, in the form of a brief and masochistic postwar marriage, he was never immobilized by the classical symptomatology. I therefore assumed that there were no residua of the war and that it was not a significant contributor to his present difficulties. My error was to underestimate the psyches' reaction to trauma. It is never not there. It merely lies dormant and encapsulated, sealed in by deep character-deforming defenses. This masking process drains energy from the creative potential of each person. The passage of time by itself does little to reclaim that lost bit of life. However, when the defensive structure is exposed to a treatment modality that peels away layer upon layer of resistance, the traumatic past is reexperienced. There is then the unique opportunity to rework the original solution. The old compromises, derived from the infantile history, can give way to more realistic and life-affirming adaptations. The guilt, the fear, and the aggression can all be reexperienced through the transference. Not only does this allow the adult ego to observe and mourn the past at its own tolerable pace, but it does this in a new context.

The traumatic history is now reenacted in the context of an "auxiliary object": one that is accepting of regressive tendencies, protective of overstimulation, and devoted to progressive adaptation. This therapeutic condition derives from the traditional stance of empathic neutrality. This "holding," when a product of the doctor's genuine unconscious acceptance of the patient, creates a reparative environment that uniquely permits the safe recovery of drive organized (transference) fantasies. The deep commitment to the patient's healing is essential in treating those who have suffered massive trauma.

To focus on the intrapsychic impact of adult trauma, as this volume does, will strike some as a misguided effort. There is a point of view that sees any adult stress as deriving pathogenic power *only* from its infantile meaning. Posttraumatic disability is understood to result from a reawakened infantile neurosis or psychosis. Present day stress is studied strictly for its symbolic value. The affectual material from adult trauma is seen solely as a derivative of deeper childhood traumas, and is considered by some merely to be a resistance to the earlier experiences. This perspective is well stated by Brenner (1953): "It seems likely that an external stimulus creates neurotic anxiety rather because of its relationship to the unconscious conflicts of the individual it affects, than because of its psychological intensity."

On the other hand, there are those who study posttraumatic disorders and see them strictly as a psychobiological response to stress. They point to the similarities in symptoms across a wide range of populations and stressors. They note the stereotyped nightmares and conclude that this is a simple cause-and-effect relationship involving autonomic overactivity, REM overstimulation, and learned behavior. They see no need for concepts of latent meaning, childhood neuroses, or unconscious conflict. Many go further and declare that any effort to look at an individual's childhood is done to avoid the present. Additionally, such digging up the past is seen as an attempt at blaming the victim for his disability.

In my view these are two polarized perspectives. The first approach fails to appreciate *any* generic power of overwhelming trauma to disrupt psychic functioning. Regression, the inevitable response to massive stress, can in and of itself lead to altered ego (and superego) functioning. To claim that all regression derives from infantile predisposition is, I believe, to misunderstand the organism as a physiologic entity whose primary motive is survival.

On the other hand, to state that patients' emotional conflicts begin only at the moment of trauma and that they bring none of their past distortions to that event is, I believe, to be naive about psychological functioning. Stressful events can only be perceived through the veil of everyday parapraxes. To totally disregard the fantasies that are stimulated by a stressor is to further traumatize the patient. A strictly behavioral concept of stress response has the potential to reinforce the primitive and concrete perceptual apparatus that the patient has regressed to. As well, the notion of blame being associated with genetic uncovering is disturbing and suggests a significant, but unfortunately not infrequent, misunderstanding about developmental vulnerabilities and analytic exploration.

The abbreviated patient vignette I mentioned earlier is a good example of a common clinical situation. To see the patient's sense of me as deriving only from his actual humiliating relationship with his commander is to fail to appreciate the extent to which it was perceived through his earlier real and fantasied relations with his father. On the other hand, to see it solely as an aspect of the erotized father transference is to miss the importance of his disturbing and unintegrated war experiences.

A "bifocal" therapeutic perspective is essential. This is nothing new. We often view intra and extrapsychic forces simultaneously and we try to help the patient learn to do the same. The layering and fluidity of defenses and associations is a usual encounter in our work. At any one moment one theme may be a resistance to a deeper one and vice-versa. Present-past, real-fantasy, shock trauma-screen trauma are always in dynamic flux. Following the unconscious thread that is most meaningful and has the greatest proximity to consciousness is the task with all patients in analytic therapy. With trauma patients, distant childhood memories may be a resistance to terror-filled combat experiences. As well, the gratification in abreaction can be an avoidance of the pain and guilt of the past, as well as a retreat from the future. (At any one moment, these all may serve as a resistance to the transference.)

Simply stated, my experience has led me to believe that we are dealing with a spectrum of pathology. There are those patients who clearly were ripe for stress-induced conflict, and there are those whose matured defenses were overwhelmed by massive trauma. Freud spoke of this concept in his "complementary series" (1917). Jaffe (1968), in a related context regarding posttraumatic symptoms, concludes:

> The pathological attacks are imbued with preconscious imagery, consisting of real and/or fantasied situations. Of course such traumata can become linked associatively with infantile material and thereby receive an affective reinforcement. Such connections could be demonstrated in some of our cases where guilt-feelings were clearly related to infantile conflicts. But infantile conflicts are ubiquitous, and it is presumed here that no psychic illness need have occurred without the subsequent massive traumatization. Freud's concept of the "complementary series" should be remembered in this context according to which subsequent traumata are capable of heavily outweighing adverse constitutional and infantile factors.

In *select* cases it seems that severe and sustained trauma carries a pathogenesis of its own.

For some patients the experience of battle, or indeed any trauma, does become fixed in the unconscious to the extent that it reawakens and crystallizes underlying unconscious conflicts. In these cases, the traumatic event so unconsciously resembles a forbidden wish, or omnipotent punishment, that the superego responds as if, via magical thinking, the patient committed a childhood crime. As the outside world is defensively invested with his own warded-off impulses (a condition exacerbated in a regression-inducing environment), the patient becomes unable to discern where his will ends and fate begins. The ensuing pervasive guilt, often in the form of restitutive self-punishment, is testimony to the ambiguity between internal and external reality. Accordingly, understanding the personal symbolic and genetic meaning of a trauma is essential to freeing the patient from a life of chronic self-blame. The traditional method of making the unconscious conscious, by establishing and working through at least partially an analyzable transference neurosis, will ultimately enable the patient to acknowledge his own impulses and thereby be able to perceive external reality as separate from himself. Through the technique of interpretation across the repression barrier, restimulated drive derivatives can be integrated and unconscious guilt resolved, permitting the patient to meaningfully put the past behind him. With this type of pathology it is mostly the *content* of our interventions that furthers the therapeutic process. I address this level of illness and treatment in Chapter 3.

There is another degree of disturbance that can result from massive stress. This situation differs from the above and demands a qualitatively different treatment form. (In reality these two conditions coexist in varying proportions, but for conceptual purposes it is best to study them separately.)

When the intensity of trauma reaches overwhelming proportions (perhaps a biologically determined point), the ego loses its synthesizing and symbolizing abilities. The issue becomes less the content of the terror than the process of being terrorized. The resulting molecular disorganization of executive functioning heralds a crisis not of isolated inhibition but of psychic integrity. There is a breech in the survival barrier.

With the regression of battle, the advanced forms of development give way to a hypercathexis of primitive survival reflexes. The confidence in physical intactness, the basis for structural maturation (and signal anxiety), is no longer a given. *Actual* abandonment, mutilation, and death are an everpresent reality.

Additionally, the internal parental images that are unconsciously relied upon for safety become helpless before the onslaught of massive terror. The good enough environment is replaced by a life-threatening unpredictability that reawakens the most primitive fears and aggression of the organism. The interpersonal structure that allows for the establishment of basic trust is undermined by a reality that reifies early paranoid preceptions. Niederland (1968) conceptualizes these events as "orally-regressed . . . situations . . . [that foster] . . . regression to archaic and, more specifically, oral incorporative levels."

The childhood model for this level of pathology, and by implication its treatment, has been suggested to be the early mother-child relationship. Anna Freud wrote (1967):

> Potentially, after his first weeks of life, the infant . . . is constantly traumatized, that is, his ego is, at the very beginning of its development, helplessly exposed to overwhelming influences

of the internal and external world. Under normal conditions it is the intervening aid of the mother that comes to his assistance and prevents a real traumatization.

Lorenzer (1968) concludes from the above and from his work with concentration camp victims that extreme stress exposes its victims to "primary traumatization and the structures built up in the early mother-child relationship are annihilated."

Were it not for the possibility (however remote) of repairing this traumatic forced regression, the following thoughts would be academic. However, through the power of the primitive transference (in the broadest sense of the term) that emerges in working with these patients there is reason to hope for some psychological maturation.

This is a most delicate matter and involves subtle forces of unconscious communication, through mutuality of fantasy, between patient and doctor. What often occurs in these situations, after the patient's early resistances to the transference have been worked through, is that the therapist begins to appear to the patient not *as if* he were the dangerous persecuting object, but as the *real* dangerous persecuting object. Accordingly, interpretation of his distortions, and of the usually underlying aggression, is meaningless to the patient for it seems to come from the devil himself. My sense is that at these moments a crucial variable becomes, as Glover put it in 1937, the "true unconscious attitude" of the doctor. As words have lost their therapeutic power we are left with, as Nacht says (1962), not what the therapist says, but who he is.

There is a danger of being heard here as advocating charismatic cures or minimizing the conflictual basis of much of the transference. I mean to do neither. What I simply wish to stress is that for some patients, and for others at some times, the *process* of the analytic relationship becomes decisive in the furtherance of the treatment. The doctor's presence, steadiness, and unconscious resonance are all aspects of this therapeutic coexistence. The physician's holding attitude, the *sublimated countertransference*, and his ability to make that available to the patient in service of progression not resistance, allows for an important new experience. Theoretically, this can be understood as altering, via introjection, the traumatically induced regression that has allied the superego with "the unreconstructed remnants of latent infantile rage" (Erickson, 1950). It can also be conceptualized as minimizing, through external positive supports, the power of the primitive aggression to intrude into the neutralized cathexes that support perceptual integrity, past-present discrimination, and a consistent sense of self.

However, returning to Anna Freud's comments, there is a clarity to viewing this phase of the analytic relationship metaphorically through the mother-infant paradigm and its stages. The affective bonding, the "complimentary regression," the stimulus regulation, the nonpossessive acceptance of clinging and separating, and the satisfaction in mastery all become facilitators of healing. This process can lead to an enhanced self-hold ability, which is the function most often damaged by sustained massive trauma.

Additionally, there is the interesting possibility, and for the many suffering patients the hopeful probability, that there are other arenas within which this healing can occur. To dissect out the nuances of the transference relationship is of course a valuable and necessary enterprise. It does however have serious limitations regarding its applicability to the large number of disabled patients. If we can use the insights garnered from our study of the therapeutic-analytic relationship to deepen our understanding of potentially healing *social forces*, we will have advanced our culture and our own science. It is toward this admittedly grand goal that a part of this volume is devoted. That is, both Chapters 9 and 10 study the role of the "attitude" of society, the larger group morale, to be an accepting, soothing, and repairing force.

HISTORICAL AND INTRAPSYCHIC DEVELOPMENT

Present concepts of treatment draw upon not only the work of Freud, but also on the many lesser known thinkers who lay the groundwork for his ideas. From a broader perspective, it was the complex evolution of Western civilization that brought man to the point where he could acknowledge his inner being and impulses. This self awareness replaced the perogatives of demons and witches. Able to safely observe our own unconscious functioning, we no longer needed to create and fear the devil outside.

Abse, in his chapter, "Brief Historical Overview of the Concept of War Neurosis and of Associated Treatment Methods," traces the intellectual and cultural currents within Western civilization and, in particular, within psychiatry as it progressed from demonology to psychoanalysis. We see the evolution from concrete somatization to self-destructive excoriation to metaphoric symbolization.

This historical backdrop sets the stage for our study of trauma victims. The long cultural tradition of externalizing conflicts resonated with individual tendencies to do the same. The presence of actual external stressors makes introspection and awareness of inner fantasy even more difficult. Self-observation and self-empathy lay beyond the reach of many traumatized patients.

Even given our culture's evident progress, we still contain the tendency to concretize and project. In the clinical situation when the therapist is faced with stress, in the form of the patient's traumatic memories and overwhelming affects, it is difficult to maintain an introspective and intimate presence. An out-growth of this, with its inevitable closing off of empathic contact, was the concept of therapeutic catharsis. While this treatment concept was a significant advance, given its recognition of unconscious functioning, it served to rationalize keeping the patient "out there" with the doctor a sanitized distance from him. Transference and working through were overlooked. As Abse points out, it is important that we fully appreciate the complex role that the doctor-patient relationship plays in treatment. He comments on a facet of this multilayered relationship when he states "his [the doctor's] loving attention to the patient enables them both to face those terrible moments; and this serves to exorcise their lingering traumatic power, while acknowledging their powerful role in shaping what we become." Building on centuries of human development, we can now not only cognitively understand our patients' metaphorical imagery, but can empathically experience it as well. This transient sharing of unconscious fantasy is an additional source for intrapsychic data.

THE RETURN OF EARLY OBJECTS

The existence of "internalized objects" has become an important theoretical and clinical construct in psychoanalysis and psychotherapy. Enriching sometimes incomplete formulations based on pure instinctual conflict, object relations psychology has emphasized the intended recipients of the drives—the early objects. These figures though do more than just receive the infant's impulses; they also metabolize them. The sensitivity of their digestive apparatus and the nutrient value of their breakdown products determines to a great extent whether they will later be perceived as whole or part objects. If they can accept and contain the infant's primitive aggression and feed back an empathic nonintrusive hold, the future bodes well for the child. He will have an inner well-spring of self-soothing that will serve him good stead through the vicissitudes of the oedipus and later life. If the parental figure distorts and magnifies the infant's aggression and projects his own fantasies of magical destructiveness, the infant is left with a seed of malignancy that will inevitably metastasize. The resultant character will contain an internal fragility born of unstructuralized rage and self-annihilatory guilt (more properly, guilt precursor).

It is during periods of trauma and regression that the internal objects are turned to in search of consistency, safety, and self-affirmation. As DeFazio discusses in his chapter, "Psychoanalytic Psychotherapy and the Vietnam Veteran," the stress of war is often the precipitant of this turning inward. For many it is the first time that their genetic programming asserts itself. For some, the traumatic regression initiates what Fairbairn calls (1954), "the return of the bad objects." This becomes part of and itself exacerbates a general contraction of ego functioning. Splitting, debilitating anxiety, and loss of sublimation predominate. Guilt emerges less from actual crimes committed than from a defensive turning against the self to protect the precious good object. The frequency with which many combat veterans reach this "point beyond which regressiveness is never fully reversed" is a tragic and humbling state to witness.

THE CONTENT AND FORM OF TRANSFERENCE

The transference is that ethereal thread to the past that reveals itself through the unique human relationship that is created in the "talking cure." When unraveled, it declares the timeless presence of even the earliest childhood experiences. Through the metaphor that is transference, we come to know the historical events and their interpretation that shape our patients' lives. Patients can free themselves from repeating their history by seeing the past live in the present through the as-if quality of transference.

Psychotherapeutic work with combat veterans teaches us that not only is the distant past relived in the transference, but also the recent traumatic past. We learn that transference presents in ways other than the usual slowly developing illusion. It seems that the regression induced by actual trauma leads to an inability to symbolize. Without this ally of the therapeutic alliance, transference becomes real. This results in the common finding that traumatized patients rapidly and concretely perceive the transference object to be actually malevolent and threatening. The therapist's recognition and successful management of this state poses significant technical and emotional challenges.

Shapiro, in his chapter, "Transference, Countertransference and the Vietnam Veteran," details his approach to this difficult problem. He suggests deflecting the early negative transference, focusing on extra therapy relationships, and accepting patients' early identifications with the therapist. In particular, he outlines an approach that delicately titrates the patient's ability to tolerate work directly on the transference. This process of education around the doctor-patient relationship is a useful method of slowly bringing in material which if mishandled could disrupt a treatment.

The importance of monitoring the countertransference is stressed by Shapiro. Therapists' intrusive sympathy and self-protective displacements can further traumatize the struggling patient. The doctor needs to be able to accept and contain disturbing affects. In addition, in working with these patients the therapist must be prepared to face a disturbing view of humanity at its worst.

PHYSIOLOGY AND FANTASY IN THE TRAUMATIC DREAM

The physiology of the unconscious intrigues clinicians and neurochemists alike. The discovery of the molecular underpinnings of intrapsychic functioning would lead to great advances in our conceptualization of the mind. While major strides have been made in the past two decades, our tools at this point remain crude. Clinically, we are limited to hit-or-miss methods of reducing gross symptomatology. While this is an important goal in and of itself, its greater value lies in the elucidation of the underlying mechanisms of consciousness.

A small but significant step in this direction has been the recent work on sleep physiology and architecture. This rich area of research brings together the organic and dynamic perspectives on the dream. The traumatic nightmare, given its ubiquitousness and stereotyped presentation, becomes an important topic for study. Its central place in the symptom picture of all posttraumatic conditions underlines its value as a barometer of both pathophysiology and unconscious fantasy.

Cornfield, in his chapter, "Traumatic War Neuroses: Some Pharmacologic and Psychophysiologic Observations," acquaints us with some of the recent research on REM cycles and their role in the posttraumatic stress disorder. In particular, Friedman's work (1978) on the 24 hour "REM State" raises the interesting hypothesis that flashbacks as well as nightmares may be related to underlying disturbances in the REM cycle. There is also the possibility that many of these patients fall within the descriptive category of "atypical depression." These thoughts may explain the early but promising results that Cornfield and others report with phenelzine in treating many of the intractable symptoms of the posttraumatic stress disorder. Although further study with sleep laboratory documentation is needed, this is an intriguing area of research that may yield new modalities of treatment for many otherwise unreachable patients.

The traumatic nightmare has of course also been the subject of psychoanalytic study. From this vantage point as well, differing theories abound. Blitz and Greenberg in their chapter, "Nightmares of the Traumatic Neuroses: Implications for Theory and Treatment," walk us through the conceptual history of this symptom. They begin with Freud's original work that emphasized drive discharge, preconscious censoring, and the classical dreamwork. They note that for Freud, the traumatic dream seemed to lay outside this paradigm and instead represented efforts at "mastery."

The authors next refer to Mack's work which places the nightmare in an ego psychology frame. This outlook underscores the variation in individual capacity to tolerate erupting impulses. Mack continues tradition, however, in identifying aggression as the major conflictual drive.

Following this, recent sleep laboratory research is described. From Greenberg's own studies, they derive the concept of the integrative function of REM dreaming. In the process, they deemphasize the importance of conflict and stress the meaning contained in the surface dream.

It is finally in the self-psychology perspective that Blitz and Greenberg find the richest understanding of the traumatic nightmare. They conclude that the nightmare represents a "failed dream." This is "hypothesized to be related to the dreamer's experience of a threat to his self-cohesion with the accompanying intense anxiety which awakens the dreamer and interrupts the dream function."

From this theoretical orientation, the authors underscore the therapeutic importance of empathy in the clinical situation. They see the narcissistic injury sustained in combat and the fragile self-structure that results as the major clinical issue in psychotherapy. The repair of this damage through the empathic doctor-patient relationship is seen as the hallmark of treatment.

REMEMBERING AND WORKING THROUGH
IN BRIEF TREATMENT

In recent years, psychoanalytically derived short-term psychotherapy has become an important therapeutic modality. Many clinicians have found that working on a focal conflict with carefully selected patients can lead to significant change in a relatively brief time. The beauty of the method lies in its careful hypothesis formulation and precise interpretive focus.

In many ways the posttrauma patient is ideally suited to short-term psychotherapy. Motivation is high, symptoms are discrete, and conflicts often revolve around a specific, albeit multilayered, stressor. As McKinnon demonstrates in his chapter, "Brief Psychotherapy of the Vietnam Combat Neuroses," the art of the procedure is in the judicious titration of anxiety and the creative *use* of the transference.

Effective short-term work is not based on simple abreaction. Neither is time limitation synonymous with manifest level conceptualizations. While one does not have the opportunity for lengthy psychic excavation, McKinnon makes clear the importance of tracing the patient's associations to his trauma. These lead to "echoes in the more recent past" which include the patient's "latent self-images." Becoming conscious of these repressed fantasies and their partial working through is a fundamental aspect of this treatment.

The content of the case material presented reveals themes common to many survivors of combat. Self-destructive guilt, retaliation fears, undoing of damage, loss of ideals—these are the psychological scars of war. They emerge whenever a meaningful therapeutic encounter takes place, independent of its length. Short-term therapy, through incisive verbal interventions and use of the doctor-patient relationship, can begin to heal some of these chronic wounds.

GROUP PROCESS ON A DEVELOPMENTAL CONTINUUM

The rap group was the first therapeutic effort developed specifically to treat Vietnam veterans. This modality emerged from the freedom that a few creative clinicians assumed in not being apologetic for utilizing parameters. It was a treatment form that did not prejudge its effectiveness or respectability on the basis of its proximity to the classical paradigm. Early notions of therapist self-revelation derived from a different model of doctor-patient relating.

The rebelliousness of the veteran patient was paralleled by the radical nature of this new treatment.

As with many revolutionary ideas, this one also contained a creative seed. With time it has refined itself. Through the inevitable evolution of ideas there has been an integration of these new techniques with more established concepts of treatment. Clinicians have begun to study the unconscious forces that are active in this group setting. In his chapter, "The Role of Psychodynamic Group Therapy in the Treatment of the Combat Veteran," Parson details the historical development of rap groups and their present role in the overall context of group psychotherapy.

Parson presents a "multiple-group developmental treatment model." He sees different types of groups being indicated and useful for different levels of pathology. These groups sit on the supportive-insight continuum familiar to many psychotherapists. He begins with the rap group, progresses to the second phase group, and continues to the psychoanalytic group. These group types differ according to the extent of transference interpretation. In particular, they vary to the degree that they accept or displace the negative transference. In addition, Parson details the many other important variables that make each group distinct. Unique membership selection, leadership style, repressing-derepressing goals, and cohesion-differentiation processes characterize each form of group treatment.

In placing the rap group on a developmental continuum, Parson demonstrates the theory underlying rap group technique. Rather than the haphazard approach feared by some, the experienced rap group leader pursues a course informed by complex intrapsychic and interpersonal constructs. The leader adapts to the evolving phase-specific unconscious needs of the group and its members. Terminating in the traditional psychoanalytic group, the leader has by then traveled a long journey with his patients. He has opened himself to being different transference objects, accepted and contained affects from all developmental stages, and carried the group from defensive cohesion to differentiation to high level cohesion. While this path is known to many from intensive individual work, it is particularly arduous in the group setting and calls upon the most profound intellectual and emotional resources of the leader.

THE CULTURAL SETTING OF CONFLICT

The context within which a trauma occurs is considered by many to have a major impact on a victim's adjustment. Just as there often is a dynamic interplay between a patient's childhood history and the traumatic circumstances, so too is there an interweaving of the individual and group experience. In studying the war neurosis, we need examine the milieu of battle and of the homefront. We are, however, limited in our ability to view ourselves as a collective. We cannot assume that because we can analyze our countertransference that we can also evaluate our culture.

To help us better see ourselves, Moses and Cohen's chapter, "Understanding and Treatment of Combat Neuroses—The Israeli Experience," is included in this volume. Viewing them study their society gives us the opportunity to be outsiders looking in. We can then bring this observing eye back home. However, their study of the Israeli experience does more than just sharpen our cultural vision. The content of their analysis bears directly on the American experience. Moses and Cohen take us through each Israeli war. They describe for each conflict the at-large social conditions and intra-army morale. The differing political environment at each occasion leads the authors to conceptualize different types of wars. Each is created from a unique matrix of national consensus, identification with leaders, and social preparedness. These factors determine the "identification threshold"—the level of psychopathology that can be contained by the unit and individual.

Moses and Cohen describe the identification threshold as deriving from a number of intra and extrapsychic conditions. Early traumata, tendencies to identify with the aggressor or victim, and fragile self-esteem result in an unconscious predisposition to combat stress. In contrast to this "readiness to develop trait anxiety," is *state anxiety*. This is "the anxiety which is related not to the traits which the soldier brings with him to the situation, but rather to the situation itself, to the state in which the soldier finds himself."

The social matrix that defines state anxiety consists of more than the intangibles of group morale or respected leadership. The authors stress the importance of society's concrete expression of concern and caring for its combatants. Their "gifts," derivatives of parental love, include trustworthy equipment, accurate information, time to sleep and good enough food.

This synthesized perspective addresses genetic conflict and environmental failure. To insist upon one or the other as *the* cause of combat neuroses is, as Freud stated (1917), to take sides "in a quite unnecessary dispute." I believe only by simultaneously recognizing the continuity of infantile instinctual life and acknowledging the function of the environmental hold will we deepen our understanding of the traumatic neuroses. Fortunately, the transference encompasses both these elements of experience. In appreciating both the archaic and current aspects of this relationship, and the experience contained in their contrast, we have available to us a broad and powerful instrument for the study and treatment of this multifaceted condition.

REFERENCES

Brenner, C. (1953). An addendum to Freud's theory to anxiety. *International Journal of Psychoanalysis* 34: 18-24.

Erikson, E. (1950). *Childhood and Society*. New York: Norton.

Fairbairn, W. (1954). *An Object Relations Theory of the Personality*. New York: Basic Books.

Figley, C. (1978). *Stress Disorders Among Vietnam Veterans*. New York: Brunner Mazel.

Freud, A. (1967). Eine distussion mit Rene Spitz. *Psyche* 21.

Freud, S. (1917). Introductory Lectures on Psycho-Analysis. *S.E.* XVI: 347.

Friedman, S. (1978). A psychophysiological model for the chemotherapy of psychosomatic illness. *The Journal of Nervous and Mental Disorders* 166(2): 110-116.

Glover, E. (1937). Symposium on the theory of the therapeutic results of psycho-analysis. *International Journal of Psychoanalysis* 18: 125-132.

Jaffe, R. (1968). Dissociative phenomena in former concentration camp inmates. *International Journal of Psychoanalysis* 49: 310-312.

Lorenzer, A. (1968). Some observations on the latency of symptoms in patients suffering from persecution sequelae. *International Journal of Psychoanalysis* 49: 316-318.

Nacht, S. (1962). The curative factors in psychoanalysis. *International Journal of Psychoanalysis* 43: 206-211.

Niederland, W. G. (1968). Clinical observations on the "survivor syndrome." *International Journal of Psychoanalysis* 49: 313-315.

Acknowledgments

First and foremost I wish to thank the contributors to this book. They applied themselves conscientiously to the difficult and time-consuming task of putting their ideas and experiences on paper. We are all the more learned for their efforts.

For my own work, I would like to express my appreciation to my colleagues who offered guidance and helpful criticism of my thinking and writing. They include Drs. Salman Akhtar, Daniel Gesensway, Richard Hole, Stephen Ring, Kenneth Weiss, and Thomas Wolman. I would like to add a special note of thanks to Dr. Paul J. Fink for his support and encouragement. I wish to also extend my appreciation to Mrs. Debra Kohler for her invaluable secretarial assistance.

Finally, I would like to acknowledge those whose psychoanalytic vision has been instrumental in my development. Without my exposure to their wisdom and humanity, my work would not have taken form.

Psychotherapy of the Combat Veteran

1
Brief Historical Overview of the Concept of War Neurosis and of Associated Treatment Methods

D. WILFRED ABSE, M.D.

FROM THE PAST TO WORLD WAR I

Certain disease phenomena attend, or they may follow with a variable latent interval, overwhelming mental excitation. The intensity and duration of the impacting excitation becomes definably excessive when it exceeds the tolerance of the psyche so that it can no longer shield itself for major functions, and in short, it can no longer (immediately or later) maintain adequate inner integration and expedient outer adjustment for healthy survival of the organism. The response of the organism is not only related to the quantity of outer stimulation, but to its meanings for that particular individual, with resultant self-generated inner excitation of greater or lesser amount. The concept of massive and overwhelming psychic trauma and that of cumulative traumata developed and evolved from consideration and investigation of such disease phenomena as conversion reactions, states of hypervigilance, multiple phobias, periodic alterations of consciousness with later amnesia, recurrent nightmares, personality changes (often of impoverishment), and other symptoms which were observed to attend and follow, sometimes episodically, traumatic

Copyright © 1984 by Spectrum Publications, Inc. *Psychotherapy of the Combat Veteran*, edited by H. J. Schwartz.

experiences in both war and peace. In this century, such consideration as applied to mental imbalance and nervous symptoms related to extreme experiences in war was influenced powerfully by the knowledge gradually gained from the investigation and treatment of psychoneurosis usually unrelated to wartime events. Thus, it is necessary to address the history of the emergence of concepts of dynamic psychiatry in general which were only later applied to the problems of military psychiatry in World Wars I and II, in Korea, and in Vietnam. Ellenberger (1970) has traced the derivation of modern dynamic psychiatry from primitive thaumaturgic medicine, demonstrating an uninterrupted continuity between exorcism and magnetism, between magnetism and hypnotism, and between hypnotism and our present knowledge and practice of psychotherapy. This development from exorcism is embedded in the matrix of the overlapping cultural movements that succeeded the Middle Ages in Western Civilization—the Renaissance, Baroque, Enlightenment, and Romanticism, centered to begin with successively in Italy, France, and Germany.

Of course, only in recent times has man been able to mitigate, if not to banish, many of his fears of the unseen which for thousands of years had kept him in perpetual torment and continuous apotropaic activity. During the Middle Ages certainly, malicious and cunning disembodied spirits, lurking in every shadow, seemed for most of humanity to have been a constant menace. Especially prominent were witches with burning eyes who cast malevolent glances from the darkness as they swung through the air. Every calamity that had befallen friend or neighbor was regarded to be the result of the malicious design of some demon of some shape, or indeed of a changing form. It was thought that life would come to a frightening end but for the guardianship of friendly spirits who waged perpetual warfare against innumerable monsters. Although written after notions cultivated during the Dark Ages had begun to yield to some degree of enlightenment in the Renaissance, the *Malleus Mallificarum* (Sprenger, 1486) is saturated with the medieval quality of wild and gloomy superstition. Moreover, the invention of printing only served to enable the "Witches Hammer" to achieve widespread influence. This influence reinstated in some considerable measure the belief in demoniacal possession that had dominated large populations of the Western World during the Middle Ages. "Demon—possessed" persons were accused of making storms at sea, of being responsible for periods of drought, of causing hailstones on land, of stunting the growth of children, and of thousands of other crimes. Because of frightened superstition and ignorance, thousands upon thousands of men, women and children suffered the most excruciating tortures. They were suspended to ceilings by their thumbs, starved in dungeons, stretched on the rack, and broken on the wheel. Death alone brought deliverance. So horrible was the torture often preceding execution, many confessed to being guilty of impossible deeds. They were, of course, the victims of a traumatic neurosis and psychosis which often mobilizes self-hatred.

Thus, it was a great cultural advance when, in the treatment of the mentally deranged, exorcism without punishment evolved in a religious setting. Of course, it too was preceded by punitive methods such as starving and searing with hot irons, under the belief that the demons would find the human body an undesirable abode and vacate the premises, as it were. But in the religious setting, gradually not only was punishment without death achieved, but exorcism without severe punishment. If the world advances only as it becomes more humane, then in this perspective, we must appreciate the value of exorcism in the alembic of the progressive historical process. The religious exorcist often became consciously benevolently concerned with the health and welfare of the distressed supplicant; this was an advance in attitude not to be underestimated, setting the stage for further development of psychotherapy.

Unfortunately, it is only too easy to draw parallels between the structure of medieval thinking and that of modern industrial masses, including many of those belonging to the political leadership in a world beset by thermonuclear threat. It is, however, not immediately relevant to elucidate the common sources in severe narcissistic disorder and the unconscious dynamisms of gross splittings and distorting projections with which we are all now only too familiar. It is here pertinent to point to the year 1775, little more than two centuries ago, as a turning point for the emergence of scientific concepts of dynamic psychiatry from the phenomena of religious exorcism.

A fateful event of this year was the clash between Johann Joseph Gassner, the exorcist and faith healer, and Franz Anton Mesmer, the physician (Zimmerman, 1879). In the early months of 1775, hordes of people, rich and poor, nobles and peasants, swarmed to the small town of Ellwangen in Württenberg to see Father Gassner whose fame as a faith healer had spread far and wide. In the presence of physicians, noblemen of all ranks, members of the bourgeoisie, and church authorities both Catholic and Protestant, and before skeptics as well as believers, he exorcised the evil demons. His every word and gesture and those of his subjects were recorded by a notary public, and the official records of his activities were signed by distinguished eyewitnesses. Although Gassner was but a modest country priest, soon after he donned his ceremonial garments and had the subject kneeling before him, astonishing events occurred. Ellenberger quotes the account given by the Abbé Bourgeois:

> The first patients were two nuns who had been forced to leave their community on account of convulsive fits. Gassner told the first one to kneel before him, asked her briefly about her name, her illness, and whether she agreed that anything he would order should happen. She agreed. Gassner then pronounced solemnly in Latin: "If there be anything preternatural about this disease, I order in the name of Jesus that it manifest itself immediately." The patient started at once to have convulsions. According to Gassner, this was proof that the convulsions were caused by an evil spirit and not by a natural illness, and he now proceeded to demonstrate that he had power over the demon, whom he ordered in Latin to produce convulsions in various parts of the patient's body; he called forth in turn the exterior manifestations of grief, silliness, scrupulosity, anger, remorse and so on, and even the appearance of death. All his orders were punctually executed. It now seemed logical that, once a demon had been tamed to that point, it should be relatively easy to expel him, which Gassner did. He then proceeded in the same manner with the second nun.

Even this short excerpt conveys to the psychoanalyst over two centuries of time an impression of intuitive skill embedded in the idiom of demonology. Gassner clearly knew how to use institutional charisma and a sacred language, how to reinforce his personal prestige as a healer through impressive exhibitionism and its respondent acclaim, and how to obtain through his rituals both emotional release and the taming of affects. As a young priest Gassner had suffered from violent headaches and dizziness; these attacks occurred or worsened whenever he was celebrating the Mass, preaching or hearing confession. This circumstance led him to suspect that he was under attack from the devil, and when he resorted to churchly rituals of exorcism, his condition improved. He then began exorcising rich people within his parish; he enjoyed considerable success in this, and his fame spread. After he exorcised—and cured—a well-known hypochondriacal countess, he received invitations from many distant places where he performed further cures by exorcism. His spreading fame brought him many impassioned enemies, however, including notably various representatives of the Enlightenment. Rumors were circulated that cases of possession were sure to manifest themselves wherever a visit from Gassner was announced. At the University and Medical School in Vienna animated controversies, both for and against him, took place. In church circles, belief in possession found its chief critic in Johann Saloman Semler, the founder of the new Protestant theology (Oesterreich, 1974). Semler was among the first—if not the first—Christian theologian to undertake a survey of the Bible from the historical point of view, and he felt that the authors of the New Testament shared ideas common to their time. By 1767 he concluded that a complete exposition of the history of possession would contribute greatly to the destruction of an anachronistic belief. He wrote:

> If I desired to collect the thousands and thousands of stories of possessed persons and their cure, it would labor and would constitute a history of the devil in the Middle Ages. It would be of relatively large proportions, but would infallibly produce a happy, profound and lasting impression on all readers, inasmuch as they themselves, however simple-minded and credulous, would judge that it must be far from the truth. The frightful superstition which still brings forth many dark fruits would be very rapidly and generally weakened thereby (Quoted in T. K. Oesterreich, 1974).

He evidently believed in the efficacy of education rather than the efficacy of prayer.

The opposition to Gassner, largely inspired in Europe by the new philosophy of the Enlightenment, which proclaimed the primacy of reason over ignorance, superstition, and blind tradition, was consolidated in commissions of inquiry. One such commission, appointed in Munich by the Prince of Bavaria, invited Dr. Mesmer, who claimed to have discovered a new principle called animal magnetism, to appear before it, thus bringing into confrontation a representative of medicine. On November 23, 1775, Mesmer gave demonstrations in Munich, eliciting in subjects the appearance and disappearance of various symptoms, including convulsions. Ellenberger (1970) writes:

> Father Kennedy, the Secretary of the Academy, was suffering from convulsions, and Mesmer showed that he was able to bring them forth in him and dispel them at will. On the following

day, in the presence of Court members and members of the
Academy, he provoked attacks in an epileptic and claimed he
was able to cure the patient through animal magnetism. In
effect, this amounted to Gassner's procedure, without involving
the use of exorcism. Mesmer declared that Gassner was an
honest man, but that he was curing his patients through animal
magnetism without being aware of it. We can imagine that,
upon hearing of Mesmer's report, Gassner must have felt like
Moses when the Egyptian wizards reproduced similar miracles
in the Pharoah's presence. But, unlike Moses, Gassner had not
been permitted to witness Mesmer's performance or to reply to
his report.

Gassner's fate was eventually sealed by an order of the Imperial
Court requiring the Prince Bishop to banish him to the small community of Pondorf. After the investigation of Gassner's activities
Pope Pius VI issued a decree defending the practice of exorcism, but
insisting on discretion and strict adherence to Roman ritual.
Gassner's absolute piety was never questioned, his unpretentiousness
and unselfishness were indeed quite clear but he was caught up in the
struggle between the new Enlightenment and forces of tradition. His
eclipse led to the honoring of a healing method without any religious
ties, one that would satisfy the requirements of a so-called enlight-
ened time. It is, of course, never enough to have a cure for the sick;
in curing them one must use methods of which the community ap-
proves. This observation is all too applicable today, when fashions of
treatment change rapidly or oscillate between one mode and another.
Mesmer, who lived from 1733 to 1815, was in time faced with the
hostility of the medical community. Ilza Veith (1965) has described
the public clamor that arose in his defense, and notes the resultant
appointment by Louis XVI of a Royal Commission to examine the
validity of the concept of "animal magnetism." It is interesting that
this Commission included the then American Ambassador, Benjamin
Franklin, as well as other illustrious men of the time in France such
as the chemist Lavoisier and the astronomer Bailly. Charged with
determining whether or not such a phenomenon as "animal magnetism" truly existed, they reported in the negative and perspica-
ciously attributed Mesmer's cures to the workings of the imagination.
It remains true, however, that the fateful turning point from
exorcism to dynamic psychiatry was reached in 1775 by Franz
Anton Mesmer. He has been compared with Christopher Columbus
inasmuch as each of these two men discovered a new world the

true nature of which he did not fully grasp, and both died bitterly disappointed men. Certainly Mesmer may be singled out as the link between methods of treatment and modern psychotherapy.

His clinic in Paris was unique; patients entered a darkened room filled with soft music and gathered around a low oaken tub or *baquet* in which iron filings were immersed in water. The patients applied to the ailing parts of their body iron rods that projected from the tub. Then Mesmer would appear in a colorful silk robe, holding a large iron wand. The ecstatic or convulsive crises manifested by some of the patients no doubt impressed and encouraged the others. A disciple of his, Puységur, found that instead of the usual mesmeric crisis a trance-like state could be induced during which the subject was highly suggestible. He first called this altered state of consciousness "somnambulism" and used it to further the cure. Mesmer, working with his baquet, was engaged in group psychotherapy as well as work with individuals and Puységur also became involved in group therapy as we shall see.

In the 19th century, the Abbé Faria, a Portugese priest in Paris, showed that the mesmeric trance described by Puységur was largely the result of the somnambulist's own expectations. Later, in 1843, James Braid, a British physician, investigated further and concluded, as had the Royal Commission of Louis XVI, that there was no mysterious fluid involved at all. Braid coined the word "hypnotism" and used the term "suggestion." As is well-known, Liébault and Bernheim, in Nancy, and Charcot, in Paris, later used hypnosis in the treatment of hysterical disorder. Incidentally, the word "psychotherapy" became fashionable under the influence of disciples of Professor Hippolyte Bernheim at the University of Nancy.

Puységur was the eldest of three brothers of the highest French nobility who were among Mesmer's enthusiastic disciples. Armand Marie Jacques de Chastinet, the Marquis of Puységur, divided his time between his military duties and his castle in Buzancy. One of his first patients was a 23-year-old peasant named Victor Race whose family had been in the service of the Puységur family for several generations. He had respiratory symptoms and was easily magnetized. While magnetized he exibited a peculiar crisis, going without convulsions or jerking movements of any kind into an altered waking state of consciousness in which he was talkative and responsive to questions. His relationship with his magnetizer was intensified in this condition, and his responsiveness concentrated only on him. He retained no memory of this experience. Puységur regarded this phenomenon as "the perfect crisis," and its similarity to natural somnambulism suggested the term "artificial somnambulism" for what was subsequently to be known as hypnotism. Soon there was a growing rift between orthodox mesmerists who clung to the value of producing any sort of crisis, and to the theory of the part played by the mysterious fluid, and the followers of Puységur, who concentrated on producing the special "perfect crisis" and adopted a psycholgical theory instead of taking a literal view of "animal magnetism"; that is, they became liberated from a disturbance of metaphoric symbolism in their thinking.

Puységur soon had so many patients that, like Mesmer, he introduced collective treatment. The public square of the village of Buzancy, surrounded by trees and thatched cottages, was not far from the majestic castle of the Puységurs. In the center of the square stood a large and beautiful old elm tree, now famous as the Buzancy tree, near a limpid spring. Peasants sat on the surrounding stone benches, with ropes hung around the branches of the tree attached to ailing parts of their bodies. They "felt" the magnetic fluid circulating through their bodies. Sometimes the master would put some of them into a "perfect crisis" one by one, and enthusiastic onlookers reported remarkable cures that they had seen result from this procedure. In all of this we readily recognize the exploitation of the primitive phallic symbolism of sacred trees and springs no doubt considered magical still in the folklore of the country people treated by the Marquis. Such magical notions are seen to this day in the resort of the wealthy to spas for treatment. Ancient myths often associate trees and springs with the healing gods.

Mesmer held that to effect healing a magnetizer must first establish *rapport*, a kind of psychic "tuning in" with his patient, and Puységur certainly understood this prerequisite. Although he did not share the illusions of his peasant clientele, and did not organize his collective treatments around a baquet as Mesmer did with his wealthier patients, but around a tree he had "magnetized," this was for him a scientific procedure utilizing popular beliefs and customs. Forests and sacred trees had been for so long considered divine by the Gauls that Christians missionaries and bishops had for centuries had difficulty eradicating tree-worship among the peasantry. Sébillot (1906), in his monumental work *The Folklore of France* describes how the sick attached themselves to trees with ropes in order to transfer their disease to these inexhaustible bearers of life.

Puységur's treatment of Victor during the phase of "perfect crisis" often went beyond using rapport for the direct suggestion of symptom abatement. In the state of altered consciousness, of heightened concentration and uncommonly alert and disinhibited consciousness, a dialogue between the magnetizer and the magnetized became possible, one of special quality within which the patient made important contributions. Thus the dialogue acquired a much more patient shared emphasis. Moreover, as Puységur's experience with Victor disclosed, a second, somnambulistic, personality can emerge in this state, one less inhibited and more brilliant than the ordinary one. The appearance of such phenomena in the trance state engendered a new model of the human mind, one based on a duality of consciousness and of inferred unconscious psychism, since one personality remained unconscious while the other dominated.

In this necessarily sketchy account of the background of the depth-psychology evolved later by Sigmund Freud, a depth-psychology which then enormously influenced the development of dynamic psychiatry, it is important to take into consideration the increasing awareness and understanding of the phenomena of multiple personality. The phenomenon of possession came to be understood as one variety of divided selfness. In "lucid possession" the subject feels within himself two souls struggling for domination and describes this conflict to his priest or physician. In "somnambulistic possession," which might follow "lucid possession," an "intruder" takes over the subject's body and shows in speech and behavior a personality which the subject knows nothing about when he returns to his normal state. As cases of possession became less frequent, case histories of other kinds of multiple personality began appearing in mesmerist literature and other medical reports. Gmelin published a case of "exchanged personality" as early as 1791, in which a 20-year-old German woman, impressed by the influx of aristocratic French refugees into Stuttgart at the outset of the French Revolution, suddenly "exchanged" her own personality for the manners and ways of a French lady, imitating them and speaking French perfectly; her own tongue she spoke then with a French accent. These "French" states recurred. While in her French persona, the subject had complete memory for all she had said and done during her previous French states, but as a German, she knew nothing of her French personality. With a motion of his hand Gmelin was able easily to make her shift from one personality to the other. Reil was greatly interested in this case, elaborated on it, and connected it with the duality sometimes evident in the contrast of waking life and dream phenomena, when the dreaming and waking personalities are in evident contrast (Veith, 1965).

A more searching study of multiple personality was inaugurated in France by the publication of the story of "Estelle" in 1840 by

Antoine Despine (Pére), a general medical practitioner who some-times practiced magnetic treatment. Another important early study was published by the professor of surgery at the Bordeaux Medical School in 1887. Eugene Azam (1887) worked with the woman Félida X for many years, beginning in 1858, and Jean-Martin Charcot wrote the introduction to his report. There is also the famous case of the Reverend Ansel Bourne, which was published by Hodgson (1891) and examined by William James (1890) in the last decade of the 19th century. In addition, notably, there is Morton Prince's case, the Miss Beauchamp about whom he wrote his monograph *The Dissociation of a Personality* in 1906. In the same connection we must mention in passing the work of Flournoy (1900) and Janet (1897).

Theodore Flournoy's work is especially interesting because it demonstrates how the rigorous application of scientific method to parapsychology could yield useful concepts for the development of dynamic psychiatry. Flournoy (1854–1930) was enamored to two maxims: "Everything is possible" and "The weight of evidence must be in proportion to the strangeness of the fact." He worked with the spiritistic mediums of Geneva, one of whom told him accurately about past events concerning his own family. A lengthy inquiry un-covered a long past relationship between the medium's parents and his own that might have made it possible for her to have heard about the events in question, which she had subsequently forgotten. This medium, Catherine Muller, widely known under the name of Hélene Smith, claimed in her "second cycle" of three to be a reincarnation of Marie Antoinette; in her first, she reenacted her supposed previous life as a 15th century Indian princess. Flournoy was able to identify much of this Hindu material as having come from a book she had read as a child. In brief, the results of Flournoy's five-year investi-gation of the medium (1900) showed that her revelations were romances of the subliminal imagination based on forgotten memories and that they expressed wish-fulfillments. Her guiding spirit, Leopold, was an unconscious personality of her own. It was Flournoy who coined the term "cryptamnesia" to help explain the caprices of memory; he clearly showed that Hélene Smith's cycles could be explained by reversions of her personality to experiences she had had at different ages: early childhood, the age of 12 and the age of 16. Similarly, he demonstrated the psychological albeit uncon-scious origin of some spiritistic messages. He was a pioneer in the exploration of the mythopoetic functions of the unconscious—that is, those unconscious tendencies to weave fantasies with which Freud came to grips with so much initial difficulty later in his study of hysteria. In this respect, present-day parapsychologists are apt sometimes to share their subjects' fantasies embedded in, or stimulated by, early forgotten experience.

It is here necessary to mention the important influence on Freud of the work of Pierre Janet of Paris. Although a few years Freud's junior, Janet was nevertheless the first to found a 20th century system of dynamic psychiatry, one to replace the 18th and 19th century probings just described. He drew heavily and consciously from the earlier explorers of the unconscious, of whom the pioneers of psychoanalysis apparently took but little note; this neglect has unfortunately often been compounded in the psychoanalytic writing of recent decades, resulting in a blemished scholarship. Here I will mention only that Janet's several studies of hypnotic suggestion, including the early article "L'influence somnambulique et le besoin de direction" (1897) were masterly, and extended earlier studies of rapport in the direction of the identification of transference phenomena subsequently accomplished by Freud.

In Vienna Freud abandoned hypnosis as a means of treatment, partly because of its relative unreliability; he was not always able to induce hypnotic trance. Moreover, it had turned out that patients improved by means of hypnosis often remained in the improved condition only as long as they remained in contact with their physician and on good terms with him. This impermanent result was often true as well of patients treated by direct suggestion while in the waking state. Freud discovered that communicated propositions were accepted by the patient with conviction because of the prestige with which the therapist was endowed through the transference to him of emotion pertaining to prestige-endowed parental figures of the patient's past. He came to show that in the dependency relationship so characteristic of hypnotic rapport, the patient reverts mentally to the earliest few years of life when he had felt his parents to be omnipotent; thus, he once again experiences the lost omnipotence of his own earliest months of life. When the patient's active mastery of his own problems fails, hypnosis makes possible a type of passive-receptive mastery which is provided also in some degree, although less intensely, by all other methods of suggestion. In sharp contrast to suggestive therapy and persuasive therapy, which employs reason heavily colored by suggestion, psychoanalysis is concerned with demonstrating to the patient the nature of his transference emotions and obtaining his collaboration in this investigative undertaking. Freud wrote in 1912:

In following up the libido that is withdrawn from consciousness, we penetrate into the region of the unconscious, and this
provokes reactions which bring with them to light of the characteristics of unconscious processes as we have learned to know
them from the study of dreams. The unconscious feelings strive
to avoid the recognition which the cure demands; they seek instead for reproduction, with all the power of hallucination and
the inappreciation of time characteristic of the unconscious.
The patient ascribes, just as in dreams, currency and reality to
what results from the awakening of his unconscious feelings;
he seeks to discharge his emotions regardless of the reality of
the situation. The physician requires of him that he shall fit
these emotions into their place in the treatment and in his life
history, subject them to rational consideration, and appraise
them at their true psychical value. The struggle between intel-
lect and the forces of instinct, between recognition and strivings
for discharge, is fought-out almost entirely over the transfer-
ence-manifestations. This is the ground on which the victory
must be won, the final expression of which is lasting from neurosis. It is undeniable that the subjugation of the transference-
manifestations provides the greatest difficulties for the psychoanalyst; but it must be forgotten that they, and they only, render the invaluable service of making the patient's buried and
forgotten love-emotions actual and manifest; for in the last resort no one can be slain *in absentia* or *in effigie.*

As Erik Erikson (1964) pointed out, the concept of transference
analysis, including the concomitant necessary understanding of countertransference, involved for Freud the relinquishment of the usual
role of the physician as the all-knowing father—a role which, at the
turn of the century, was quite safely anchored in the whole contemporary cult of the paternal male's mastery of all human enterprise
outside of the nursery and the kitchen. Indeed, in the *Studies in
Hysteria* (1895), an evolutionary change in the doctor-patient relationship becomes gradually, although unevenly, evident. From the
beginning of their studies, Breuer and Freud were bound to respect
the sometimes outstanding talents and characters of their patients
rather than adopting the prevalent global notion that degeneracy was
the hallmark of hysteria. In *The Gift of Anna O*, Bram (1965) shows
that the primordium pf psychoanalytic thinking and technique did
not develop simply as a matter of chance but involved the patient's
intensive relationship with Breuer in which she participated in a joint

investigative and creative approach to her problems and symptoms. Breuer stopped her treatment prematurely because of its assault on his own sense of identity as a physician and his fear of departing too far from the orthodox doctor-patient relationship. This is an example of noxious countertransference which causes treatment to founder. It remained for Freud to develop the physician's offer to the patient of a conscious partnership in which the healthy part of the patient's mind collaborates in their common understanding of those unhealthy parts that are immersed in conflict. Thus a basic principle of psychoanalysis (that of mutual enterprise) was established as a method of scientific investigation as well as of treatment. The human mind can be studied adequately only by engaging the fully motivated partnership of the observed individual and by entering into a sincere contract with him.

Freud, as Janet, drew his early inspiration partly from the Salpêtrière, the elegant 17th century hospital, built on the site of a former gunpowder factory. The earliest important work in the field of the neuroses to issue from this famous hospital in Paris was the *Traité Clinique et Therapeutique de L'hysteria* by Paul Briquet (1859). When, later, hysterical conditions were studied on Charcot's service the ground had been prepared by various descriptive clinical contributions of high quality, notably that of Briquet.

There is now in this country a pronounced tendency to return to this base (1963) and to ignore, or crowd out, the vast advance made by the studies of Charcot and his associates and followers. It is a widespread fallacy, especially among neurologists, that Charcot remained exclusively focused on organic disease of the nervous system in these cases of hysteria. Certainly, organic predisposition is never slighted, but careful perusal of Charcot's lectures (1889) yields the ineluctable conclusion that there is a progressive conceptual change from an initial exclusive interest in the organic aspects of this nervous disease to a broadening view in terms of "functional" disease and psychodynamic causes, so that in retrospect Janet could reasonably assert that his mentor Charcot had held the view that hysteria had psychic origins (1907). Owen (1971) notes, "What is surprising in Charcot's development is not his devotion to the organic and the material, but his emancipation therefrom—an orientation that more than the contributions of any other school opened the door to the era of psychological interpretation of the neuroses."

Like Charcot himself, the hospital of the Salpêtrière occupies a unique place in the history of mental healing. The institution has come to be a presiding symbol of a revolution in attitude of many physicians toward mental illness, and a refutation of both the demonological approach and that of a one-sided materialism. Since ancient Graeco-Roman times the supernaturalistic and the naturalistic approaches had competed. The naturalistic concepts of the Corpus Hippocraticum did not reach into the understanding of the overwhelming majority of the people of ancient Greece who remained close to their gods. For physical and emotional disturbances they had recourse to the temples of Aesculapius. Some elements of their practices are homologous with those based upon the concepts of modern dynamic psychotherapy. The temples were usually situated in places of considerable natural beauty, conducive to rest and relaxation. After an initial period of sacrifices, ablutions, and fasting, no doubt facilitating considerable relief from guilty self-oppression, the patient was enjoined to rest on a couch in a small room. There the god would appear in a dream. Since the ancient Greeks were much concerned with their dreams which were generally a considered portentous, the appearance of the god at this time was not too surprising. Ilza Veith writes (1965):

> A number of votive tablets found at the temple sites tells of the dreams and the visions the patients experienced during their temple sleep. In most cases, it seems Aesculapius appeared to them and brought about their recovery by words alone or manipulation at the site of the malady. The god carried a staff and was often accompanied by one or more of the large snakes which abounded in the temples. Sometimes the patients felt they were touched or licked by these snakes. According to the tablets, cure was the almost invariable result of these dreams. It was a distinctly psychotherapeutic atmosphere in which these cures were undertaken with rudiments of many of the procedures that were to endure through the millenia to the present day. Even the couch, of a fame then scarcely forseeable, was in evidence.

At the Salpêtrière, the polar categories of "organic" and "functional" replaced notions of the ancient supernatural and the medieval demonological. These categories were, however, well within the naturalistic sphere of thinking of early elite Greek scientific medicine. As I have shown elsewhere (1971), the conceptual framework of the ancient Greek physicians conflated the psychological and anatomical, on account of a defect in metaphoric symbolism. This was to a considerable extent remedied in Paris towards the end of the 19th century by Charcot and his associates. It must be added that while at first these polar categories of "organic" and "functional" were clarifying they also soon became a source of error as some physicians took a crude "either-or" view of nervous disease, a pitfall which Charcot himself avoided. Indeed, Charcot insisted that central nervous pathways were always involved in functional diseases, and sometimes these pathways were, he acknowledged, unknown at the time of his investigations. These same polar categories, though continuing to be useful, continue also to impede and obscure further conceptual development as long as an either-or fallacy is maintained and cultivated. A rigid one-sided approach to treatment can result from this.

Henri Ey quotes Pitres' five propositions defining mental and physical disturbances of an hysterical nature (Hurst, 1940):

1. They are functional disturbances of the nervous system.
2. They are labile and can be suddenly brought on, modified, or suppressed.
3. They rarely exist in isolation, and generally occur with other manifestations of a neurotic condition.
4. They develop irregularly.
5. They do not cause deterioration of the general physical condition.

Traumatic neuroses fulfill these criteria, except that very often they do cause deterioration of the general physical condition, especially when associated with alcohol and drug abuse as is frequently the case today.

In the time of Charcot, with the beginning expansion of industry in France and the increasing organization of the working class, physical injuries resulted in claims for compensation. Similarily, as the railways burgeoned across North America and Europe, accidents on them resulted in claims for damages, and there was, as there now is, much legal dispute. Charcot showed that nervous disorder often derives from "psychonervous commotion," even when the victim sustained little or no physical injury; he found that such disorders were produced or occasioned by mechanical accident even if their appearance was delayed. Later, in the War of 1914-1918, there was a considerable incidence in soldiers of all the nations involved of "battle neuroses." Valiant attempts were made to provide some respectible organic explanation for the curious phenomena which occurred with such frequency. The term "shell shock" was coined and expressed the general medical belief that in some way these conditions were the result of structural disturbance. Some physicians, notably Sir Arthur Hurst (1940) in Great Britian, demonstrated the functional nature of several conditions which had hitherto been regarded as organic, including paralyses, contractures, abnormal postures and gaits, tremors, seizures, disorders of speech, vomiting, deafness and blindness, stupor and amnesia, and "soldier's heart," all of which were differentiated from "true shell-shock." The latter diagnosis Hurst reserved for cases in which the patient had been exposed "to the forces generated by the explosion of powerful shells in the absence of any visible injury to the head or spine." "In such cases," he added, "there is an organic basis, which consists of the more or less evanescent changes in the central nervous system resulting from the concussion caused by aerial compression, to which is often added concussion of the head or spine caused by the sandbags of a falling parapet or by the patient being blown into the air and falling heavily on to his head or back. On this organic basis, hysterical or anxiety symptoms are often superposed."

FROM WORLD WAR I TO THE PRESENT

The three physicians whose works most influenced psychiatrists at the beginning of World War I were Herman Oppenheim, Jean-Martin Charcot, and Sigmund Freud. Oppenheim, who studied many patients suffering nervous sequelae of physical injuries caused by industrial accidents, recognized four conditions: hysteria, neurasthenia, organic syndromes and traumatic neurosis (Strauss, 1934). Hurst (1940) based his view of true shell-shock, noted earlier, on Oppenheim's opinion that the etiology of traumatic neurosis resided in molecular disturbances "due to electrical changes in the central nervous system." Charcot had dissented from this view, emphasizing psychogenesis; he noted that some of the symptoms of traumatic neurosis such as alterations of consciousness resembled those observed in hypnosis, and that some symptoms could be removed by hypnotic suggestion. He held the view that "nervous shock" in accident cases caused an alteration of consciousness which included an exceptionally heightened suggestibility when autosuggestion could readily produce symptoms. He used the phrase "une condition seconde" which was originated by Eugene Azam (1887) in his study of the successive states of Félida X. Freud (1895) agreed with Charcot that the altered state of consciousness was related to the hypnotic trance and called it the hypnoid state. At that time, he concluded that it was from the emotions generated and suggestions conveyed during this state that neurosis developed. As regards the traumatic neuroses of war, following in this path, were W. H. R. Rivers (1924), William McDougall (1926), as well as Freud's followers Ferenczi, Abraham, Simmel and Jones (1921), and Eder (1917).

Charcot himself refused to admit an essential distinction between traumatic neuroses which comprise conversion phenomena and conversion hysteria without a history of a recent evident and severe traumatic event or for that matter, of prolonged antecedent traumatic stress. Of course, later Freud and others showed that adult psychoneuroses were associated with forgotten traumatic situations in childhood, and now there is much controversy as to the etiologic roles of actual trauma and associated fantasies of self-generated fantasy in early life masquerading as memories of psychic trauma. In any case, as Fenichel (1945) insists, there is not traumatic neurosis without psychoneurotic complications. He writes:

> After the individual has experienced too much influx, he is afraid, cuts himself off from the external world and therefore blocks his discharges; and experience of a trauma creates fear of every kind of tension, sensitizing the organism in regard even to its own impulses. If, on the other hand, discharges are blocked [psychoneurotic defense] a little influx, otherwise harmless may have the effect of one much more intense, creating a flooding. A neurotic conflict creates fear of temptations and punishments and also sensitizes the organism in regard to further external stimuli. "Trauma" is a relative concept. . . .

After World War I there were many victims of chronic traumatic neurosis; Abram Kardiner (1947) explored the discombobulations of ego function evident in these chronic cases. He emphasized the attempts at adaptation, and the attempts of the organism to achieve psychic equilibrium after trauma. He wrote: "The traumatic experience can precipitate any of the well-known types of neurotic or psychotic disorders. However, irrespective of the nature of the resulting clinical picture, the distinctive features of traumatic neurosis are always present." This view is in accord with that expressed more recently by Krystal and Niederland (1968), who recognized a syndrome resulting from massive psychic trauma characterized by persistence of symptoms of withdrawal from social life, insomnia, recurrent nightmares, chronic depressive and anxiety reactions, and far-reaching somatization.

In war neurosis in general, the etiologic emphasis is on the role of the immediate stress and the actual conflict engendered by it, whereas in peacetime neurosis the emphasis is on unsettled infantile and childhood situations. As is illustrated with case examples from World War II in *Hysteria and Related Mental Disorders* (Abse, 1966), there is always an etiologic constellation of conditions within the field of medical observation. In one case, the relevant conditions may obtain more in constitution or in developmental maladjustments, and in another in the degree of recent stress to which a person was subject. Psychoanalytic work has revealed that the amount and type of stress which can be tolerated without symptoms of illness depends in large measure on individual experiences and reactions during the early years of life.

In discussing the war neuroses, Freud (1921) referred to "parasitic doubles of the superego" which for a time could usurp the power of regulation of the superego acquired in childhood. Not only does a "war superego" permit the expression of impulses otherwise forbidden, but it may even make demands which continue to be tempting, which the reinstated superego of peacetime may find difficulty defending against.

Both Jung (1928) and McDougall (1920) point out the limited therapeutic value of abreaction in the traumatic neuroses engendered in the "unique psychic atmosphere of the battlefield," to quote Jung. The dramatic rehearsal of the traumatic moment, its emotional recapitulation in the waking or in the hypnotic state, certainly often has a beneficial therapeutic effect. On the other hand, McDougall points out that in quite a large number of cases simple abreaction can worsen the patient's neurotic disturbance. He argues that in such refractory cases, an essential factor, that of dissociation, has been overlooked. It is this dissociation in the psyche and not only the existence of a highly charged affective complex that has to be reckoned with in treatment; the therapeutic task must include the facilitation of integration. As Jung observed, "the typical traumatic affect is represented in dreams as a wild and dangerous animal—a striking illustration of its autonomous nature when split off from consciousness." Abreaction is itself an attempt to reintegrate the autonomous complex, but this attempt at incorporation and belated mastery, by reliving the traumatic situation repeatedly, can be effected adequately often only with the active support, and in the presence of the doctor. As Jung insists, this curative process requires something more than a feeble rapport in many cases. These considerations amply demonstrate the application of key concepts forged during decades of psychotherapeutic work before World War I and afterward. The work of the therapist in such instances may be stated figuratively; his loving attention to the patient enables them both to face those terrible moments. This serves to exorcise their lingering traumatic power, while acknowledging their powerful role in shaping what we become.

At the onset of World War II, the concepts of dynamic psychiatry were much better understood and accepted, and further studies such as those of Grinker and Spiegel (1945) extended our knowledge of the effects of trauma upon the ego. Moreover, later, the effects of prolonged traumatic experiences were explored. In their account of clinical observations on the Survivor Syndrome, Krystal and Niederland (1968) show that the problems of survivors of massive destructive assault are many and complex. They describe far-reaching disturbances of personality that can be traced directly to the oppressive threatening milieu in which the survivors were forced to dwell for so long. An identification with the bad image attributed to them by their oppressors ("devil-identity") may become a life-long burden—or a reversal and reprojection may sometimes take place as in the "white devils" theory of the American Black Muslims. Commonly, however, the victim assumes a "slave" identification or a "slave house-boy" identity. The former involves a constriction of human capabilities, the latter an ambivalent ingratiating stance associated with a turning against fellow sufferers. These authors discuss the consolidated masochistic and paranoid character deformations engendered by the need to maintain repression of reactive hostility, including murderous rage, toward their oppressors for a prolonged period. Krystal and Niederland further introduce consideration of the dimension of social pathology, especially the later formation of abnormal families and communities. For besides such symptoms as hypervigilance, conversions, phobias, sleep disturbances, disorders of memory, spells of disorientation, dreams merging into hallucinosis and dream-like experiences in the waking state, muscle tensions and other psychosomatic disorders, very serious schizoid and paranoid and depressive disorders were engendered in these survivors of prolonged stress; their families and communities were later adversely affected. Lifton (1970) also emphasizes social pathology, including the dehumanization of invaders and those invaded in war. It is obvious that the concepts developed from the early treatment of individual traumatic neuroses can only convey some hints of what may be necessary for people who have been exposed to extreme situations for long periods, often *en masse*, including "death immersion." Of course, wars between nations now create conditions which quickly facilitate collective regressive attitudes—dehumanization of the enemy, disowning projections onto him, rationalizations, and license to murder him. Some of these regressive mental changes stick with many of the survivors in the ensuing peace with distressing social consequences.

In 1973, Van Putten and Emory discussed and gave case histories to illustrate, the earlier ignoring of traumatic neuroses in Vietnam returnees. These patients, because they reject authority and mistrust institutions, came for medical help to the Veteran's Hospital only out of desperation, years after discharge from service. Explosive aggressivity, "flashbacks" of combat scenes, and phobic problems of a paranoid type had led to mistakes in diagnosis such as psychomotor epilepsy, schizophrenic disorder, or attribution entirely to substance abuse. Such patients in my experience have not received early effective treatment with emphasis on cathartic psychotherapy. On the contrary, they received, while in Vietnam, treatment which emphasized massive psychotropic medication, followed by crowding out with sundry recreational activities any focus on their essentially traumatic and pathogenic experiences. Such temporarily suppressive treatment invited the reinforcement of dissociation though it may have worked for the while, while the soldier was in active service overseas. Van Putten and Emory rightly insist that early recognition of the syndrome is really essential. Even in these cases, with delayed recognition of combat neurosis, appropriate treatment resulted in much genuine improvement. As they state, "The current emphasis on the 'here and now' in psychotherapy, in conjunction with the combat veteran's reluctance to discuss his traumatic experiences and the therapist's wish to be done with the war, may easily create a tacit agreement between therapist and veteran to avoid the subject, although desensitization through abreaction may be more helpful."

Hendin et al (1981) have shown that the individual "meanings of combat" require elucidation in an adequate psychotherapy. Two veterans, for example, had similar experiences of witnessing a prisoner of war pushed to his doom from a helicopter. For one, the event aroused an identification with the helplessness of the victim; for the other, a sense that he could have prevented it. To eventually secure adequate psychotherapeutic leverage, these meanings obviously would require an understanding of their connections by both therapist and patient. Schwartz (1982) has shown that in such cases of posttraumatic stress disorder, the building of a trustful relationship with the patient is achieved only by great patience and quiet perseverance. These patients suffer from deep-seated guilt related to the unconscious mobilization of primitive, destructive fantasies and they are apt to disown and project the wish to destroy upon the therapist, making the handling of the transferences a difficult but not usually insurmountable problem. Only as a more positive dependent transference is achieved can the patient gradually recover memories of traumatic events, discuss their meanings for him and his feelings and notions about his own involvement, and achieve progressive integration.

REFERENCES

Abse, D. W. (1966). *Hysteria and Related Mental Disorders*. Bristol: John Wright and Sons.

Abse, D. W. (1971). *Speech and Reason*. Charlottesville: University of Virginia Press.

Azam, E. E. (1887). *Hypnotism, Double Conscience et Alteration de la Person-alite*. Paris: Balliere.

Bram, F. M. (1965). The gift of Anna O. *British Journal of Medical Psychology* 38: 53.

Briquet, P. (1859). *Traite Clinique et Therapeutique de L'Hysterie*. Paris: Balliere.

Charcot, J. (1889). *Clinical Lectures of the Disease of the Nervous System*. London: New Syndenham Society.

Eder, M. D. (1917). *War Shock*. London: Heinman.

Ellenberger, H. F. (1970). *The History of Evolution of Dynamic Psychiatry*. New York: Basic Books.

Erikson, E. (1964). *Insight and Responsibility*. New York: Norton.

Fenichel, O. (1945). *The Psychoanalytic Theory of Neurosis*. New York: W. W. Norton and Company.

Ferenczi, S., Abraham, K., Simmel, E., Jones, E. (1921). *Psychoanalysis and the War Neuroses*. London: International Psychoanalytic Press.

Flournoy, T. (1900). *A Study of a Case of Glossolalia*. New York: Harper.

Freud, S. (1895). Studies in hysteria. *S. E.* 3.

Freud, S. (1912). The dynamics of transference. *S. E.* 12.

Freud, S. (1921). Psychoanalysis of war neurosis. *S. E.* 17.

Gmelin, E. (1791). *Materialen fur die Anthropolgie*. Tubingen.

Grinker, R., Spiegel, J. P. (1945). *Men Under Stress*. Philadelphia: Blakiston.

Guze, S. B., Perley, M. J. (1963). Observations on the natural history of hysteria. *American Journal of Psychiatry*. 119: 960.

Hendin, H., Pollinger, A., Singer, P., Ulman, R. B. (1981). Meanings of combat and the development of post-traumatic stress disorder. *American Journal of Psychiatry* 138: 11.

Hodgson, R. (1891). A case of double consciousness. *Proceedings of the Society of Psychical Research*. VII: 221.

Hurst, A. (1940). *Medical Diseases of War*. London: Edward Arnold and Company.

James, W. (1890). *The Principles of Psychology.* New York: Holt.
Janet, P. (1897). L'influence somnambulique et ie besoin de direction. *Revue Philosophique* I: 113-143.
Janet, P. (1907). *The Major Symptoms of Hysteria.* New York: Macmillan.
Jung, C. G. (1928). *Contributions to Analytical Psychology.* London. Routledge and Kagen Paul.
Kardiner, A. (1947). *War, Stress and Neurotic Illness.* New York: Paul B. Hoeber.
Krystal, H., (Ed.). (1968). *Massive Psychic Trauma.* New York: International University Press.
Lifton, R. J. (1970). *History and Human Survival.* New York: Random House.
McDougall, W. (1920). Discussion of the revival of emotional memories and its therapeutic value. *British Journal of Psychology.*
McDougall, W. (1926). *Outline of Abnormal Psychology.* New York: Charles Scribner and Sons.
Oesterreich, T. K. (1974). *Antiquity, the Middle Ages, and Modern Times.* New York: Causeway Books.
Owen, A. G. (1971). *Hysteria, Hypnosis and Healing, the Work of J. M. Charcot.* New York: Garrett.
Prince, M. (1906). *The Dissociation of a Personality.* Green and Company.
Rivers, W. R. (1942). *Instinct and the Unconscious.* London: Cambridge University Press.
Schwartz, H. (1982). Vietnam veteran: handle with care. *Medical Portfolio for Psychiatrists* (audiotape) 3: 1. Ossining, New York.
Sébillot, P. (1906). *Le Folk-Lore de France.* Paris: Guilmoto.
Sprenger, J., Kramer, H. (1486). *The Malleus Malificarum.* Cologne.
Strauss, I., Savitzky, N. (1934). Head Injury, neurologic and psychiatric aspects. *Archives of Neurology and Psychiatry.* 37: 893.
Van Putten, Emory, W. H. (1973). Traumatic neuroses in Vietnam returnees: a forgotten diagnosis? *Archives of General Psychiatry* 29: 695.
Veith, I. (1965). *Hysteria, the History of a Disease.* Chicago: University of Chicago Press.
Zimmerman, G. A. (1879). *Johann Joseph Gassner, de Berumte Exorcist.* Kempton: Jos. Kosel.

2
Psychoanalytic Psychotherapy and the Vietnam Veteran

VICTOR J. DEFAZIO, PH.D.

INTRODUCTION

The second Indochina War, as the political scientist and economist Bernard Fall (1963, 1972) called it, was the longest war in American history. The first of almost 59,000 Americans killed in action died there in 1960 and the last in 1973. The American military was there in some force in 1954 (not counting OSS missions during World War II) and U.S. Marines were killed in the area as late as 1975 (Mayaguez casualties).

The nature and style of the war contributed to psychological difficulties experienced by its veterans although not always directly to those syndromes noted as traumatic psychopathology. It was not a "classic" 20th century war. Much of it, but by no means all, was fought as a clandestine guerrilla war. This gave it a particularly insidious and almost fiendish character. The sense of danger was omnipresent since even the most innocent looking civilian (including children) might be a guerrilla double agent or informer. The American soldiers' sense of being an alien was exacerbated by the striking differences in language and culture. Morale was undermined by the rotation system and the soldiers' easy access to news of antiwar demonstrations and sentiment back in the "world."

Copyright © 1984 by Spectrum Publications, Inc. *Psychotherapy of the Combat Veteran*, edited by H. J. Schwartz.

In the early years of the war the operations of the U.S. Army Special Forces was controlled by the Central Intelligence Agency (CIA). Assassination and murder, begun by the communists during the first Indochina War, became an accepted style of warfare by both sides. The CIA fought a secret war in Laos with its own airforce and mercenary army. Brutality was too often commonplace. One should keep in mind that matters were made worse because to the Vietnamese it was a civil war. It brought out the talionic (Masterson, 1981) impulse in both sides.

The war was often a conglomeration of small unit actions with endless patrols, ambushes, and more than the usual amount of close combat. While tours of duty for individual combatants were only 365 days, which theoretically kept down the number of psychiatric casualties (Bourne, 1970; Figley, 1978; Borus, 1974), actually many men spent almost the entire time in combat, ie, in contact with or attempting to contact the enemy or under shell fire. Months of "humping" through the "boonies" was broken by a week or two of R and R and then a return to the same savage routine. The war was a mix of many wars: the overt and the covert. There were those who held support positions but were subject to periodic attack and those who had especially dangerous positions, eg, long-range reconnaissance units. In some years the fighting was especially intense (1967–1971) and whole American units were wiped out almost to the last man. However, all had in common the elements of some physical danger, alienation from the indigenous population, physical fatigue (from heat and exertion), and separation from home and loved ones.

The Second Indochina War was fought largely by a young and working class army. The average age for soldiers was 19 compared with 26 for World War II. Two-thirds of those killed in action were 21 years of age or younger. Of the possible pool of men available for the draft from 1964–1973, only 9.7 percent actually served in Southeast Asia (Kolb, 1982). This included about 3.5 million men and women of whom about half a million were naval personnel serving off shore. Two-thirds of all possible draftees served no active duty time at all. Besides the dead, some 303,704 men were wounded, 75,000 of them severely. Some 2,448 men remain missing in action and unaccounted for.

A much higher proportion of combat deaths were due to small arms fire, booby traps, and mines than in either of America's other major 20th century wars (Musser and Stenger, 1972). The nature of the combat (frequently at close range), the type of wounds (a high proportion to head, neck and thorax), especially multiple wounds, combined with excellent medical care resulted in a higher incidence of complicated disabilities, including multiple amputations, paraplegia, and hemiplegia. The percentage of Vietnam veterans who suffered severely crippling wounds was 300 percent higher than in World War II and 70 percent higher than in Korea.

The psychiatric casualty rate for all branches of the service has been reported as being much lower for the Indochina war. Overall, it was purported to be 12 per 1,000 as compared with 37 per 1,000 during the Korean conflict and as high as 101 to 250 per 1,000 in World War II (Bourne, 1970). The statistic for the Indochina veterans is a matter of much contention (Figley, 1978; Goodwin, 1980). The probability of this figure reflecting the real extent of the problem seems unlikely. Mental health professionals in the Armed Forces are faced with a chronic dilemma. While on one hand they are charged with healing the injured, on the other, they are charged with a partial responsibility for manpower. One view of this was provided by Johnson (1967). He wrote,

> There have been criticisms of such statistics . . . and that the individuals treated by the described methods and returned to duty do not do good duty. It has been further said that sending such individuals (psychiatric casualties) back to duty will only fix their neurosis so that they can never be cured. It may be pointed out initially in answering these criticisms that, even if they were true, the action was justified since in combat whether an individual is ill, injured or psychiatrically disabled, the criterion for return to duty is not comfort or complete absence of symptoms but rather the ability to perform (p. 44).

A contrary view was presented by Glasser (1971). Of the issue he wrote,

> We used to believe that conversion anxiety reactions removed without sufficient uncovering techniques would only go on to re-establish themselves in other ways . . . In Vietnam the psychiatric patients go back to duty. One hundred percent of the combat exhaustion, 90 percent of the character disorders, 90 percent of the alcoholic and drug problems, 56 percent of the psychosis, 85 percent of the psychoneurosis, 90 percent of the acute situation reactions . . . at least that's the official belief. But there is no medical or psychiatric follow up on the boys after

they've returned to duty. No one knows if they are the ones who die in the very next fire fight, who miss the wire stretched across the tract, or gun down unarmed civilians (pp. 147–148).

It was precisely because of this suspicion, later partially born out (Egendorf, Kadushin, Laufer et al, 1981) that the whole Veterans Outreach Program was started (Blank, 1982). The purpose of the program was to contact the estimated 800,000 veterans who were suspected of suffering from some sequela of the war.

BRIEF HISTORY OF COMBAT PSYCHOPATHOLOGY

Some of the very first observations as to the effects of combat on men were laid down by Homer in the Odyssey (1937). He wrote of the grief, anger, and tears which Odysseus displayed at a banquet given in his honor by King Alcinoos. Those syndromes labeled as war neurosis or the special characteristics associated with war related stress disorders may very well be a peculiarly new phenomenon coincident with the advent of modern warfare (generally agreed to date from either the Crimean or American Civil Wars). Appel (1966) and Glass (1958) cited data which indicated a correlation between total number of days of combat exposure and psychiatric break-down. After 80 to 100 days of combat exposure, psychological vul-nerability of the soldier increases sharply with a probability that his performance will decline significantly. Before the mid-19th century, the supply and transportation of large armies for prolonged periods of time was very difficult such that, with the exception of seiges, sus-tained combat was virtually impossible.

Extensive and detailed accounts of the effects of modern war on the psyche began with World War I. Observations from the major political antagonists in the struggle as to the consequences were practically identical (Ferenczi, 1916; Freud, 1919; Kardiner, 1941). Since front line psychiatry did not exist at the time, attention to early symptom development was not well documented. The initial theory that the "shell shock" syndrome was a result of an insult to the central nervous system was quickly abandoned when psycholog-ical casualties appeared who had little or no direct exposure to combat.

In most instances the symptoms were alarmingly persistent and resistant to the treatments of the time. Generally, symptoms in-cluded night terrors, tremor (variously described as being Parkinson-like), hyperaesthesia of various senses, paralysis, muscle spasms, hyperalertness, incoherent speech, anxiety, and amnesia. These existed in various combinations depending on the individual and to some extent on the precipitating factor and circumstances. Undoubtedly, physicians at the time were dealing with a variety of diagnostic categories, ie, hysterical conversion reactions, schizophrenia, and traumatic neurosis, which were lumped together.

Close observations as to the effect of combat stress on the individual soldier were made first during World War II (Menninger, 1963; Grinker and Spiegel, 1945). Breakdown was viewed as a three-stage process: the incipient stage, stage of partial disorganization, and the stage of total disorganization. The incipient stage was characterized by irritability and sleep disturbance. The second stage was characterized by a number of symptoms, not all of which were present simultaneously, ie, difficulty in concentration, a tendency to become reclusive or morose, an apparent affective flattening, increased apprehensiveness, an increased dependence on comrades, a reluctance to accept responsibility, a tendency to become confused, and various psychosomatic symptoms such as tremor, diarrhea, etc. In the stage of complete disorganization, all the previously mentioned symptoms became worse. Soldiers acted erratically. They cried uncontrollably or babbled like children. At various points in the process the soldier tended to often become absolutely oblivious to danger, as in failing to take cover or the like.

The "experienced soldier" became "hardened" by successive combat experiences up to a point. However, there are assaults on his psychic integrity, the most powerful of which is the experience of losing comrades. "In the opinion of many observers, this is the most destructive influence bearing upon personality integrity in the battle situation. The maintenance of the psychic equilibrium, the defense against yielding to fear and chucking the whole business has its chief emotional anchorage in personal attachments and unit identification" (Menninger, 1963, pp. 159-160).

PSYCHIC TRAUMA IN PSYCHOANALYTIC THEORY

Psychic trauma has, at different times, held a key place in the psychoanalytic theory of the development of neurotic symptoms. At first, traumatic events in childhood of a sexual nature, including seductions involving genital stimulation as well as outright rape, were viewed as the casual agents in the etiology of neurosis. Most often, these appeared to be of an incestuous nature. This idea, espoused in *Studies in Hysteria* (Breuer and Freud, 1895) was supplemented by the notion that the trauma had its effect by happening during a mental state of special vulnerability, such as a hypnagogic or hypnoid-like state. This view was modified such that Freud conceived of the mental state as being relatively unimportant compared with the opposition of the ideas (of the real event) to the conscious mental life, leading to its repression and accompanying affect. The repression of the cathected ideation was then viewed as the mechanism whereby the symptoms developed. Gradually, Freud became aware that the reports of childhood seductions by patients were often more fantasied than real and from other observations it seemed to him that these fantasies were a means of deflecting memories of forbidden autoerotic activities. One of the effects of this early conclusion on the developing theory was to emphasize the (symbolic) meaning an individual attributed to an experience rather than to emphasize the importance of the event itself. Thus, the problem as to why similar events had different effects on different patients was partially resolved theoretically. As psychoanalytic theory continued to evolve, the concept continued to change slightly. Each time the emphasis on trauma shifted, a different place in the causal chain of pathological and normal development was implied. As the theory progressed, the emphasis became more and more on internal mental processes and certain phylogenetically determined critical periods and less on external events including obvious trauma.

In the *Introductory Lectures* (Freud, 1917), trauma was defined as an "excessive magnitude of stimuli too powerful to be worked off in a normal way." Before that time it was merely viewed as any experience involving "uncomfortable" affect. As World War I burst upon the scene the need to understand the psychopathology concomitant upon trauma became imperative. Freud (1919) viewed the "war neurosis" as resulting from an ego conflict. He wrote, "The conflict is between the soldiers' old peaceful ego and his new warlike one, and it becomes acute as soon as the peace-ego realizes what danger it runs of losing its life owing to the rashness of its newly formed, parasitic double. It would be equally true to say that the old ego is protecting itself from a mortal danger by taking flight into a traumatic neurosis and that it is defending against the new ego which it sees as threatening its life. Thus, the precondition of the war neurosis, the soil that nourishes them, would seem to be a national (conscript) army; there would be no possibility of them arising in an army of professional soldiers or mercenaries" (p. 67).

Freud (1920) commented further on those neurosis incidental to war. He noted that, "The symptomatic picture presented by traumatic neurosis approaches hysteria in the wealth of its similar motor symptoms, but surpasses it as a rule in its strongly marked signs of subjective ailment (in which it resembles hypochondria or melancholia) as well as in the evidence it gives of a far more comprehensive general enfeeblement and disturbance of the mental capacities. No complete explanation has yet been rendered either of war neurosis or of the traumatic neurosis of peace. In the case of the war neurosis, the fact that the same symptoms came about without the intervention of any gross mechanical force seemed at once enlightening and bewildering" (p.132).

The symptoms endemic to the war neurosis (the traumatic dream) presented some contradictions to the then current theory. It was observed that the repetitive dreams whose contents are endless variations of the traumatic situation occur in all cases in which the recollection of the actual trauma is not available because of an amnesia.

Freud gave a teleological explanation for such dreams. He stated that,

> Those dreams are endeavoring to master the stimulus retrospectively, by developing the anxiety whose omission was the cause of the traumatic neurosis. They thus afford us a view of a function of the mental apparatus which, though it does not contradict the pleasure principle, is nevertheless independent of it and seems to be more primitive then the purpose of gaining pleasure and avoiding unpleasure (p. 32).

Thus, the "absence of fright" and the "break" of the stimulus barrier are held responsible as important etiological components in the traumatic neurosis. The posttraumatic dream has as its purpose to retrospectively master the stimulus while stimulating anxiety generated by the dreamer's ego. The ultimate aim is to degenerate the stimulus which leads to a "death instinct" theory; the repetition compulsion is the expression of the "instinct" and represents a principle which phylogenetically is antecedent to the pleasure principle.

With the development of the structural model, Freud used the expression "traumatic situation" to relate to experiences of nonsatisfaction and helplessness where stimulation attained unpleasurable levels which could not be mastered or discharged. This definition along with the interpretation of anxiety (signal anxiety) appeared in *Inhibitions, Symptoms and Anxiety* (1926). Later in

Moses and Monotheism (1939), Freud reaffirmed his belief in the importance of trauma in the development of neurosis but left open the question as to whether all neurosis have a traumatic origin.

Psychic trauma was highly significant in the initial conception as a component in the etiology of neurosis. It played a role in the development to a larger extent in the topographic model and to a lesser extent in the structural model, of the theory of the etiology of neurosis. Out of it grew the concept of repetition compulsion, ie, in the need to explain the special qualities of the traumatic dream, as well as "thanatos" and the development and revamping of the conception of anxiety.

PSYCHOANALYTIC THEORY FROM WORLD WAR II

Psychoanalytic observers played key roles in combat psychology in World War II. Of the various metaphychological positions, the adaptive point of view was most heavily relied on for explanations (Rado, 1942; Kardiner, 1941; Grinker and Spiegel, 1945).

Rado (1942) basically held the position that the traumatic neuroses of war consisted in the establishment of a new adaptation or style based on limited psychic resources. His main concern was control systems and he stressed the secondary gain as a motivation for the persistence of the pathology.

Grinker and Spiegel (1945) consider the war neuroses as a syndrome which is essentially similar to those which occur in peacetime and resulting from unconscious conflicts around self-esteem, pride, etc.

Kardiner (1941; Kardiner and Spiegel, 1947) regarded the symptoms as an outgrowth of conflicts between the individual, his inner resources and the relation to the group. He described the traumatic syndrome as having "altered" the veteran's conception of himself in relation to the world, ie, a fixation on the trauma. There is a general irritability as well as a proclivity to aggression and even violence which can be carried out in fugue states with diminished states of awareness. There is a "typical" dream life which includes repetitive nightmares and later dreams of failures to consummate successful actions. Lastly, and perhaps most important, is the contraction of the level of ego functioning including intellectual functioning. The individual suffers from a kind of delusion that the world is an unbearably hostile place. Affect becomes constricted and there is a kind of deterioration which resembles the kind seen in chronic schizophrenics. Ego functioning becomes regressive.

Essentially in this scheme the trauma is viewed disrupting the old previously effective adaptations and resulting in a new adaption to a hostilely renewed world with a constant attempt to shrink from it.

To Kardiner (1959), the operational system used in the Freudian system is not as applicable to the traumatic neurosis as to the neurosis of peacetime. "We cannot isolate any instinct or component instinct that is disturbed, nor can we account for the pathology on the basis of substitutions" (p. 252). Kardiner uses the prototype of "fatigue" as a model of the operation of the traumatic war neurosis.

Essentially the symptoms which develop out of trauma are still viewed by analysts like Furst (1967) as an experience in which the ego is overwhelmed and the individual is forced back to pre-ego mechanisms for dealing with internalized external environments. Furst put it succinctly when he wrote that the "traumatic experience confronts the ego with a 'fait accompli,' so that the ordinary and available defuses and adaptive devices are of little value" (p. 10). Similarly, Solnit and Kris (1967) define trauma as "phenomena that reflect a reaction of the individual to an inner or outer demand or stimulus that is experienced as overwhelming the mediating functions of the ego to a very significant degree" (p. 123). The concept of "overwhelming" characterizes the stimulus as being sudden. With respect to the individual's reaction to the demand, characteristically it "rends the stimulus barrier, is disruptive, renders the individual in some manner helpless while disorganizing feelings, thoughts and behavior and promoting regressive phenomenon" (p. 123).

Anna Freud (1965) made clear the notion that a painful event by itself is not traumatic. That is, it becomes so when its meaning for the person is understood in relation to the level of ego development and the "critical" period during which it occurs. Thus, exposure to surgery might be a trauma in a seven-year-old boy but merely unpleasant to a 12-year-old child. Ernest Kris (1956) differentiated between what he called "shock" and "strain" trauma. Shock trauma reflects the effect of a single, powerful experience while strain trauma represents the effects of long-lasting situations which cause symptomatic effects by the accumulation of undischarged or unassimilable frustrating tensions.

Waelder (1965) preferred to limit the term "trauma" to the acute shock type in order to maintain its meaning more clearly.

PROBLEMS OF TRAUMA IN PSYCHOANALYTIC THEORY

In spite of the massive literature on trauma and its importance in psychoanalytic theory, the actual treatment of those who have been exposed to massive psychic trauma, ie, concentration camp survivors and war veterans, by psychoanalysis has been relatively unsuccessful (Krystal, 1968; Winnik, 1967; Wexler, 1972). Among the Holocaust survivors those who fared worst experienced the trauma during adolescence or were badly sexually abused. This relative failure of the analytic process has been attributed to the results of the ensuing regression which reinstitutes traumatic ego adaptive devices, a failure in the synthetic functions of the traumatized ego and the inevitable negative transferential difficulties in which the analyst is viewed as a malignant, even persecutory figure.

It should be kept in mind that the American army in Vietnam was basically made up of adolescents. The military experience (especially exposure to modern warfare) has a tendency to disrupt character formation by working against individuation (Blos, 1968), increasing superego punitiveness (which generates increased aggression), interrupting the development of ego continuity, inhibiting a clear-cut sexual identity based on normal heterosexual contact, and preventing the working through of childhood trauma (DeFazio, 1975).

In spite of the explanations, theoretical as well as more practical difficulties arise in an orthodox psychoanalytic framework. The original conception of the etiology of the traumatic neurosis was born out of an economic metapsychological point of view which represents a closed system model no longer considered particularly useful in terms of its explanatory power.

There has always been controversy as to whether the traumatic neurosis of war is really a special case of often seen peacetime traumatic neurosis, or is in a special category representing a very different phenomena with a different etiology. Theoretically, it is more parsimonious if the one theory can explain the war neurosis as being like the peacetime neurosis in terms of etiology. This is, no doubt, the reason that efforts are constantly made to discover certain predisposing personality styles or factors which would explain the debilitating effects of war and its trauma. Psychoanalytic theory, after all, stresses the factors in early development and only since the advent of the neo-Freudians have other (later) life cycle phases come to be seen as having any importance.

When considering the special case of concentration camp survivors, analytic writers tend to agree that character development and prior styles (genetic factors) tend to be dominated by the massive trauma itself. That is, that it is not merely that the trauma provides a trigger to set off dominant but preexisting pathology, but rather that it initiated new conflicts and new psychopathology (Waldhorn and Fine, 1974; Niederland, 1981).

Niederland (1981) noted that,

> The guilt feelings and guilt anxieties in an unresolved grief situation, psychoanalytically speaking, are usually considered as being based on early hostile and death wishes with regard to the family members wiped out in the course of the holocaust. In the patients under scrutiny (during the past 35 years I observed and studied close to 2000 survivors of the holocaust) *I cannot accept this explanation.* It is true that masochistic tendencies are operative in many of them, but in the great majority it is the survival itself that stands at the core of the inner conflict (pp. 420-421).

There is the objection voiced by Kardiner (1959) that psychoanalytic theory has less explanatory power in dealing with traumatic pathology of war because,

> the neurotic syndrome cannot be accounted for on the basis of interference with the instinct of self-preservation or ego instincts. There is no unitary instinct of self-preservation and ego instincts have no standing in pathology. Why talk of instincts in a creature whose adaptability depends not on inherited patterns of behavior but on learned and integrated systems of action?" (p. 252).

In order for any theory to properly explain the psychopathologies concomitant with war, such a theory must be able to explain a number of widely agreed upon observations and notions. These have been developed since World War I and include observations from World War II, the Korean War, and the Vietnam War. They include observations from most Western armies.

1. Everyone exposed to the extreme stress of war develops some symptoms no matter how transitory or fleeting. Perhaps the most common of these symptoms are the traumatic nightmare and

the sensitivity or an alertness to loud noises. The persistence of some symptoms for as long as 30 years after the traumas is well documented (Klonoff et al, 1976).

2. A very wide variety of psychopathologies is seen in warfare. These range from full blown psychotic episodes to the transient symptom just mentioned. This is particularly a very old issue, ie, of symptom or even disorder selection.

3. Apparently some of the manifestations of the disorders just appear many years later. In some cases, new, apparently fresh cases of the traumatic neurosis occur as long as 15 years later (Archibald et al, 1962).

4. The manifestations of the psychopathology of war differ over time. Hysteria-like disorders were common during World War I and relatively rare even by the advent of World War II. Character disorders were rarer during World War II and diagnosed as relatively common for veterans of the Vietnam War (Lumry and Brantz, 1972).

5. Lastly, and perhaps most importantly, is the observation that soldiers with apparently excellent premorbid adjustment histories develop serious and intractable psychological disorders. This is well documented among concentration camp survivors (Niederland, 1981).

OBJECT RELATIONS APPROACH

The incorporation of an object relations approach with the current theory adds a dimension which has broken ground for a possible explanation for some of the widely observed phenomenon previously mentioned.

VARIATIONS

Winnicott (1958) and Fairbairn (1952) of the English school in their revision of Freudian libido theory, view the whole course of development as depending on the extent to which objects are incorporated and the natural techniques which are employed to deal with these incorporated (introjected) objects. Psychological development is essentially conceived of as a process whereby infantile dependence upon the object (breast and then mother) gradually proceeds to mature dependence upon the object by the gradual abandonment of an original object relationship based upon primary identification, and the gradual adoption of an object relationship based upon differentiation of the object. The most prominent characteristic of infantile dependence is primary narcissism which is defined as an early state of identification with the object. Secondary narcissism is the state of identification with an object which is internalized. Identification is defined as a primarily unconscious process by which the subject takes over aspects of the object and then behaves as if they were his own. Moreover, the process of identification involves blurring of boundaries, so that thinking and actions that are characteristic of the object upon whom the subject depends, are internalized.

Briefly, in this scheme, objects and/or part objects are incorporated by the ego. There are splits in which gratifying (good) objects are separated from nongratifying or rejecting (bad) objects. Unconscious aggression is directed against internalized objects. The "true self" tends to be hidden and the whole complex universe of dynamic action is surrounded by a false self (that self which deals with the outer world in compliance).

Fairbairn (1952) noted that,

> All must recognize, of course, that no individual born into this world is so fortunate as to enjoy a perfect object relationship during the impressionable period of infantile dependence, or for that matter during the transition period which succeeds it. Consequently, no one ever becomes completely emancipated from the state of infantile dependence, or from some proportionate degree of oral fixation; and there is no one who has completely escaped the necessity of incorporating his early objects. It may consequently be inferred that there is present in every one either an underlying schizoid or an underlying depressive tendency (p. 56).

Thus, to Fairbairn (1952) the traumatic or war neurosis is precipitated by the return of the "bad" objects; ie, rejecting objects, and is intimately connected with issues involving dependence and separation anxiety. In this view *everyone* is subject to the development of neurotic symptoms and breakdown depending on the amount of stress and the degree to which infantile dependence has persisted. Stress becomes a factor in that, simply put, the more unsatisfactory the outer reality, the more the individual is forced inward to internalized fantasies and gratification from already incorporated objects. Also with increased stress there is a lessening of the ability of the ego to repress, and thus a "release" of "bad" objects ensue. Early conflicts (infantile ones) may become prominent again. The early infantile conflicts involving incomplete development revolve around issues of love and hate (ie, hate destroying the loved object as in the depressive position, and love destroying the loved object as in the schizoid position), while the distintegration of the self becomes the ultimate feared outcome.

An object relations point of view can be used to account for phenomena widely observed in a simple but global fashion. The observation that soldiers with good premorbid adjustment can develop pathology as well as the observation that no one seems immune from some symptomology, even if temporarily, can be understood in this framework.

To reiterate, splitting as a defensive operation is present in all individuals, if only at the deepest levels of psychic structure. It is a given in psychological development. Thus, the pathology evident in such a process can be seen under conditions of stress. The degree of stress required to demonstrate the pathology varies from individual to individual and the pathology is also determined by the degree to which infantile dependence has persisted. Thus, all persons are subject to separation-anxiety and the psychopathology of the unrepressed, unsatisfying libidinal objects, their derivatives or part objects.

So far as Fairbairn (1952) is concerned separation-anxiety is the universal feature of the "war-neurosis." Morale and group integrity become the only real bulwarks against breakdown. This simple contention is borne out by the often cited observation that the most destructive event to occur in combat is the loss of close comrades in a unit, the dissolution of other close interpersonal ties (eg, death of family members while the soldier is in action), or the witness of death—a reminder of the ultimate separation (Lidz, 1946; Menninger, 1963; Fairbairn, 1952). This way of looking at events begins to explain the high rate of psychiatric casualties before intense combat is even experienced (Tischler, 1969) and psychiatric casualties which occur merely by being transferred to a combat zone (Egendorf et al, 1981). That is, the mere separation (or in some instances the mere threat of separation) from familiar surroundings and benign supportive relationships can precipitate intense anxiety and symptom development.

Thus, the less fused the introjects, the more aggression available and the weaker the ego, the less the adaptive and integrative functions of the ego operate optimally and therefore the more quickly the individual succumbs to even minor stress. Regardless of which system of character classification is used, ie, Fenichel (1945) or Kernberg (1976), those individuals with the severest pathologies fall victim fastest. In a sense, the stress of military life and combat become a "shaking out" or "sifting" process.

I have treated a half dozen men who were clearly schizophrenic before service. Several had received treatment before being drafted. One man had succeeded in controlling the more obvious symptoms of his disorder prior to service with heavy drug use. Interestingly, his initial period of service had a compensating effect partially based on the strong identification with his comrades. He used drugs during the transitional period. In his first combat action, his unit came under fire from a single sniper. He moved forward and hurled a hand grenade which accidentally slightly wounded a man from his unit. Immediately upon discovering what had happened he became guilt stricken and quickly decompensated. Within a day after the incident florid symptoms of psychosis appeared and he had to be medically evacuated.

Regression becomes a key concept in understanding the effects of traumatic situations. Once one accepts the notion that, even in normal psychological development, regression is always present as a reaction to unpleasant stimulation (Freud, A., 1965), the elements of the stress disorder begin to fall into place. Regression allows pre-oedipal psychic organization to be touched.

Perhaps the most disturbing aspect, in terms of long-term consequences, of the stress disorders is the general contraction of ego functioning first described by Ferenczi (1916) and elaborated by Kardiner (1941). This "alteration in life course" is characterized by a chronic underachievement and instability. It is often punctuated by a wandering life style and even antisocial acts (Lipkin et al, 1982). In the worst cases it resembles severe borderline character disorders or chronic schizophrenic deterioration. It is concomitant with a general alienation, social isolation and very poor interpersonal relationships.

Parson (1982) was among the first to point to the similarity between the stress disordered veterans of the Vietnam War and the more common difficulties associated with borderline and narcissistic character disorders. That is, the prominent problems are in the areas of impulse control, lack of anxiety tolerance, the failure of sublimatory channels, and narcissistic regulation (Kernberg, 1975).

Ordinarily an individual ostensibly normal or with a high level character disorder (Kernberg, 1976) is exposed to stress in a war situation. The more prolonged and severe the stress the more likely regression is to take place as an ordinary adaptive mechanism. Up to a point the process is reversible. Beyond that point the individual regresses to preego or early ego mechanism of defense and structure along with the release of hereto repressed "bad objects." Fairbairn (1952) notes that,

> . . . the release of repressed objects of which I speak is by no means identical with that active externalization of internalized bad objects, which is the characteristic feature of the paranoid technique. The phenomenon to which I specially refer is the escape of bad objects from the bonds imposed by repression. When such an escape of bad objects occurs, the patient finds himself confronted with terrifying situations which have hitherto been unconscious. External situations then acquire for him the significance of repressed situations involving relationships with bad objects. This phenomenon is accordingly not a phenomenon of projection, but one of transference (p. 76).

This transference converts the world into a malevolent atmosphere to be guarded against. By their nature "bad objects" have a valence which is heavily tinged with aggression. Such a valence increases experienced anxiety. At this level splitting is a primary defensive mode and exacerbates the situation since by its nature it weakens ego boundaries, interferes with the refusion of introjects and the differentiation of self and objects. Splitting is reinforced as a basic protection of the positive introjects and a general protection of the ego against diffusion of anxiety.

At this point the victim becomes trapped by the cycle. The outside world, including personal relationships, appears malevolent. The weakened ego is unable to recognize the falsification. The individual is embroiled in attempting to deal with high degrees of anxiety and aggression. Attempts to break out are foiled by the diminished synthetic functioning of the ego. Mastery in almost any endeavor is bound to fail since the delay of gratification and necessary sublimation are simply not available. Self esteem suffers and attempts at regulation are sought through fantasy or drug use which only diminishes reality testing further.

In this context such dramatic symptoms as "flashbacks" (the reliving and reexperiencing of traumatic events) are interpreted to be a blurring of concepts of past and present as a result of profound ego weakness. This notion is reinforced by the observation that frequently these "flashbacks" are precipitated or exacerbated by drug or alcohol use.

The victim of the stress disorder often tends to react with rage and guilt. The rage exists simultaneously at many levels. It is partly the result of the narcissistic injury at contemporarily being an incompetent individual. In the syndrome the individual is vaguely aware of no longer functioning as he once did or could. The regression and object splitting have caused a return to more primitive idealizations (unrealistic all good and powerful object images) such that ideals now become impossible to attain and by internal comparison the individual indeed seems puny. Thus, there is a constant self-flagellation and sadistic attack by the now more powerful superego. Behaviorally, the rage almost seems to take the form of a need for revenge, ie, to reverse feelings of helplessness and impotence so that another is now the victim. This is highly reminiscent of Masterson's (1981) elaboration of the talionic impulse. Masterson noted that in such persons the need to get even seemed to outweigh the need to get well. The rage is also a reaction to the transfer of bad objects to the outside world and along with them the aggressive interplay involved.

Guilt also has several sources. There is the moral guilt over real but regretted acts or omissions. However, in this approach guilt originates as a preoedipal device which is an additional defense against situations involving bad internalized objects. Guilt originates on the principle that the child finds it more tolerable to regard himself as conditionally (ie, morally) bad then to regard his parents (internalized good objects) as unconditionally (ie, libidinally) bad. Thus, in the regressed individual guilt is released regardless of the reality of acts.

Forensic issues involving diagnosis frequently surface with regards to veterans. Gratefully, the issue has been largely resolved with development of the posttraumatic stress disorder classification. However, from a theoretical point of view the concept is foggy. This syndrome is not really a character disorder. Such a designation implies a stable and consolidated impulse and defense configuration which minimizes anxiety and protects against the awareness of troubling neuroses while rendering symptoms ego syntonic. This is certainly not the case in the chronic posttraumatic stress disorder where neuroses of the trauma are intrusive, anxiety abounds, and symptoms are distressing. Perhaps Parson's (1982) designation as a "fluid character" pathology best describes the syndrome. He notes that, "The term fluid character pathology is best reserved for combatants (and other traumatized persons) who suffer delayed or chronic stress symptomology or from acute post-trauma reactions" (p. 25).

Levels of Psychopathology

Broadly speaking, combat psychopathology can be categorized (DeFazio, 1978) according to the degree of pretrauma dependence, the severity of stress and the degree of the ensuing regression. They do not imply a discontinuity but rather a continuum in terms of ego autonomy, defenses, anxiety tolerance, mastery, and aggression. They do differ in the extent of consolidation of the symptom pattern and the prognosis.

Briefly, stress in such situations can be defined. For relatively normal premorbid personality adjustments, high stress situations include individuals exposed to heavy combat where units took many casualties; those who were wounded in action; men in high risk occupations such as members of recon units or those involved in secret work in combat areas; nurses in field hospitals; persons assigned to graves registration; and prisoners of war. This is certainly not an all inclusive list, but is illustrative of the kind of activities which lead to difficulties.

For those with very poor premorbid adjustments and who were highly dependent, no matter how cleverly disguised, stressors might be as simple as receiving an order to report for advanced infantry training or seeing a comrade hurt in training.

Attitudinal Change

These men are considered well functioning and are seldom seen in treatment. However, attitudes have changed in such a way as to cause them to adopt a new style not necessarily classifiable as pathological. Wilson (1980) gives a good description of these styles using the intervention of stress during adolescence as a starting point. In any psychotherapy with these individuals the experience of the war is often neglected in favor of a concentration on earlier developmental events, an obvious omission.

Unchanged Character Disorder

These men consist of individuals who have and had (prewar) higher level borderline conditions, narcissistic personality disorders, character neurosis, etc. Of the signs of nonspecific ego weakness, many may be present with the exception that these individuals retain strong sublimatory capabilities. In addition, under ordinary conditions, impulses are controlled (ie, while not under the influence of drugs or alcohol). Their tolerance for anxiety varies but it seems to hover near or in the normal range. In one way or another their experience of the war tended to exacerbate existing conflicts or reinforce the consolidation of pathological character defenses and traits.

Harold appeared for treatment out of a sense that the war may have contributed to his current problems but he was not quite sure how. He was a successful individual in his field but secretly felt he still had to prove himself. His relationships seemed shallow and he was eager to please anyone in authority. His mother had been ambitious for him and his father appeared to be chronically depressed and disappointed. This man joined the service to get away from his family, "to get a breath of fresh air." In the army he was assigned to the combat zone and saw action but spent most of his time in supply. He did a magnificent job. His men never lacked for the small luxuries obtainable. His need to excel, to find meaning and to find narcissistic gratification in the applause of others was obvious to him as he sat before me. The war had merely proved to him that he could "feel better about (himself)" if others liked him. He was aware of his lack of empathy for the misery of the "grunts" but was also aware of the carryover into civilian life, ie, the way he regarded his co-workers. The war had not really changed him but presented a reinforcement of a reality (his own) which he expected. It merely became a new testing ground, in some ways the first since he entered right after college.

The stressors to which this group was exposed tend to be minimal to average. The war was a backdrop in front of which their style was played out.

Psychotherapy with these men tends to run a normal course. Management problems are no greater than are ordinarily encountered. Their war experiences can sometimes be used as a means of withholding or control since it is often regarded as a "secret" area of experience not to be readily shared. That is, the experience of the war comes to have a symbolic meaning within the psychodynamics of the individual. This becomes an important point to keep in mind since, at first, other categories of stress disordered individuals are not readily capable of making symbolic transformations nor do they generally show the insight of men in this group. It is not uncommon, however, to find a specific symptom related to a war experience which might not be explored in a treatment where the therapist is not sensitive to the stresses such men were subjected to. General issues of moral guilt, responsibility, relatedness, and idealizations are almost always present.

Delayed Regressed Character

The pattern of symptom development and the instigating circumstances tend to be remarkably similar in this group of veterans. The patient usually presents himself as having lived a very normal life since his return from Southeast Asia. Suddenly and with no warning he begins to have night terrors. Often at the start he is aware of having nightmares but cannot remember the content. He wakes up from a fitfull sleep drenched in sweat. After a long hiatus he once again becomes sensitive to sound and the world becomes a hostile place. He experiences high levels of anxiety and deep periods of depressiveness. Invariably, these episodes are set off by separation-anxiety as a result of real or threatened abandonment, eg, marital separation, death of a parent, etc.

The clients in this category are numerous. John was a typical example. He developed all the standard symptoms which began to develop around the separation from his wife. Since his return he had never spoken of the war. He was married before service and was old for his outfit. John had a number of severe traumatic encounters during his tour but developed a real amnesia for all of them. He could not even remember the nicknames of his closest friends. When his wife openly began to have affairs with other men he began to develop symptoms. He had to temporarily cease working a job he held steadily for almost 12 years. The therapy sessions held real terror for him. He would often have severe anxiety attacks on the way to sessions. These subsided quickly as he began to recall real events and remember the dreams. These sessions were particularly dramatic. The anxiety, depression, and guilt, however, did not completely subside until the current issues of separation were at least partially worked through.

Chronic Regressed Character

The men and women in this group find themselves trapped in the cycle of regression mentioned earlier. They present a wide variety of disorders. Those with the best reality contact often appear depressed. Upon closer examination one discovers rather that affect is flat but with no subjective experience of depressiveness. Rather they experience fatigue and literally describe themselves as being "burned out." Thinking tends to be concrete and riveted to the present. They tend to be socially isolated and relate superficially. In such individuals, good prognostic indicators are subjective feelings of depressiveness, some anxiety and even anger, to a point. The ability for symbolic transformations are absent at first such that standard interpretations seem to have little effect. The key to treatment here seems to be a preparatory period during which the therapist begins to make the most elementary connections between past and present, thought and action, and thought and feeling. As soon as affect and symptoms (usually nightmares) begin to surface, the treatment begins to become standard.

The much more difficult cases in this group involve individuals in whom reality testing is poorer and where non-specific signs of ego weakness are present, ie, anxiety, inability to sublimate, and poor impulse control. The best prognostic indicators in such individuals is the pretraumatic adjustment picture and degree of prior relatedness. The therapy here can be exceedingly difficult and an approach as that used by Masterson (1981) seems most appropriate. Setting limits becomes important as does the frequency of sessions (usually twice per week). The basics in such a situation involve standing firm against the client's manipulations and handling the considerable counter-transference difficulties which rapidly arise.

Howard, a case in point, had a fairly typical adolescence. After joining the Marines he was sent to Vietnam and spent most of his time in combat. He was wounded seriously and evacuated home. He had difficulty adjusting and never found steady employment. He was bitter and resentful when he was first referred for treatment 11 years later. He spent countless hours recounting the government's bungling on the war and the inequalities of American democracy. He felt alone but constantly made demands on the therapist for time or "favors." He drank episodically and initially appeared at sessions drunk. He made calls to the therapist at all hours.

Initially the "therapy" really consisted of confrontations about these attempts to hamper the therapy. Months were spent on merely working on the minimum requirements for therapy, ie, that he appear for sessions on time and be sober. Once accomplished, the next stage of beginning to talk about relevant matters began, ie, himself.

Also in this group one sees the most difficult cases. That is, those who appear and for all practical purposes are psychotic and badly deteriorated.

Albert was seen for a consultation and was accompanied by his older brother who brought various documentation with him. Albert had been a gregarious, athletic young man in high school. He had a regular girlfriend, was a good student and was regarded as popular.

In the service he was wounded several times in action and saw heavy combat. Upon his return home and after recuperation he became delusional and violent. He was hospitalized on numerous occasions. At the point he was seen he sat mutely.

CONCLUSIONS

In treatment one needs to keep in mind that there is no such thing as a stress proof individual. The style of treatment is dictated by the nature and force of the stressors, the premorbid personality picture, the degree of regressiveness, the ongoing conflicts and the current adaptive and character pattern. In some victims there is a point beyond which regressiveness is never fully reversed.

The stress disorders due to combat appear to be different from those of civilian life where reactivated genetic conflicts are more the rule. In military stress disorders due to prolonged exposure to combat character seems no longer immutable.

Although the war has been over for more than ten years, for some individual combatants the struggle to return to the "world" continues.

REFERENCES

Appel, J. W. (1966). In Anderson, R. S., Glass, A. J., Bernucci, S. R. J. (Eds.). Neuropsychiatry in World War II, Vol. I., Washington, D.C.: U.S. Government Printing Office, 373-415.

Archibald, H. E., Long, D. M., Miller, C. (1962). Gross stress reaction in combat: fifteen year follow up. American Journal of Psychiatry 119: 317-322.

Blank, A. S. (1982). Apocalypse terminable and interminable: Operation outreach for Vietnam Veterans. Hospital and Community Psychiatry 33: 913-918.

Blos, P. (1968). Character formation in adolescence. Psychoanalytic Study of the Child 23: 245-263.

Borus, J. F. (1974). Incidence of maladjustment in Vietnam returnees. Archives of General Psychiatry 30: 554-557.

Bourne, P. G. (1970). Men, Stress and Vietnam. Boston: Little, Brown.

Breuer, J., Freud, S. (1955). Studies in Hysteria. S.E. 2. London: Hogarth Press. (Originally published in 1895).

DeFazio, V. J. (1975). How the Vietnam Veteran Differs Psychologically from his College Peers. Paper presented at Conference on Vietnam Era Veterans. Largo, Maryland: Prince George Community College.

DeFazio, V. J. (1978). Dynamic perspectives on the nature and effects of combat stress. In Figley, C. (Ed.). Stress Disorders Among Vietnam Veterans. New York: Brunner Mazel.

Egendorf, A., Kadushin, C., Laufer, R. S., Rothbart, G., and Sloan, L. (1981). Legacies of Vietnam: Comparative Adjustment of Veterans and their Peers. Washington, D.C.: Committee on Veteran's Affairs.

Fall, B. (1963). The Two Vietnams. New York: Praeger.

Fall, B. (1972). Last Reflections on a War. New York: Schocken.

Fairbairn, W. R. (1952). Psychoanalytic Studies of the Personality. London: Routledge and Kegan Paul.

Fenichel, O. (1945). The Psychoanalytic Theory of Neurosis. New York: Norton.

Ferenczi, S. (1916). Further Contributions to the Theory and Techniques of Psychoanalysis. London: Hogarth Press, 124-141.

Freud, A. (1965). Normality and Pathology in Childhood. New York: International Universities Press.

Freud, S. (1955). Introductory Lectures on Psychoanalysis. S.E. 16. London: Hogarth Press. (Originally published in 1917).

Freud, S. (1955). Psychoanalysis and the War Neurosis. S.E. 17. London: Hogarth Press. (Originally published in 1919).

Freud, S. (1955). Beyond the Pleasure Principle. S.E. 18. London: Hogarth Press. (Originally published in 1920).

Freud, S. (1955). Inhibitions, Symptoms and Anxiety. S.E. 20. London: Hogarth Press. (Originally published in 1926).

Freud, S. (1955). Moses and Monotheism. S.E. 23. London: Hogarth Press. (Originally published in 1939).

Furst, S. (Ed.) (1967). Psychic Trauma. New York: Basic Books.

Figley, C. R. (1978). Stress Disorders Among Vietnam Veterans. New York: Brunner Mazel.

Glass, A. J. (1958). Observations upon the epidemiology of mental illness in troops during warfare. In Symposium on Preventive and Social Psychiatry. Washington, D.C.: Walter Reed Army Institute of Research. 17: 185-197.

Glasser, R. J. (1971). 365 Days. New York: Bantam Books.

Goodwin, J. (1980). The etiology of combat related post-traumatic stress disorders. In Williams, T. (Ed.). Post-traumatic Stress Disorders of the Vietnam Veteran. Cincinnati: Disabled American Veterans, 1-23.

Grinker, R. R., Spiegel, J. P. (1945). Men Under Stress. Philadelphia: Blakiston.

Homer (Translated by Rouse, W. H.) (1937). The Odyssey. London: Thomas Nelson and Sons.

Johnson, A. (1967). Psychiatric treatment in the combat situation. United States Army Republic of Vietnam Medical Bulletin. 2: 38-45.

Kardiner, A. (1941). The Traumatic Neurosis of War. New York: Hoeber.

Kardiner, A. (1959). Traumatic neurosis of war. In Arieti, S. (Ed.). American Handbook of Psychiatry, Vol. 1. 1st ed. New York: Basic Books.

Kardiner, A., Spiegel, H. (1947). War Stress and Neurotic Illness. New York: Hoeber.

Kernberg, O. (1975). Borderline Conditions and Pathological Narcissism. New York: Jason Aaronson.

Kernberg, O. (1976). Object Relations Theory and Clinical Psychoanalysis. New York: Jason Aaronson.

Klonoff, H., McDougall, G., Clark, C., Kramer, P., Horgan, J. (1976). The neuropsychological, psychiatric, and physical effects of prolonged stress: 30 years later. Journal of Nervous and Mental Disease 163: 246-252.

Kolb, R. (1982). Vietnam veteran fact sheet. Stars and Stripes, July 8, 6-9.

Kris, E. (1956). The recovery of childhood memories in psychoanalysis. *Psychoanalytic Study of the Child* 11: 54-88.

Krystal, H. (Ed.) 1968). *Massive Psychic Trauma*. New York: International Universities Press.

Lidz, T. (1946). Nightmares and the combat neurosis. *Psychiatry* 9: 37-49.

Lipkin, J. O., Parson, I. R., Blank, A. S., Smith, J. (1982). Vietnam veterans and post-traumatic stress disorder. *Hospital and Community Psychiatry* 33: 908-912.

Lumry, G. H., Brantz, G. A. (1972). The Vietnam Era Veteran and psychiatric implications. Paper presented at Workshop on the Unique Problems of the Vietnam Era Veteran. V.A. Hospital, New Orleans.

Masterson, J. F. (1976). *Psychotherapy of the Borderline Adult*. New York: Brunner Mazel.

Masterson, J. F. (1981). *The Narcissistic and Borderline Disorders*. New York: Brunner Mazel.

Menninger, W. C. (1963). *The Vital Balance*. New York: Viking Press.

Musser, M. J., Stenger, C. A. (1972). A medical and social perception of the Vietnam Veteran. *Bulletin of the New York Academy of Medicine* 48: 859-869.

Niederland, W. G. (1981). The survivor syndrome: further observations and dimensions. *Journal of the American Psychoanalytic Association* 29: 413-426.

Parson, E. R. (1982). The reparation of the self: clinical and theoretical dimensions in the treatment of Vietnam combat veterans. *Journal of Contemporary Psychotherapy* 14(1).

Rado, S. (1942). Psychodynamics and treatment of traumatic neurosis. *Psychosomatic Medicine* 4: 362-372.

Solnit, A. J., Kris, M. (1967). Trauma and infantile experiences. In Furst, S. (Ed.). *Psychic Trauma*. New York: Basic Books.

Tischler, G. L. (1969). Patterns of psychiatric attrition and of behavior in a combat zone. In Bourne, P. (Ed.). *The Psychology and Physiology of Stress*. New York: Academic Press.

Waelder, R. (1965). Unpublished contribution to panel on the concept of trauma. Annual Meeting of the American Psychoanalytic Association, 1965.

Waldhorn, H., Fine, B. (1974). *Trauma and Symbolism*. Monograph Series of the Kris Study Group. New York: International Universities Press.

Wexler, H. (1972). The life master: a case of severe ego regression induced by combat experience in World War II. *Psychoanalytic Study of the Child* 27: 568-597.

Wilson, J. P. (1980). Conflict, stress and growth: the effects of war on psychosocial development among Vietnam Veterans. In Figley, C. R., Leventman, S. (Eds.). *Strangers at Home*. New York: Praeger.

Winnik, H. Z. (1967). Psychiatric disturbances of Holocaust survivors. *Israel Annals of Psychiatry and Related Disciplines* 5: 91-100.

Winnicott, D. W. (1958). *Through Pediatrics to Psychoanalysis*. New York: Basic Books.

3
Unconscious Guilt:
Its Origin, Manifestations, and Treatment
in the Combat Veteran

HARVEY J. SCHWARTZ, M.D.

A physician had the following experience: He went on a deer hunt with a friend. They spied a buck. The friend shot and killed the animal. Immediately after, he (the hunter) grew restless, was confused, jumped around, uttered incomprehensible words, finally threw himself beside the animal and lay there as if lifeless . . . He enacted on his own person what had happened to the animal; he identified himself with it in death, repeating the crime of murder on himself and apparently punishing himself in this way.

> Herman Nunberg (1934)
> *The Feeling of Guilt*

The Vietnam war has been over for more than a decade. For many veterans however, it remains a part of daily existence. The human psyche does not adapt to political realities. The timelessness of the unconscious keeps alive the events and traumas of war's terrible moments. Political treaties mark the beginning, not the end, of the intrapsychic work of mastery.

The phenomenologic perspective has been the major orientation of the research on the psychological sequelae of battle. After a lengthy period of ignoring postcombat distress an extensive effort was begun to discover and document posttraumatic symptomology. There was a study of the epidemiology, a listing of the symptoms, a measurement of stress levels and the introduction of a new diagnosis. These efforts were essential in mobilizing attention to this forgotten illness. It led to important findings and new psychophysiologic concepts of "stress." It did not, however, offer a deeper appreciation of the combat experience. The fantasies and conflicts elicited by combat have remained essentially unstudied.

My emphasis in this chapter is on the personal meaning of battle to its combatants. I have studied the effects of combat on the unconscious. My data base is the patients' dreams, associations, and transference images that arise in the therapeutic-analytic encounter. Specifically, I address the role of unconscious guilt and the defenses against it in the mental life of the returning Vietnam veteran. This focus is not intended to minimize the many other already understood conflicts that arise after battle. War time is an awesomely complex emotional experience. It inevitably evokes reactions in the biological, developmental, interpersonal, and spiritual realms. It is the conflict over unconscious guilt though that I believe is central to chronic posttraumatic disability.

LITERATURE REVIEW

The literature on the psychological state of combat veterans has reported extensive depression (Nace et al, 1977), somatization (Strange and Brown, 1971), "problems with hostility" (Fow, 1972), and uncontrolled aggression (Yager, 1976). The dynamic basis to these and other symptoms has not been addressed in most studies. The underlying unconscious fantasies, compromise formations, and transference images have not been the focus of the work. There is the possibility that a central unconscious conflict underlies the plethora of reported symptoms.

It is veterans' conscious reactions to battle that have been the subject of the most research. There are limitations to this approach. Borus (1973) studied "adjustment issues" faced by returning Vietnam veterans. Under the category of "social adjustment" he found that "only 10 percent of the respondents acknowledged feeling guilty or significantly upset about any of their actions in

Vietnam." Under his section of "emotional adjustment" however, he reported that three fourths of his subjects experienced a major change in their temperament since Vietnam and half of them felt it was a damaging change. In addition, one half of all the veterans disliked thinking or talking about Vietnam and tried to shut it out of their mind. One quarter of the sample had recurrent nightmares and intrusive thoughts about Vietnam. These were related to witnessing the death of a friend and the killing of women and children.

In a similar investigation, Goldsmith and Cretekos (1969) interviewed hospitalized veterans of combat. The patients were asked about their "attitude toward the war" and based on their verbal reports he concluded that "many of the psychological difficulties apparent in the post-combat period and return to [the U.S.] seemed to be related to family and marital problems rather than to combat." In the case histories presented, however, there seem to be contradictory data. One depressed patient found himself "worrying about the parents of the people he killed." Another patient, admitted because of a drunken suicide gesture, had a "particularly disturbing image . . . (of) shooting a six-year-old girl when his unit was sweeping a village." He had recurrent nightmares about this shooting. Another 20-year-old patient with the diagnosis of anxiety reaction reportedly was "proud that he had killed many of them." He remembered seeing their bodies with flies about them and "laughed at them." At the time of hospitalization though, he could not tolerate noise, needed to live alone and stated that he "doesn't like to see anybody in pain . . . (I) now want to help people."

What both these papers have in common is their data base. Borus asked his subjects about their guilt feelings and Goldsmith queried his soldiers about their attitude about the war. They report the patient's *conscious* replies. Both patient groups answered without an awareness of specific stress over their combat experience. However, their disabling symptomatology reveals, in fact, the presence of severe intrapsychic conflict. I believe the concept of "unconscious guilt," guilt that the patient is unaware of, best explains these seemingly conflicting data. It makes sense of the absence of conscious guilt in 90 percent of Borus' sample and yet of the presence of symptoms that reflect severe guilt. Similarly in Goldsmith's sample, the patients' conscious answers led the investigators to conclude that guilt or any other feelings concerning combat were not contributing to their presenting difficulties. However, they ignored the data from the patients' unconscious as revealed in dreams and symptoms. Specifically, they did not study the unconscious significance to the patient of having killed a six-year-old girl. The patient though had recurrent nightmares of the murder and attempted suicide. In fact, the patient himself stated that before Vietnam, "I could understand myself . . . now I am different." I believe his confusion resides in his unconscious and specifically in his unconscious guilt.[1]

Gault (1971) spent two years as a psychiatrist evaluating scores of Vietnam returnees. His paper is addressed to the causes and results of the soldiers' experience of "slaughter" of innocent victims. He presents a case of a patient with headaches, chronic anxiety, restlessness, and insomnia, all beginning since his Vietnam tour. The patient explained his symptoms by figuring "I seen too much crap." As an example, he related how he, ten other soldiers, and a lieutenant entered a village. They demanded information from the villagers and when their inquiries were met with silence had two old women stand over a well. When further demands for information were ignored, the lieutenant "had a couple of the guys push the old women down the well, then throw a grenade in the well."

Significantly, in this brief vignette the patient does not spontaneously report on his own involvement in this or other atrocities. It is the "other guys" who commit the crimes. In fact, he is aware only of the guilt of "seeing crap" not of doing it. He reports conscious remorse and yet his symptoms are a reminder to us that his superego still holds him accountable for his as yet unspecified crimes, real or fantasied. Without this idea of unconscious guilt, this patient's treatment would be relegated to supportive efforts at helping him forget the past. The conceptual possibility of uncovering his own personal guilt, with or without attention to infantile origins, offers a more powerful therapeutic tool toward freeing this man from chronic disability. A clinical demonstration of this concept is provided by Langner.

Langner (1971) presented a case history entitled "The Making of a Murderer." The patient, a medic, was evaluated after making a suicide attempt. His conscious reasons for the attempt were his guilt feelings concerning his buddy's death, along with the feeling that he should have died in his place. Despite repeated ventilation of these

---

[1] The specifics of different investigators' conceptual frameworks have important implications for research design and interpretation. Conclusions drawn from studies of patients' conscious replies cannot meaningfully be compared with research into patients' unconscious productions. If we are to be able to profitably use different workers' findings, we must make clear the parameters used in studying patients.

conscious guilt feelings, the patient did not improve. He was given an amobarbitol interview in an effort to understand his unconscious processes. While under the influence of the medication, the patient made no reference to his dead friend. Instead, for the first time he described in detail a military assault on a village in which he participated in the killing of all living things including women, children, and livestock. Specifically, he spoke of killing an elderly injured man who lay at his feet pleading for help.

This patient's own active crimes had been repressed from memory—their only symbolic reminder was his suicide attempt. His presentation is a dramatic illustration of the importance of the concept of unconscious guilt. Without it, this patient's conscious guilt over the death of his friend would be seen as responsible for his suicidal wishes. His failure to improve would perhaps be explained by postulating an inadequate ego. However, the derepressing effects of amobarbitol revealed a complex substrata of unconscious fantasy, recent and genetic memories and potential transference distortions that make available for treatment the core of his unconscious conflict.

Other researchers have similarly found it useful to administer amobarbital to reach into the patient's unconscious and evoke warded-off material. Solomon et al (1971) presented case histories of three Vietnam veterans who were also interviewed with amobarbital and methamphetamine.

Patient 1 was admitted guarded, suspicious, and complaining that "I was framed." During his hospitalization, the patient refused to verbalize any of his thoughts and made numerous suicide attempts. Under amobarbital, he revealed the heretofore unknown precipitant to his first psychiatric hospitalization which was for psychotic depression. The patient reported that he was ordered to shoot an innocent 14-year-old Vietnamese girl who had refused the sexual advances of an officer. By chance, the patient had befriended the girl and spent the entire previous day with her without sexual involvement. Under threat of court-martial the patient killed her. He then became very upset, began a fight with the officer, and shot him, making it appear as if it had been enemy fire. Near the end of the interview the patient pleaded, "How can I ever live with myself knowing what I have done?"

After the interview, the patient improved. He began to socialize with others and began relating with his family. Ultimately though, apparently under the influence of the talionic law, the patient shot himself to death.

Patient 2 was admitted after a suicide gesture. Under amobarbitol he revealed that while high on amphetamine he mistakenly shot and killed several friendly Indo-Chinese and wounded two American advisors. Significantly, the deaths were attributed to enemy fire and "the patient's role in it [was] never questioned." After this episode the patient began a living-out atonement and "felt he could only justify living by serving others." The authors concluded that "never [having been] punished for his 'error' in shooting allies, chronically self-destructive acting out and attempts at masochistic restitutive object relationships were the only alternative." Significantly, after the interview the patient began a successful psychotherapy.

Patient 3 presented with a persistent incapacitating pain around the scar of his war wound. An amobarbital interview revealed that a few days before being wounded himself, he told another soldier to throw a grenade into a bunker. The grenade hit the bunker wall, bounced back and killed the thrower and two others. His own wounding followed soon thereafter. While being medevaced out of danger by his one close friend, the friend was shot and severely wounded in the lower extremities. The patient never found out if his friend's legs were saved. Throughout the interview the patient expressed great guilt and stated, "I deserve to suffer." After the interview, a psychotherapeutic approach based on an understanding of the patient's guilt was begun and was successful.

This work is a clear example of the explanatory power of unconscious guilt. The memory of the disturbing events and their emotional reactions to them were not consciously available to the patients. However, through the use of a medication that reduces the repression barrier (Herman, 1938; Kubie and Marcolin, 1945; Grinker and Speigel, 1944), the pathogenic force of these events was revealed. Significantly, in my experience similar data become available through the technique of free association and resistance analysis.

In all three of Solomon's cases, underlying infantile fantasies were seen as responsible for the patient's vulnerability to guilt and depression. Their understanding is helpful for the therapist to guide him through the many transference distortions that will arise in the treatment even when it is focused on the traumatic situation.

The transference and the sometimes dramatic resistances to it that emerge in the treatment of severely guilty patients commonly evoke powerful countertransference reactions. Haley has written extensively on this aspect of the therapeutic treatment of Vietnam veterans.

In her first work (1974), she presented three clinical vignettes that illustrate guilt, self-destructive acting out, and identification with the victim in veterans who had committed atrocities in Vietnam. She noted the importance of being "in touch" with the patient, which she feels requires the therapist to acknowledge their own potential for sadistic acts. In her later work (1978), she described her own dramatic countertransference reactions in the four-year treatment of a Vietnam veteran. She concluded that the therapist must maintain empathic contact with the patient in order to assist in the reworking of the traumatic past. Elsewhere (1979), Haley suggested that the paucity of social and clinical attention to these patients derives from the difficulty that the culture at large and therapists in particular have with the fantasies and transference images these men bring to treatment.

The saturation of the Vietnam combat experience with uncontrolled violence has not permitted these soldiers to live out their lives peacefully. The mechanization of the war, the dehumanization of the enemy, and the reported "psychic numbing" all have been suggested as factors enabling these men to avoid awareness of what they have done. For large numbers of them these mechanisms have not been effective once they returned to civilian life. Repeated intimate encounters demand a break in the wall of emotional isolation. It is then that the horror and guilt of the past explodes within their psyches. The meaning of having killed and sometimes mutilated another human being, *and the fantasies thereby stimulated,* haunt these soldiers no less than it would anyone else. Military training does not undo structural development. There was, so to speak, no rest and relaxation for the superego in Vietnam.

A word is in order about the two treatments I am about to present. It is intrinsically artificial to select from any psychotherapy a single theme to explain a patient's pathology. To do so is to ignore the overlapping and overdetermined elements that are part and parcel of psychic conflict. This is all the more true when presenting two very different patients. However, even given this limitation it can be useful to highlight a particular thread that, while individually determined, is common to a number of patients. It is towards this goal that I recount my initial experiences with these men and the role of their unconscious guilt.

As you will see, I had a brief exposure to Mr. A. who is a brittle man with disabling defenses of projection and acting out, as well as periods of paranoia. Significantly, he was by all accounts functioning at a much higher level before combat. Mr. B. also experienced severe and chronic postcombat symptomatology. He has however never displayed psychotic level paranoia nor required the ego support of hospitalization. His somewhat greater developed capacity for symbolic thought allowed a slightly more finely tuned psychotherapy to take place. For example, his impulsively leaving sessions in mid-hour was gradually followed by our collaborative study of his internal state before and during the acting-in.

In my experience, motor activity as a defense against painful affects, particularly those involving the transference, is the rule with traumatized patients. As demonstrated by both these men, this regressive defense also includes somatization. I have found that it is the slow and persistent "translation" of these physical discharges into coherent affects and words that is the hallmark of the work with these patients. These nonverbal remnants of an unbearable past need to be structuralized through the person and words of the therapist into ". . . memory traces, and in so doing to overcome their impediments to drive and ego development" (Cohen, 1980).

CASE PRESENTATIONS

Patient A

Mr. A. is a 32-year-old black man who came to a VA clinic with a history of two previous psychiatric hospitalizations related to his presenting difficulties. The patient's symptoms consisted of frequent nightmares of Vietnam since his discharge ten years ago, initial and middle insomnia, frequent daytime visual flashbacks of Vietnam, critical auditory hallucinations, sudden aggressive outbursts, multiple somatic pains, periods of vomiting, and feelings of anxiety and depression. The patient had been diagnosed as suffering from schizophrenia and was receiving 10 mg of haloperidol per day without significant benefit.

The patient reported that his nightmares and flashbacks began after his return from Vietnam. He was first hospitalized six years after his discharge for these same complaints. In addition, at that time he was abusing multiple drugs "in order to get rid of the nightmares." He was working at a job that he had been at for many years although with periods of very irregular attendance. At work he was then beginning to feel harrassed and reported that "They are plotting against me." He was suspended from work for threatening to kill a guard and was having financial difficulties. He described having an "urge to kill" and was fearful of hurting his wife of eight years and two children. He described conscious guilt feelings over his activities in Vietnam.

His second hospitalization was three years after his first and lasted five months. On admission his complaints were the same. In addition, he complained of extreme nervousness and was fearful for his life. Because of this fear he had bought a rifle and sat at the window of his home to protect himself, "I thought someone would come in the house to kill me and my family." He reportedly felt like he was "going to explode," and was unable to function at home or work. He had not been working for the previous three months and again was in difficult financial circumstances. At this time he reported hearing the voice of a girl whose mother he had killed in Vietnam. Also at this time he declared his conviction that the cause of his troubles was his having been exposed to Agent Orange while in Vietnam. He believed it affected himself, his wife, and, most importantly, his two children, both of whom he described as suffering from seizures. The patient's wife reported that at times he would be violent with her and that on occasion he put his hands into the gas stove flames. She as well strongly believed that origin of her husband's troubles as well as her own emotional problems was his Agent Orange exposure.

The patient had not had any major psychiatric difficulties before going to Vietnam. He described being popular in high school with many friends and many satisfying heterosexual experiences. He graduated with honors and was on the football and track teams. He is the eldest of four college attending brothers and twin sisters. He reported that as a child he use to say that he always wanted to be in the army just like his father who was injured in World War II. He described his father as hard working, religious, and strict and that he and his father did not get along although he has no memories of corporal punishment. He described his mother as the one who made the decisions in the family. The patient was told that as a preschooler he was "bad and treacherous." He would "kill the other kids' chickens" and their parents would not let their children play with him. Other than his uncle and grandfather, who reportedly abused alcohol, there is no family history of psychiatric disturbances.

Course of Treatment. Mr. A. presented to the clinic on his first visit with his wife. Upon meeting me he quickly and vociferously explained that all of his symptoms were due to his exposure to Agent Orange. As he continued what turned out to be a lengthy diatribe, he also made clear that he was enraged at those who "worry about their jobs while I'm dying."

This was a rather dramatic initial encounter. The patient created an intense moment between us before I could know anything about him or his problems. The "good guys" and the "bad guys" were in clearly separate camps and he was checking me out to see which side I was on. However compromised, I had little choice.

I allowed him to draw from me my own inclinations to view the soldiers of the war as victims. I communicated my willingness to see his symptoms as possibly organically determined and I suggested we work together to see what could be done.

My response, as well as my knowledge of Agent Orange, surprised, pleased, and somewhat confused the patient. I seemed not to be the enemy he came to do battle with, at least not yet. I was hoping that this veneer of a positive transference would enable me to eventually broaden my base of contact with him. He had no interest at that time in understanding himself and was quite vocal in his perception of his difficulties being caused by "them." He did however elicit from me a warm and interested response. I sensed a defensive quality to his rage and felt him to be tired of always attacking others. His wish to be heard, and not surprisingly, cared for, communicated itself despite his polemics. I was though prepared to be seen as one of "them" and frankly didn't know if we would be able to develop a common ground from which to view his distrust.

The patient missed his next appointment and called the following day to reschedule. He returned and began describing his nightmares of atrocities committed in Vietnam and how he was the only survivor of his unit during the TET offensive. The following visit revealed the origin of his nightmare from Vietnam. He began the hour by describing that when he heard his children crying at night he would bring them into his bed as he feared their death. He also described a repetitive intrusive thought of "Why did they do this to us?" referring to government spraying of Agent Orange.

He went on to speak of Vietnam. When he arrived there he began noticing meaningless brutality and felt confused and angered by it. He described wanton murder of entire families and recalled wondering then if it "would come back to me." He then revealed the central experience that was to crystalize all of his unconscious conflicts stimulated by Vietnam. He was returning from a firefight where many of his buddies were killed when he came upon a Vietnamese woman who offered to sell him a coke for one dollar. He became enraged and felt he was being exploited by the very people he was there to protect. Thereupon he took his rifle and pointed it at her head. The woman's daughter began to beg him not to shoot her mother. He did shoot and kill her. This is the child whose pleadings he has heard nightly since he left Vietnam. Significantly, the lieutenant who witnessed the crime "didn't say anything."[2]

I began to understand this man. In the sessions he easily returned to Vietnam as if it occurred yesterday. However, in his tales of violence he would suddenly shift from his own crimes to cry of the brutality of the government and how he suffered at their hands. It was clear that the "they" who were cruel and violent was unconsciously his own self. He protected himself from awareness of his own guilt by projecting his sadism onto others. This allowed him to feel virtuous through his identification with his superego. This mechanism also gave him the opportunity to pay for his crimes with his own and his family's well being. It also enabled him to defensively express his aggression, now from the safe helpless position. His passive wishes, powerful as they may have been, were not at this time seen as primary, but as defensive in nature and reflecting his supplication for external forgiveness.

However, despite the accumulating evidence for these silent speculations, his cancellations and severe somatic complaints suggested primitive defenses against verbal recollection. Similarly, the transference was quickly becoming filled with violence.

His wife called and cancelled his next appointment. He came in one day later requesting medication as "I don't have time for an appointment today." On the next visit he reported severe insomnia and of hearing a crushing noise in his head with "my body feeling

---

[2] The genetic meaning of this event was not made clear in this limited treatment. Underlying sadomasochistic primal scene fantasies as well as pregenital destructiveness may be responsible for its tenacity. It is notable that a chronic feminine identification occurred following this expression of violence. This defensive retreat was acted out both within and outside the transference.

In a similar vein with another patient, the terror of retaliation (castration) for the acting out of presumptively forbidden aggression in Vietnam led to a defensive regression to a feminine position. Along with powerful predetermining childhood experiences and fantasies, this was a component in his later crossdressing behavior and impotence. Interestingly, for this man the V-shape of the Vietnam War Memorial symbolized the "castrated" female genitalia that so frightened him.

like it was being crushed." When he awoke from his ordeal of night-mares he "didn't feel like going to work." He went on to describe how he feared killing others and of losing the ability to distinguish past from present. At the end of the hour he asked me for a letter excusing him from the work he missed as he was "too ill." I com-mented on the difficult position he put me in, in demanding a letter from me for his weekend infirmity. He exploded in a fury—I had instantly crossed the line and in that moment of not being his unques-tioning ally became his persecutor. It emerged that he could not tolerate me, indeed could not conceive of me, as an interested helper who would assist in his learning about himself. To him I was either an impotent, but friendly "yes man" or else a dangerous attacker.

He returned for his next session and passionately railed against all those in the world who are insensitive to the plight of the down-trodden. I pointed out how he sees everyone only as either bad society or the good guys and how his sense of me shifts rapidly from one to the other. We spoke more of his violence in Vietnam and I commented on what seemed to be his guilt and self-punishment.

At this time he was coming regularly and working at his job without problems. During his next visits he comfortably started right in reporting instances of wartime atrocities and how he felt respon-sible for the deaths of others. He spoke of his discomfort with having emerged physically unscathed from the war. While he remained somewhat confused about our relationship, he seemed to be gaining relief from his visits and expressed interest in continuing them.

He did not show for his next visit. He came unannounced one day later and complained of severe insomnia and nightmares. At this time I carefully raised for his observation his most overt expression of acted out provocation and resistance to the transference—his not calling to cancel our sessions. His response was momentary silence and confusion. It was as if he did not understand what I was saying. He then became enraged and furiously demanded to know what right I had to ask to be treated respectfully. He exclaimed how I was nothing to him. After a long and vituperous attack on me, he shouted that I just saw him as a "number" anyway.

At this point I inquired into this transference fantasy and we (with some joint effort) unearthed his projected image of me as a cold and ruthless "body counter."[3] At the same time I took

---

[3] At this time the sense of the aloof and cruel transference figure was born from a projection of his own sadistic "body counting" activities that occurred in Vietnam. There were indications later that it also contained elements of his child-hood perception of his "cold" and unavailable father. Unfortunately events precluded full exploration of this component.

pains to clarify that I did not view him as a number, but a valued person.

My interest in eliciting his fantasies of me at first bewildered and frightened him. There was a hopeful sign though of his being curious about it and of appreciating my survivability. However, his need to project his sadism and see himself as the innocent sufferer continued to drive his perception of me as the cruel oppressor. His pain served to expiate his guilt.

He missed his next two visits. He came one week later demanding a letter from me to his boss suggesting that he be assigned only light duty because of his disability. Seeing myself being forced to choose sides between the presented abuser and the abused, I attempted to raise this dilemma for our observation. My words were meaningless though for it was my hesitation to comply, and thereby affirm and gratify his helplessness, that he responded to. This was proof to him of my "not caring" and of my cruelty and insensitivity. He was enraged. He reported not coming to our sessions because he didn't want to and that he didn't call me because his home phone was disconnected since he didn't have any money. I imagined him living in a primitive hut like those of his victims in Vietnam. In a now more intensive way, I was the sadist and he my victim. His wish for the punishing, and perhaps ultimately gratifying, beating was strong.

He came in the following week and angrily demanded a new doctor. He was paranoid and agitated and felt that I was trying to hurt him just as the government did by spraying him with Agent Orange. At this time, speaking only to the guilt, I calmly but firmly spoke of his perception of me as hurting him. I pointed out that his real persecutor was his conscience and how it was not actually me who was holding him accountable for his crimes. I said how his image of me as being cruel to him came from his persistent sense of himself as evil and that he has never forgiven himself for killing the innocent woman. I also spoke of his need to see himself as my passive victim as this helped him avoid awareness of his own active violent feelings that were stimulated by combat and are frightening to him. He was afraid of his own aggression ever since it became associated with the death of the woman.

These comments were repetitions of things I had said in the past. At this time though they were highlighted by the intense and terrifying transference. It seemed that the contrast between his frightening perception of me and my accepting but challenging interpretation allowed my words to be meaningfully heard. To my surprise, there was a startling transformation from a panicked paranoid patient to a tearful trusting one. He slumped in his seat, began sobbing, and for the first time spoke of his inner pain. He slowly smiled, relaxed and described his discomfort in liking me. After a few minutes, he began to articulate some optimism for his future. He also said how he wanted to be strong to care for his family. This latter element apparently was a beginning identification with me based on my previous emphasis on surviving in order to father his children.

He returned one week later having slept well that week for the first time in years. He appeared relaxed and comfortable. He began to describe feelings of pleasure during violence in Vietnam. He also for the first time spoke of his wife, heretofore idealized platonically, and of traits of hers that annoyed him. His broader affect seemed to reflect a beginning return to his premorbid less-regressed functioning.

He called and cancelled his next visit and missed the next two. He then called to set a new appointment and failed to show for that. Three months later the patient walked into the clinic requesting a letter from me putting him back on full work duty. He reported not having missed a day's work in three months for the first time in years. He was off all medication, had no insomnia, nightmares, or flashbacks and he was not troubled by feelings of depression or obsessive thoughts. His affect was warm and broad, and he displayed a deep, good-natured laughter. He reported getting along with his family and co-workers and he expressed a profound appreciation of our work together. He also made clear that he hoped not to have to return to the clinic.

This brief encounter is difficult to draw conclusions from. I suspect that as Bak described (1946), his paranoia was "delusional masochism." That is, his feelings of being attacked represented a masochistic submission to his projected sadism (which was taken in by his superego). This defended against awareness of his aggression, punished him for it, and regressively gratified his passive wishes. I am inclined to think that the opportunity to identify with a safe but firm male figure accounted for his temporary symptomatic improvement. It is possible as well that my intervention brought to consciousness his overpowering unconscious guilt and thereby reduced its regression inducing potential.

Whatever the case (and there is insufficient information to prove a hypothesis), the follow-up data tend to support the importance of his search for punishment. This continued to be intertwined with his feminine transference wishes as indicated in the following vignette. With his return to treatment, however, there was evidence of a burgeoning perception of my trustworthiness and ability to be of help to him.[4]

Nine months after his last visit, the patient returned complaining of a recurrence of his nightmare. He had up to that point been able to work steadily at his job and relate comfortably with his family. However, the ghost of his past returned to haunt him. He had unconsciously arranged a reenactment of his crime, this time with punishment. He attempted and was arrested for a bungled robbery and faced a prison term which he felt "might be the best thing." During his capture the policeman pointed a gun at his head. At that moment he underwent a dissociative episode and reexperienced his Vietnam crime, now as the victim. He visualized the head of the innocent woman as he blew it apart and saw the same thing now happening to him. He was retreating from his aggression and attempting restitution by identifying with her. As for his own anticipated death, "I welcomed it—it's the way it's supposed to be."

Patient B

Patient B is a 33-year-old white man who presented on evaluation complaining of rage outbursts that have been plaguing him since his discharge from Vietnam thirteen years ago. He declared succinctly, "I'm destroying myself and what's around me." He also reported periods of depression as well as insomnia, recurrent nightmares, headaches, tension and severe anxiety. "I have mental lapses that are not normal for a 33-year-old to have." He described extreme social withdrawal with his only interpersonal relation being his girlfriend. The patient had completed two years of college, was working full-time and had no history of psychiatric hospitalization.

History. The patient served in Vietnam in continuous combat for ten months. He was the point man for his unit which brought him into intimate contact with the most violent and dangerous aspects of guerrilla warfare. Death and mutilation were an everyday encounter, and most of his friends were either maimed or killed.

---

[4] The chronicity of this condition has been well documented in the descriptive literature by Archibald and Tuddenbaum (1965). On a dynamic level Reich noted (1928), "Freud calls our attention to the fact that, as a neurosis progresses, it often gradually loses its painful character, because the tendencies to punishment come more and more to serve the masochistic tendencies of the ego. More and more does self-punishment become gratification."

After repeated close encounters with injury which included stepping on mines that failed to explode, the patient developed the reputation of being a talisman whose mere presence protected others from injury. He himself began to feel invincible and for a period of time felt no fear. However, on one occasion he observed the mutilated body of an acquaintance and suddenly had the realization that he in fact was not invulnerable and that he too could be damaged. He became overwhelmed by fear and told his commander that he was "fed up" and refused to fight. Ultimately, he met a sympathetic doctor who sent him home.

When he arrived home he could not adjust to civilian life. He wandered the country alone and aimless for two years with intermittent drug and alcohol abuse and conflicts with the law. He settled in a "hut" in Hawaii and lived isolated from those around him. Eventually he returned to his home town and completed two years at a junior college. He married, fathered a son, and worked without interruption. In time though, his moodiness and chronic resentments grew, and after five years his wife left him. She became afraid of his explosive anger although he reportedly never physically abused her. Numerous medical evaluations and pharmacologic interventions during this time were of no help.

The patient is the third of nine children with two older brothers. He described himself as a nervous child who was always afraid of the "monster in the closet." He was raised by his mother and father until their separation when he was 16. His initial description of his parents hinted at what would emerge as his extensive concern with comparative genital anatomy, revealed through multiple derivative symbols. "One was a male and one was a female and I don't know if they understand what was going on." He described his mother as a strong woman who would frequently beat him with a "coathanger and belt." However, he grew up feeling very close to her and felt she protected him from his father who was seen as more dangerous. The patient felt "he had it in for me." He recalled a constant level of fear during his childhood and noted that he frequently responded to this fear with laughter. This character trait was to elaborate into a defensive system that included a pseudofearlessness and arrogance. He recalled frequent beatings at the hand of his older brother to which he submitted without struggle. It was only when this brother either hit their younger brother or yelled at his mother that the patient would wildly attack him. The patient saw himself as the protector of the downtrodden.

His only memory of being beaten by his father was when he was twelve and had shot a bird with a BB gun. He recalled that his father beat him with a "pole" thirteen times and had to be stopped by his mother. He reportedly ended the beating by telling the patient, "You're no son of mine."[5]

While growing up the patient always felt small. In his constant comparisons with other boys and men, he perceived himself as deficient and held them, particularly his father, in awe. With excitement and admiration he would describe in detail the power and grandeur of his father's "tools." He saw himself though as allied with his "suffering" mother against his father. He identified his father as sadistic although in reality he (father) was often the victim of his mother's violent tantrums.

The patient recounted that his parents argued a lot, "They broke each other's nuts." He easily recalled a scene from his adolescence when his father "came after me." His mother knocked the father down with a pan and the patient responded, "I hope you didn't kill him. We have to get rid of him."

The only aggression expressed towards his father occurred after he felt his father was "putting mother through a lot," which included his having numerous affairs. In a fit of anger, he grabbed his father's finger and broke it.

His parents divorced while he was in Vietnam. He did not see or speak to his father for 12 years. During this time he spoke to his mother weekly. His most recent description of his father was of a "frail old man." This image, imbued with defensive revision, reemerged in his associations and provided an important clue to the unconscious meaning of his symptoms.

Course of Treatment. The patient's first presentation to me was of a man in great pain. He spoke of the brutality of war as a poet would. The meaninglessness, hypocrisy and cruelty of his Vietnam experience were related in an eloquent and sensitive fashion. He was

---

[5] This recollection of 'shooting off his gun' and then being beaten by his father's 'pole' (and then being abandoned) was apparently a screen memory. The limited depth of this treatment has not made possible the recovery of the specific underlying experiences and fantasies. However, it is clear that this constellation became the central metaphor of his adult life and formed the nucleus of the transference neurosis. Referring to the beating by his father, he would later comment on its displacement, "It was a good lesson in politics."

outraged at the "system." I felt myself drawn to him as I would to a friend who had been dealt a harsh blow by fate. I was being asked to join with him in his pronouncements of righteousness, and I was tempted. As I became aware though of his compaign for my allegiance, and through my trial identifications with his inner experience, I sensed his blind spot. I was being pulled into a world view that had *them* as the cruel ones and *him* as the innocent sufferer. The intensity of his indignation suggested that his real suffering lay in his need to deny and project his own aggression. I wondered what he had done in Vietnam. I also became concerned about our ability to suspend his intense manifest vision and join together in curious investigation of his latent conflicts. At that time I revealed to him my interest in his sensitivity and experiences, and we began our work on that note.

He soon spoke of the event in Vietnam that contained many of the elements of his life-long conflicts. He had been fighting in the jungle continuously; many of his comrades had been killed. He crossed a stream and stepped on a land mine. Inexplicably, it failed to explode. *He laughed.* Soon thereafter, he spotted a "frail old man" on a dike who was "just carrying a *tool.*" He fired a single shot at the man and killed him. "*No one said anything.*" That night he ate dinner in the village of the old man. He saw a six-year-old boy carrying his younger brother on his back. Through an interpreter the boy told him that his father had been killed that day. Aware that he shot the only Vietnamese, he told the boy that he had killed his father, and he offered him food. The boy reportedly responded, "C'est la guerre," and they ate together.

Notably, his lieutenant witnessed the crime. His response was to take credit for it as his own kill and he added it to his body count.

The meaning to the patient of these events gradually emerged. The next session was delayed ten minutes due to an unavoidable emergency of mine. The patient assumed I arranged the delay on purpose in order to study his reactions. His casual approval of such a therapeutic approach barely concealed his fury and feelings of humiliation. Upon my careful encouragement of his fantasies, he elaborated on his feelings of helplessness with specific castration imagery, "It's like someone took my gun away." Parallel to this theme and driven by it was his difficulty in separating the present from the past. In response to my lateness he instructed me, "People die if you're late; you must be able to depend on others." I intervened by commenting on the reality behind my delay and carefully explained how I consider his assumed form of manipulative treatment to be highly disrespectful and counterproductive. He seemed relieved.

I began to silently speculate that the murder of the "frail old man" symbolized and reactivated the struggle with his father. This would lead to intense unconscious guilt and fear of retaliation. The actuality of the event would imprint his underlying infantile fantasies and aggression with the magical "stamp of reality." This would intensify the back pressure from his castration fear. As it also distorts the ego's repression barrier, which leads to decreased ability to discriminate outer reality from inner drive-fantasy, the therapeutic regression with its instictual reliving would become a frightening and resisted experience. The transference relationship would become the trial ground to enlarge his ego's capacity to experience fantasy and thereby create an "arena" (external then intrapsychic) to tolerate and explore now safe aggressive and submissive wishes.

Specific defensive self-images began to emerge in his tales of Vietnam. He spoke of how he gave away all his food to the Vietnamese and that his buddies would have to feed him. He recalled going into a hut and seeing a young girl with infected skin sores. He began teaching her parents how to care for her condition, when suddenly the lieutenant burst in and reprimanded him, "This ain't no Red Cross station." At another time he described crying from a distance as his unit was burning a village and killing all the inhabitants. His Vietnam stories portrayed himself as a bloody but innocent bystander. He saw himself as only wanting to help people while the "others" hurt them.

His relationship to me began to take two forms. He began to idealize me; he complimented my on my clothes and admired my education. At the same time he would mockingly laugh at some of my comments, just as he laughed at his father, and the mine that almost destroyed him.

Characteristic of his efforts to avoid the transference was when he told me that he was getting Valium illegally on the street to control his temper outbursts at his girlfriend. He saw this woman as representing the only loving aspect of himself that remained since the war.[6] I commented on his not asking me for the Valium. He was surprised and taken aback. "I don't want to ask you for anything!" he exclaimed four times. His character defenses were emerging as a resistance to the transference, "If you say no, I'll laugh and go get it

---

[6] In reality this girlfriend masochistically provoked and manipulated the patient's sadism and guilt. It required extensive work for him to recognize the self-punishing elements in his unsatisfying relationship with her. As well, his oedipal inhibitions led him to avoid women with whom he could share a deeper intimacy.

on the street." His resisting my becoming an object of his wishes revealed his perception of me as the cruel lieutenant/father whose "presence" led to the defensive memories of feeding civilians and healing the young girl. I was becoming the feared retaliatory father and alternately the orally longed for father with whom he could feel safe and be strengthened by. (His grandeur suggested a defensive identification with the idealized paternal power [phallus] that he wished to steal and ingest.) He in turn was discovering the small, frightened and envious boy that lay behind his defensive phallic grandiosity. "I don't want to go back to being a scared, *beaten* little dog. I built myself up to be rock on my own. I don't want to have those memories and feelings again."

He soon thereafter began to become aware of the intense fear that underlie his laughter and aggression, "I feel left bare, susceptible—I have to defend myself in an aggressive way." Concerning his fear and wish of asking me for diazepam, he said he felt like a "little kid with his hand in the cookie jar." His guilt led him to assume that I was "suspicious" of him and that I would "ambush" him for "trying to get over" on me. This was a transference fantasy created from the imagery of wartime, yet derived from symbolic infantile aggression and guilt.

His paralyzing unconscious guilt became the theme for a long time to come. As his associations in the following session revealed, he would go to great lengths to defend against his own aggression and guilt.

He opened the hour by explaining that he began watching a television show on Vietnam and observed a Vietcong soldier being shot. He became acutely anxious and could not sleep. He said it re-awakened his fear. He quickly explained that due to group firing he never really knew if he or one of his friends was responsible for a kill. This denial was not sufficient and he went on to project his guilt by speaking of the government's hypocrisy in lying about the Cambodia invasion. I commented on his own pain in having taken a life. He sadly admitted to having killed unnecessarily. He then quickly dealt with the guilt by projection and rationalization by adding that there was peer pressure for higher body counts. This defense also was not sufficient and he then intellectualized and generalized as he mused about the "death of it all." Seeking absolution (as well as an identification), he reminded himself and me that the son of his victim simply said, "Such is war." My further comments on the pain of his own guilt brought him to realize how much the murder affected him, "After that I started to help these

people . . . I let some North Vietnamese go . . . I became against it."
The genetic meaning of his act was elaborated in his next two associations. "I admired The Man . . . he was very smart . . . I admired The
Man I was fighting . . . I was getting letters from home . . . mother
was being divorced from father." The life-long results of his guilt
were revealed when he spoke of how it has taken him ten years to
earn an adequate salary. "I go one step forward in life . . . I feel
depressed and take three steps back . . . I wish I were dead . . . to
forget the year that never ended . . . I killed the little boy in me"
[the little boy killed The Man].

He began to report that the fog in his thinking was lifting and
that he no longer was losing his temper at his girlfriend. He also
returned to school and was taking a night course in chemistry. His
return to education contained many levels of meaning. It was both
a therapeutic identification with me as well as a defensive identification. He was trying to accrue as much "educational power" as he
felt I had so he would be safe with me, my assumed judgments, and
from his fear of retaliation. He was also attempting to undo his awe
of my "power" which evoked his castrating wishes. He imagined
getting his degree and leaving the country to "avoid being identified
as a violent American. I might leave, or destroy myself." He began to
cry for the first time and painfully revealed his guilt, significantly
though as a projection, "I forgive the government and people of this
country, they don't forgive me." He further commented on the
results of his guilt, "I don't care about myself, I just want to be kind
to other people."

In another session he angrily described attacking a lieutenant
who killed an "innocent pregnant woman." To my asking for his
associations to this memory, he immediately referred to the peasant
man he shot. His now intermittently more tolerant conscience
allowed him to recognize the power (if not the wish) in his acted out
aggression, though this recognition was limited to the wartime "old
man." He struggled with tearfully experiencing internalized sorrow
for having killed him. He then haltingly described previously
unspoken of acts of genuine heroism in Vietnam. While these activities were to some degree restitutive and life-endangering, they also
drew upon and emerged from his quite competent leadership skills.
I commented on how he minimized and hid this facet of his Vietnam
experiences. It seemed that the genetic power of his guilt clouded
his ability to realistically appreciate his strength as a fine soldier.
He defensively retreated from seeing himself as the able leader
he was.

He continued to become aware of his fear of me. "You're like the dink—you just sit there and watch. I want to sit in your chair and you in mine." This suspiciousness and fear of me waxed and waned throughout the initial phase of treatment. There was a long testing period in which he studied my consistency and safety. At one point he became panicked and saw me as a dangerous exploiter who could not tolerate his aggressiveness. At the height of this perception, he required a real encounter with me to feel safe. In the midst of a tirade against the "cruel government," he frightfully asked me if I knew the author of a radical political treatise. I did and told him so. He felt relieved.

A significant event in the patient's treatment occurred when he reexperienced one of his ongoing symptoms. He was in chemistry class and the teacher dropped a test tube on the table top. The patient became startled at the noise and jumped away drawing the attention of the class. He fought off an overwhelming urge to run out of the room and found himself in the midst of a severe anxiety attack. The patient by this time was able to associate to the event. To the teacher's "accident" he recalled that in Vietnam he felt that an accident is equivalent to someone's death. His next thought was that his shooting of the old man was also an accident. This then led to vivid recall of his buddy's mutilation in battle. The immediacy of his symptoms, along with his associations to violence and then injury, led him to become conscious for the first time of his present day sense of constant danger. This was a turning point in his treatment as he began to be aware of the forces of retaliation that so much of his character and symptoms were created to deal with. The patient's aggression and fear of retribution were the unconscious link between the noise of the test tube and his startle response.[7]

---

[7] The hypersensitivity to loud sounds—the startle response—is a frequently reported symptom in trauma victims. It has generally been thought of as a learned response. An interesting additional hypothesis is suggested by Roiphe and Galenson's work with children who suffer from noise hypersensitivity (1973). They speculate that when the regressed ego is flooded with unneutralized aggression, a common experience in battle, there is a deterioration in object representations. "We propose that the ensuing object loss anxiety and fears of dissolution of the self may evoke the primitive mechanisms we have described in these children: *anxiety becomes manifested in the auditory sphere* . . ." This strain in the relations with the object evokes disruptive amounts of aggression "which is dealt with by this primitive forerunner of defense—*the somatization of aggression in the auditory sphere*" (my italics).

The central importance of the feeling of ever-present danger further evolved in our work. He began the next session by anxiously describing his rage at sloppy and careless co-workers at his job. He then recalled battle scenes where a friend had his foot cut off because of the incompetence of another soldier. He continued to describe the workings of his "sixth sense" for danger that he became aware of in Vietnam and that now operated reflexly as if he were in Vietnam. In fact, when I questioned whether the real danger now was the same as then, he said it was, "I don't think to stay ahead of the danger, I just do it; it's the same as in Vietnam." The fantasy of mutilation was so pervasive, it didn't matter that actual injury was possible there and unlikely here.

As we isolated his fear for study, he was able to make a therapeutic split in the ego and allow the feelings of fear to emerge under the safety of our alliance. When it grew to the point where it contrasted with the newly perceived (and transitory) safety with me, he smiled, relaxed and softly said, "I'm calm now because I realize about the danger." He again became anxious and said, "If I slow down I feel that they'll nail me." Letting the "they" stand as is for now, I commented on his living in a "*psychic* Vietnam." He immediately smiled, relaxed and for the first time spontaneously associated to his adolescence. He spoke at length of how he avoided any competition in sports, "I never played to win—I would lose on purpose." His thoughts then returned to Vietnam as he again alluded, through displacement, to the presence of these violent struggles in the transference, "I survived the best fighter in the world, the North Vietnamese soldier—I have respect and fear of him." He then said that it was and is his "manhood" that was on the line, "Someone wants to challenge me as a man or a woman."

This patient went to war afraid of his aggression and fearful of talionic retribution. His exposure to symbolic castration fixed his unconscious fear and clouded his ego's ability to evaluate the real world. The infantile struggle with the powerful "best fighter in the world" father was acted out in Vietnam. The unconscious guilt over the murder/castration of "The Man" led to the constant fear of retaliation.

Throughout this period of his associations to the struggle with the violent and powerful "father," the patient wore daily the prominent beltbuckle of a dead North Vietnamese soldier. This was an everpresent reminder of his cravings for the idealized paternal "power." The passive wishes in this desire remained for a considerable time in the acting out sphere, both within and outside the transference situation. They were expressed through dangerous provocations to be beaten. Massive resistances blocked conscious awareness of derivative wishes for transferential/father love—even as these served defensive purposes to a significant degree. Affectionate male friendships carried this charged valence and also were avoided. The libidinal elements in this submissive conflict remained prominent in his ceaseless battle with the "cruel government."

The patient's global fear of vengeful attack slowly began to be drawn into the transference relationship. It became more discrete and coherent as it was repeatedly explored and tested in the burgeoning transference. This lessened its intensity outside the consulting room and freed the patient to relate somewhat more comfortably to those around him. It also drained some of the frightening violence from his relationship with his real father and enabled the patient to experiment with a potential conflict-free identification with him. He called his father for the first time in 12 years. Revealing both his infantile wish and nascent capacity for sublimation, he explained, "I'm a businessman like him . . . I want to buy stock in his company."

Follow-up on this patient, after 18 months of *vis-à-vis* therapy, reveals that his Vietnam experiences have receded in importance in his associations. His nightmares, startle responses, and rage reactions have resolved. He has begun an intimate relationship with a kind and loving woman. In the treatment his primary conflicts remain an interplay between his paternal masochistic longings and his guilt-ridden competitive phallic strivings. These feelings have withdrawn themselves from the battlefield and are now being worked through with his present day family and, increasingly, in the transference.

Throughout his associations there has continued to be images of sickly and helpless "old men." Repeatedly, his restitutive and defensive efforts to care for them, especially at personal sacrifice, emerges. Within the transference these forces express themselves through submissive idealization. Although these wishes are not entirely defensive, increasingly his aggression toward the transference object is beginning to become recognizable and tolerable to him (our earlier displacements notwithstanding). A growing neurotic level alliance has allowed these urges to be reexperienced with me in a meaningfully affective fashion. He is simultaneously internalizing a safe version of the doctor and has begun to recognize and identify with the real shared work of introspection.

DISCUSSION

Freud introduced the concept of unconscious guilt in 1907 (p. 123) and elaborated on it in 1923 (p. 50). At that time he observed that some patients deteriorated in response to therapeutic progress. He understood this to be the result of latent guilt that forbade growth and satisfaction. The patient however was unaware of this undermining force. Accordingly, Freud understood the therapeutic task to be "unmasking its unconscious repressed roots, and of thus gradually changing it into a conscious sense of guilt."

Later (1924, p. 166), Freud refined the term unconscious guilt to a "need for punishment" as it is psychologically incorrect to describe a feeling as unconscious. The former term though has remained a part of psychoanalytic parlance.

The presence of unconscious guilt in patients has been an important area of clinical and research attention. Its origins have been traced to oedipal wishes as well as earlier separation-annihilation impulses. Its manifestations include subtle success-phobias as well as dramatic self-destruction. Its malignant presence has been noted throughout the years in the form of the negative therapeutic reaction.

In all these situations the patient is not consciously aware of his guilt or of the forbidden fantasies that elicit it. There is a vast array of defenses erected to maintain such unawareness. These intense counter cathexes can lead to the development of what Fenichel called the "counter-guilt" character (1945, p. 496). He found that in this condition "The various attempts to deny guilt feelings may even contradict one another, as in the anecdote by Scholom Aleichem. The woman who failed to return a borrowed pot excused herself: "I never borrowed the pot; furthermore, the pot was broken when I borrowed it, and, moreover, I returned it long ago" (p. 497). Therapeutic attention to the many defenses with working through can relieve much of the suffering that derives from the unconscious dimension of the guilt.

From my work with trauma victims, I have observed a number of defensive systems that are frequently utilized. For example, projection onto a scapegoat is one of the more commonly used mechanisms. Through this defense the *other person* is seen as evil and in need of condemnation. Asch noted (1966), "In such situations, one finds that the unacceptable impulses of the attacker are being projected onto the victim. In addition, there also occurs a displacement of that part of the self representation which would otherwise be assaulted by the superego as the source of these disowned impulses."

In severe cases, the projection of guilt may lead to actual violent attacks on others. Reik (1941) found that "the subject's perception of his guilt has in these cases assumed such an exceptionally severe and acute form that he must drive his aggressiveness outwards if his ego is to remain intact." Ultimately, it is the fear of retaliatory punishment that drives the defensive hostility.

Fenichel (1945) highlighted a number of other defensive structures. For example, persistent declarations of being unfairly treated often are a means to avoid feeling that the punishment was deserved. It also ensures that the sufferer continues to be in pain. Similarly, a search for power can derive from a need to "identify with the persecutor" (p. 500) in an effort to escape from feeling judged by that persecutor. This process often becomes endless as the patient fails to perceive that the judgement he seeks to avoid is from his own superego. There is also the commonly known ingratiation through suffering whereby a patient becomes the victim of unconsciously arranged mishaps. This is a trading off of lesser punishments "in the hope of paying an installment that may be accepted in lieu of the full sum" (p. 500). It also serves to "distract the judge" from the more serious crime.

This distraction is an important element in Freud's "Criminals From a Sense of Guilt" (1916). In this brief but major paper, Freud noted that the very act of committing a crime can derive from an underlying sense of unconscious guilt for a deeper repressed "crime." The latent state of ill defined distress can paradoxically be relieved by committing an actual (or repeat) crime for which the patient can then consciously feel guilt. In such cases "his sense of guilt was at least attached to something" (p. 332). In addition, through real criminal activity the punisher becomes the state instead of the omniscient and inescapable superego. This defensive activity is often interminable unless the patient is helped to become conscious of the earlier guilt that plagues him.[8]

This fleeing from the conscious awareness of guilt becomes tragic when "the mastery of guilt feelings becomes the all-consuming task

---

[8] In the treatment situation, the transference object often is seen as the judge. The intermittent acting out of "forbidden" behavior, often in the form of failed payments or illegal activity, is frequently an unconscious effort to "distract the judge" from emerging guilt-ridden transference "crimes." This is both a provocation of lessor punishment and a resistance to the deeper transference related impulses and retaliation fears.

of a person's whole life . . ." (Fenichel, p. 496). The now instinctually driven need to suffer infuses and misshapes the ego leading to syntonic "living out" atonement. It is only when the character deforming defenses become observable "foreign bodies" and the latent guilt is brought to consciousness that the self-induced suffering is relieved. This diminishes the ego-weakening pressure from the sadistic superego which in turn enables further work to proceed on the drive elements of the experiences and fantasies.

The intensity of the suffering that the ego experiences is in large measure determined by the developmental level of the superego. There seems to be a difference in the quality of the guilt that derives from a mature superego from that of a regressed one. Grinberg (1964) and Modell (1965) have, from their own theoretical models, investigated levels of superego development and their consequent guilt. Their findings bear directly on our study of guilt elicited by regression inducing trauma.

Grinberg posits the existence of two types of guilt, persecutory and depressive. The persecutory guilt, modeled on the paranoid position, is the result of an immature or regressed ego and superego. He describes it as beginning very early in life and accounting for later masochistic patterns. Clinically, it manifests as extreme resentment with paranoid feelings, hypochondriacal and psychosomatic disorders, as well as an inability to mourn. Depressive guilt, on the other hand, is seen as emanating from the depressive position and developmentally is a more advanced form of guilt. It can contain "sorrow, concern for the object and the self, nostalgia and responsibility." He reports that patients presenting with persecutory guilt can, in a treatment situation where recollections and subjective experiences are systematically elaborated, show a gradual transformation to depressive guilt. Similarly, he states that "There always remain elements of persecutory guilt which, *under traumatic circumstances* . . . are intensified" (my italics). When the depressive guilt becomes unbearable, a regression may result in an increase in persecutory guilt.

Modell similarly describes two types of guilt, primary and secondary. Primary guilt derives from an earlier developmental stage and is the result of a partial developmental arrest of the superego. This results in a diffuse unconscious guilt which "pervades the entire personality structure . . . all pleasure that can be experienced with dignity and self respect is undone and negated." Secondary guilt, however, tends to be more circumscribed and limited, with only partial ego inhibition and limited to only a sector of the personality.

This more mature guilt emerges from an "adequately structuralized" superego. Significantly, Modell finds that *it is the experience of a successful identification with the father that leads to a more functional and structuralized superego.* In the absence of this successful identification, there follows a developmental failure of the superego with its pathological sequelae. Modell as well notes the possibility of regression to primary guilt, vestiges of which exist in everyone.

The aforementioned qualities of persecutory and primary guilt well describe the internal life of the post combat patient. The pretrauma superego (of whatever maturity) was exposed to a violence-ridden environment that respected none of the fragile sublimations of adolescent life. It was inevitable that conflicted infantile impulses would become attached to the pervasive acting out of violence, especially as it involved civilian families. The most generic fantasies of incorporation, annihilation and mutilation were acted out *without any apparent limit.* The ensuing regression to oral-sadistic levels heralded the unrelenting primitive superego.[9] The consequences of this primitive superego (or more accurately, superego precursor), as stated, infect every nuance of the personality. Sorrow and mourning, the necessary prerequisites for working through the past become impossible. Instead of experiencing and verbalizing these developmentally advanced affects, the regressed character amalgamates them

---

[9] Dramatic evidence of the predominence of oral level introjective-projective mechanisms brought on by the regression of battle comes from a Vietnam death ritual. In the jungle it was common for the foot soldier to carry in his pack the most prized and sought after food item among all available—a "can of peaches" in sweet syrup. If the soldier was killed, it was understood that his best friend would open the dead man's pack and eat his "can of peaches." To this day numbers of combat veterans keep an unopened and untouched "can of peaches" in their closet—a semisymbolic "linking object" (Volkan, 1981).

While this behavior can be examined from many perspectives, in particular its implication for the form of the transference, I mean to introduce it here as an indicator of the extensive regression that was widely experienced and shared in combat. The importance of the introjection-identification process at this regressed level, and in particular its function as a precursor of symbol formation, has theoretical and technical implications for the treatment of the severely disturbed patient.

as preverbal sadomasochistic somatic discharges—"resomatization."
Paranoia, masochism and psychosomatic illness ensues.[10]

In Neiderland's short but seminal paper on the "Survivor Syndrome" (1968) he reported:

> In order to understand more fully the pathogenesis of the
> survivor syndrome, I repeatedly stressed the need for a sharper
> focus on the all-pervasive guilt of the victim as well as the need
> for a sort of *hyperacusis to guilt* on the part of the analyst who
> has to be aware of the difficulties because of repression, elabo-
> rate defenses, and denials that tend to obscure the guilt. The
> patients' guilt-ridden fear of emotional closeness, their frequent
> attempts to assuage guilt, their repetitive guilt-ridden fantasies
> and dreams about death, violence, destruction and their lost
> love-objects, not only demonstrate the marked ambivalence
> toward the latter (intensified by the parents' apparent failure to
> protect the victim from the persecution), but also result from
> the sadistic incorporative fantasies leading directly to guilt in
> orally-regressed personalities and situations.

In my experience, the defensive unawareness of unconscious guilt
is often the major clinical problem in the chronic cases of the war
neuroses. Attention to the elaborate defenses against it, its transference manifestations, and its potential for a negative therapeutic
reaction are the constant work for the treating analyst or therapist.
Conscious denials or confessions of guilt are of little therapeutic
value as the unfolding of the transference through free association

---

[10] As noted in the clinical material presented, and in numerous other cases, the
traumatic regression has major implications for the reactivation of conflicted
passive wishes. As Bak reported (1946), "The failure of sublimation and the
direct threat of castration [the classic conditions of battle] lead to a retreat
from phallic activity and induce a masochistic regression (homosexuality) where,
according to the phallic and anal-sadistic organization, the desires to be castrated,
beaten and anally abused are reactivated." Seen in this light, post combat
paranoia and violence may be viewed as a defense against reemerged passive
longings.

An additional point is that the specifically *visual* shock of combat traumata
may resonate with and reactivate scoptophilic impulses from childhood. The
visually overstimulating scenes from *both* periods may together contribute, as
Greenacre pointed out (1947, 1949), to superego regression and screen
'flashbacks.'

(and acting out) reveals the latent strata of unconscious hostility and guilt. The neutralized energy made available by becoming conscious of these two warded off affects is the fuel for the therapeutic alliance. Despite some recommendation to the contrary, I find that persistent attention to "forgotten" deeds and unconscious fantasies (often revealed through behavior) yields important therapeutic progress. Outbursts of rage are almost never the 'bedrock' of conflict. In my experience they give way to therapeutic consistency and defense interpretation. It is not unusual for violent and self-destructive veterans of combat to become verbal and self-reflective when their unconscious guilt is made conscious. Incisive interpretive attention to warded off guilt is a powerful yet tolerable therapeutic tool when combined with the respect inherent in the holding environment. Grinker and Speigel (1945) similarly report an "amazing change" (p. 297) in patients when their unconscious guilt is made conscious. They go on to report the therapeutic benefit of focusing on this guilt even as it effects the traumatic dream:

> In the depressed individual, catastrophic battle dreams are punishment dreams with a strong masochistic coloring. The patient attempts to renew his good relations with his ego-ideal by suffering, in order to atone for the guilt attributed to his unconscious hostility. These dreams, in which there is so much suffering, disappear as guilt feelings abate (p. 304).

As I've indicated, the ubiquitous primitive guilt and the disruptive defenses against it derive from the traumatically regressed superego. As Modell has suggested, in these situations there is an absence of a successful identification with the father. Similarly emphasizing the presence of libidinal forces in superego development, Nunberg (1934) pointed out, "With identification, not only the hated but also the *beloved father* was absorbed by the ego" (my italics) (see also Kramer, 1958).

This often overlooked aspect of the superego plays an important role in its pathology and has implications for the treatment of many of these patients. The good and dependable father is a necessary ingredient for a matured and 'autonomous' superego. The internal presence of this father allows for the development of crucial self-observing abilities. Specifically, as Rothstein stated (1982), "self-observing function of the ego necessary for successful analytic work derives, in part, from an identification with a 'Loving and Beloved Superego' introject. . . . "

I believe it is useful, though not customary, to study the actual traumatic situation and the response to it by the immediate parental figures in order to better understand potential reinforcers of neutralized self-observation. More precisely, there is reason to suspect that there were certain conditions in the jungle war of Vietnam that exacerbated individual tendencies to regress. The absence of the all important good-enough and admired "father" has had major unconscious implications.

Almost all of the patients I've evaluated or treated (including the two reported in this chapter) who reported committing self-defined atrocities in Vietnam have immediately followed their recital with "and no one said anything." Indeed, most stated that their superior officers looked the other way or took credit for the crimes themselves. This abandonment of the expected disciplinary stance by the "father" failed the soldier in his need for a dependable and fair superego. Without this just parent, the primitive aggression remained untamed and the archaic retaliatory fears flourished. There existed no path out from the regression of combat. As Schafer stated (1960):

> Both by imposing meaningful limits on behavior and by administering real punishment, the parent corrects the terrifying archaic fantasies of punishment introduced by the child in his struggle with his own impulses. As a result, the child will experience less alienation from real objects, less damning up of impulses, less devious discharge or sudden eruption, and less sense of guilt and need for punishment.

Schafer specifies that it is the child's identification with the consistent and unambivalent parental superego that leads to the taming of the "terrifying archaic fantasies of punishment." This is also true for the adult survivor of trauma. The good-enough "father" contains the combatants' moral precepts while he temporarily takes leave of them to engage in battle. This admired figure then need be available for reidentification when the trauma has subsided. The possibility of identification after combat with the beloved, yet phallic, father is essential to allow a de-regression of the sadistic superego. This permits a return to pre-combat functioning.

The "containing" function of the dependable object leads to the reestablishment of benevolent self-observation—the function that is otherwise lost through the regression induced by massive trauma. This allows the mourning process to take place without the interference of a retaliatory superego. If this reparative process has not occurred, either individually or through group ritual, therapeutic-analytic treatment is indicated. It then becomes the analyzing function of the doctor that provides the model for benign self study. The therapist's unique combination of personal presence and professional reflection can fulfill the post trauma patient in his quest for dependability and identification. The 'testing' that these patients frequently go through with their therapists partly represents this search for the realistically predictable and therapeutic object. The childhood need for a consistent and moral model rebegins after severe trauma.

Through the therapeutic encounter with a person who is both genuinely benevolent and, in addition, utilizes a technique of neutral observation, the patient becomes able to utilize his (the physician's) more matured ego-superego alignment as a transitional template for his own eventual structural progression. This is related to, but somewhat different from, Glover's thoughts when he stated (1955, p. 370), "The dosed introjection of good objects is regarded as one of the most important factors in the therapeutic process." Whether it is the object per se that is internalized or instead a depersonified abstraction is an often debated question. This issue, hairsplitting to some—of fundamental concern to others, bears on our study of the treatment of patients who suffer from severe unconscious guilt (see also Greenson, 1945).

One perspective is that the genuine qualities of the therapist together with his analytic functioning serve metaphorically (and transiently) as the beloved father. This nidus for maturation acts as a foil for the regressive superego with which the patient is struggling and often externalizing. This new auxiliary superego, a component of the analyzing stance, becomes available for initial global introjection and later selective identification (Ticho, 1972). The analyst's or therapist's unambivalent and consistent emotional attitude allows for the interpretation of layers of resistance and the unfolding of the transference regression with its safe reexperiencing of infantile wishes and distortions. This secure frame is the medium that permits the interpretations of unconscious guilt and aggression to be perceivable.

It is ultimately the therapist's personal manner of "even hovering attention," so unexpected by the patient in its benevolence, that allows for the patient's affectful yet safe recognition of his "need for punishment." The evolving *therapeutic* regression (in contrast to the traumatic one) through the transference, with its simultaneous yet coherent experience of the past-in-the-present, leads to a more securely permeable repression barrier which results in greater access to the creative use of drive energy. This develops the possibility of an *inspiring* relationship with one's conscience—now the ego ideal.

It is Freud's early version of this ego ideal (1914, 1916-17, before it became synonymous with the superego), what Jacobson called "a pilot and guide for the ego" (1954) that offers a counterpoint to the unforgiving superego.[11] In addition to becoming conscious of the conflicted drive wishes that lead to the reinstinctualization of the punitive superego, there are other factors that also contribute to the amelioration of its severity.

It has long been recognized that while early identifications are crucial, postoedipal models play a significant role in the evolving ego ideal. As Fenichel noted (1945, p. 469-70), "In addition to the construction of the superego, the formation and modification of ideals in later life, too, are of importance in forming the character. Sometimes certain persons, who serve as models, or certain ideas become "introjected into the superego" in the same manner as the Oedipus objects have been introjected in childhood . . ."

As Karush stated (1967), the nonresistant elements of the transference become the vehicle for ideal formation:

> Infantile regressive tendencies live side by side with infantile progressive capacities in the transference relationship. Among these progressive capacities are forces essential to successful working through; *these are the identifications out of which the ego ideal evolves and which help to strengthen the ego's tolerance for frustration and threat.* The transference therefore includes psychic structures and functions that work for recovery and freer development, as opposed to regression and fixation. These segments of the transference transcend the role of reason and understanding in bringing about fundamental changes in behavior. (my italics)

Through the persistent clarification of the resistant elements of the transference, and in particular by the tolerance of and genetic reconstruction through the negative transference, the patient begins to experience the therapist not only as the original transference object, but in addition as "the object who helped resolve the transference" (Viederman, 1976). The nondefensive "emulative identification" (Karush) with the doctor's actual qualities of patience and introspection, the *analytic ideals*, leads to the emergence in the

---

[11] The ego ideal, as "heir of the negative oedipus complex" (Blos, 1965) also serves to bind the restimulated homosexual libido.

patient of an ego ideal and an ideal self ("the self-I-want-to-be," Sandler et al, 1963). Ongoing exposure through the regression to the therapist's analytic integrity, usually revealed through his honest study of the material and nonpossessive dedication to progression, helps advance the internalizing process from mimicry to self-directed striving and sublimated goal setting (Lampl-de Groot, 1956). The process of identifying with the physician's analyzing stance, in parallel with the interpretive analysis of self-esteem reducing conflicts such as unconscious guilt, leads to a matured ideal self and autonomous superego. This enables the patient to control his acting out and tolerate further exploration of the *deeper* transference fantasy. This sets the stage for and is itself a part of the cycle whereby the transference fantasy is repeatedly relived and tested against the current analytic context which in turn permits further unraveling of resistances with exploration of broader and deeper transference imagery. Through this working through there develops a growing cathexis of the observing portion of the ego and an expanding capacity to neutralize drive energy. This is of major importance in "survivors."

The question can be raised, what may be in the substrate of the transference experience that aids this progressive adaptation? Is it mere suggestion and compliance? While this is a complex question, in my view the stimulus for this process of maturation derives from the tension inherent in the doctor's stance of 'empathic reflection.' The paradox contained in this state of intimate observation yields for the patient a therapeutic vacuum that leads to affective insight. Both what it is not—gratification, and what it is—a dependable arena of titrated frustration, results in a unique cognitive and affective experience. The selective emptiness within this space as well as the "walls" around it make it a nidus for developmental recovery and ego mastery.

The size and shape of this space, while different for every patient, bears the unique stamp of each clinician's life history. As individual as a fingerprint, the shading and texture of each doctor's vision of "neutrality," while meeting some minimum for nonintrusiveness, is a particular synthesis of their unconscious history, personal analysis and professional training. This personal creation of the therapist is for the patient a delicate yet potent force for recovery after traumatic arrest.

I bring up the concept here of the analytic space not only to emphasize its nonverbal containing and hence therapeutic function, but also to recognize the impingements on this space that arise when working with severely traumatized patients. I also underscore the importance of the personal history of the treating analyst or therapist because in transiently identifying with the experiences of our more disturbed patients, and one must to work affectively, we may be exposed to "anxieties that belong to the earliest developmental stages in which our own physical and mental survival once depended literally upon the continuous presence of a good-enough, protecting object" (Grubrich-Simitis, 1982).

While Grubrich-Simitis' work deals with concentration camp survivors, and there are important differences between that experience and combat, it beautifully studies and describes the countertransference reactions that can emerge in working with severely traumatized patients in general. The regressive pull of *actual* massive violence can lead the therapist as well as the patient to a state of withholding of empathy. To resist the narcissistic withdrawal into fantasy (the frequently employed defense of trauma victims) as well as the equally dangerous temptation to act (in the form of inappropriately medicating or rejecting the patient) demands that the therapist tolerate potentially severe countertransference reactions. The result can be that

> reaction formations, sublimations, mature superego structures may come under pressure, *deeply repressed sadomasochistic drive impulses become activated*. It is as though we too were to fall under the sway of the preambivalent split between persecutor and persecuted and . . . to catch a glimpse not only of the earliest stages of our drive development but also of our earliest ego organization. (my italics)

Through our trial identifications we may become exposed to the "extreme helplessness of the oral phase" and the introjective-projective mechanisms derived from that stage. The resulting tendency to place all unpleasurable experiences "outside" can lead to a "contemptuous rejection" of the patient. This can take the form of moralizing, interpreting war horrors as fantasies and engaging in political debates. The tendency to "despise the sufferer" can derive not only from the patient's projection of their own sadism (and their frequent provocation, often successful, to be rejected [see Model, 1965]), but also from our own reactivated projective tendencies (Grubrich-Simitis).

Ongoing self-analysis may be essential to resist this identification with the aggressor. Neither that nor the defensive acceptance of the patient's sadism, an identification with the victim, will further the therapeutic process. It is the maintenance of the aforementioned personal creation of each therapist that will deter both our own and the patient's unconscious attempts to act out the sadomasochistic paradigm. It is this complex creation and the unique relationship it forms that leads the patient to discover that contrary to his internal notions he does have a "right to a life" (Modell; Sharpe, 1950).

Through our ability to keep part of our ego in the observing position despite powerful transferential pulls in the direction of the experiencing ego, we can help our patients both feel and reflect. In experiencing the therapist's empathic identification with his primitive sadism and guilt (which validates his experience) *and* the therapist's freedom to return to the analyzing position (which organizes his experience), our patients will sense that they too are allowed to be creative (and by implication, sexual). This state, from which emerges the timing and content of our interpretations, is an important component in the working through of unconscious guilt and of patients becoming able to "justify their existence to themselves" (Sharpe).

REFERENCES

Archibald, H. (1965). Persistent stress reaction following combat: A twenty-year follow-up. *Archives of General Psychiatry* 12: 475-481.
Asch, S. S. (1966). Depression: three clinical variations. *Psychoanalytic Study of the Child* 21: 150-171.
Bak, R. (1946). Masochism in paranoia. *Psychoanalytic Quarterly* 15:285-301.
Blos, P. (1965). The initial stage of male adolescence. *Psychoanalytic Study of the Child* 20: 145-164.
Borus, J. F. (1973). Reentry I: adjustment issues facing the Vietnam returnee. *Archives of General Psychiatry* 28: 501-506.
Cohen, J. (1980). Structural consequences of psychic trauma: a new look at 'beyond the pleasure principle.' *International Journal of Psychoanalysis* 61: 421-432.
Fenichel, O. (1945). *The Psychoanalytic Theory of Neuroses.* New York: W. W. Norton and Company.
Fox, R. (1972). Post-combat adaptations problems. *Comprehensive Psychiatry* 13(5): 435-443.
Freud, S. (1907). Obsessive actions and religious practices. *S.E.* 9.
Freud, S. (1914). On narcissism. *S.E.* 14.
Freud, S. (1916). Criminals from a sense of guilt. *S.E.* 14.
Freud, S. (1916-1917). Introductory lectures on psychoanalysis. *S.E.* 16.
Freud, S. (1923). The ego and the id. *S.E.* 19.
Freud, S. (1924). The economic problem of masochism. *S.E.* 19.
Freud, S. (1930). Civilization and its discontents. *S.E.* 21.

Gault, W. B. (1971). Some remarks on slaughter. *American Journal of Psychiatry* 128(4): 82-86.

Glover, E. (1955). *The Technique of Psychoanalysis.* New York: International University Press.

Goldsmith, W., Cretekos, C. (1969). Unhappy odysseys—psychiatric hospitalizations among Vietnam veterans. *Archives of General Psychiatry* 20: 78-83.

Greenacre, P. (1947). Vision, headache and the halo. *Psychoanalytic Quarterly* 16: 177-194.

Greenacre, P. (1949). A contribution to the study of screen memories. *Psychoanalytic Study of the Child* 3-4: 73-84.

Greenson, R. (1945). Practical approach to the war neuroses. *Bulletin of the Menninger Clinic* 9: 192-205.

Grinberg, L. (1964). Two kinds of guilt—their relations with normal and pathological aspects of mourning. *International Journal of Psychoanalysis* 45: 366-372.

Grinker, R. R., Spiegel, J. P. (1944). Brief psychotherapy in war neuroses. *Psychosomatic Medicine* 6(3): 123-131.

Grinker, R. R., Spiegel, J. P. (1945). *Men Under Stress.* Philadelphia: Blakiston.

Grubrich-Simitis, I. (1982). Extreme traumatization as cumulative trauma. *Psychoanalytic Study of the Child* 37: 415-450.

Haley, S. A. (1974). When the patient reports atrocities. *Archives of General Psychiatry* 30(2): 191-196.

Haley, S. A. (1978). Treatment implications of post-combat stress response syndromes for mental health professionals. In Figley, C. (Ed.). *Stress Disorders Among Vietnam Veterans.* New York: Brunner/Mazel.

Haley, S. A. (1979). Countertransference toward the Vietnam veteran: a case presentation read at the American Psychiatric Association Meeting, May 14, 1979, Chicago, Illinois.

Herman, M. (1938). The use of intravenous sodium amytal in psychogenic amnesic states. *Psychiatric Quarterly* 12: 738-742.

Jacobson, E. (1954). The self and the object world: vicissitudes of their infantile cathexes and their influence on ideational and affective development. *Psychoanalytic Study of the Child* 9: 75-127.

Karush, A. (1967). Working through. *Psychoanalytic Quarterly* 36: 497-531.

Kramer, P. (1958). Notes on one of the preoedipal roots of the superego. *International Journal of Psychoanalysis* 6: 38-46.

Kubie, L. S., Margolin, S. (1945). The therapeutic role of drugs in the process of repression, dissociations and synthesis. *Psychosomatic Medicine* 7: 147-151.

Lampl-de Groot, J. (1956). The role of identification in psychoanalytic procedure. *International Journal of Psychoanalysis* 37: 456-459.

Langner, H. P. (1971). The making of a murderer. *American Journal of Psychiatry* 127(7): 126-129.

Modell, A. H. (1965). On having the right to a life, an aspect of the superego's development. *International Journal of Psychoanalysis* 46: 323-331.

Nace, E. P., Meyers, A. L., O'Brien, C. P., Ream, N., Mintz, J. (1977). Depression in veterans two years after Vietnam. *American Journal of Psychiatry* 134: 167-170.

Niederland, W. G. (1968). Clinical observations on the "survivor syndrome." *International Journal of Psychoanalysis* 49: 313-315.

Nunberg, H. (1934). The feeling of guilt. *Psychoanalytic Quarterly* 3: 588-604.

Reich, W. (1928). Discussion on the need for punishment and the neurotic process. *International Journal of Psychoanalysis* 9: 227-246.

Reik, T. (1941). Aggression from anxiety. *International Journal of Psychoanalysis* 22: 7-16.

Roiphe, H., Galenson, E. (1973). Object loss and early sexual development. *Psychoanalytic Quarterly* 42: 73-90.

Rothstein, A. (1982). The implications of early psychopathology for the analyzability of narcissistic personality disorders. *International Journal of Psychoanalysis* 63: 177-188.

Sandler, J., Holder, A., Meers, D. (1963). The ego ideal and the ideal self. *Psychoanalytic Study of the Child* 18: 139-158.

Schafer, R. (1960). The loving and beloved superego in Freud's structural theory. *Psychoanalytic Study of the Child* 15: 163-188.

Sharpe, E. (1950). Variation of technique in different neuroses. In: Brierley, M. (Ed.). *Collected Papers on Psychoanalysis* (1931). London: Hogarth.

Solomon, G. F., Zarcone, V. P., Yoerg, R., Scotte, N. R., Maurer, R. G. (1971). Three psychiatric casualties from Vietnam. *Archives of General Psychiatry* 25: 522-524.

Strange, R. E., Brown, D. E. (1970). Home from the war: a study of psychiatric problems in Vietnam returnees. *American Journal of Psychiatry* 127(4): 130-134.

Ticho, E. A. (1972). The development of superego autonomy. *Psychoanalytic Review* 59: 217-233.

Viederman, M. (1976). The influence of the person of the analyst on structural change: a case report. *Psychoanalytic Quarterly* 45: 231-249.

Volkan, V. (1981). *Linking Objects and Linking Phenomena.* New York: International University Press.

Yager, J. (1976). Post-combat violent behavior in psychiatrically maladjusting soldiers. *Archives of General Psychiatry* 33: 1332-1335.

4
Transference, Countertransference, and the Vietnam Veteran

ROBERT B. SHAPIRO, PH.D.

INTRODUCTION

The war in Vietnam posed unusual difficulties for American soldiers. They were engaged in a battle that had little popular political, or moral support at home. Traditionally society views the soldier as a heroic representative of the political, moral and religious institutions of the country. Society usually debriefs its warriors by celebrating their return, listening to their exploits and proclaiming the righteousness of their struggle. Those in authority (officers) are there to help the soldier move from the position that killing is sinful to feeling that it "achieves honor, fellowship, something close to a state of grace" (Lifton, 1973). The officer defines what is right or wrong. The army attempts to relieve the soldier from feelings of personal responsibility. The Vietnam era soldier was instead confronted by diverse and conflicting messages from the government, officers, families, and antiwar groups. These men could not sustain an identity as the good and moral warrior.

The war and its aftermath was very disruptive to many of these men. Their ability to trust others was profoundly shaken. As symbols of an unpopular war they were left to fend for themselves when they returned. There were few avenues of expression for their feelings of guilt, rage, and helplessness. Some of these veterans sought psychotherapy to help them deal with their resentment, confusion, and difficulty in adapting to civilian life. How did their experiences in Vietnam impact on their view of the therapeutic situation?

This chapter focuses on a number of assumptions and fears about psychotherapy and the therapist that often emerge in work with Vietnam veterans. Such common transferential themes as distrust of authority, the tendency to withdraw from close relationships, and the expectation that they will be rejected need to be understood in terms of both the Vietnam experience and the individual history of the veteran. We also consider typical reactions of therapists in dealing with these men. The nature of this transference-countertransference relationship suggests the need for important modifications in therapetic technique.

TRANSFERENCE

"Transference is the experiencing of feelings, drives, attitudes, fantasies and defenses toward a person in the present which do not befit that person but are a repetition of reactions originating in regard to significant persons of early childhood unconsciously displaced onto figures in the present" (Greenson, 1967).

Psychoanalytic psychotherapy relies on this re-creation of the patient's past to help him recognize how early experiences continue to influence contemporary perceptions and relationships. The therapist works to clarify how the patient's adult behavior is still dominated by the child he once was. The analysis of the transference focuses attention on the early source of the present tensions and stress that the patient is experiencing in his life (Saul, 1972). The patient, by reenacting the past, brings memories, fantasies, and family mythology into the treatment setting.

The decisive part of the work is achieved by creating in the patient's relation to the doctor—in the "transference"—new editions of the old conflicts; in these the patient would like to behave in the same way as he did in the past, while we, by summoning up every mental force [in the patient], compel him to come to a fresh decision. Thus the transference becomes the battlefield on which all the mutually struggling forces should meet one another (Freud, 1917).

Psychotherapists rely on three major allies in the war against the patient's neurosis:

1. The therapeutic alliance (Zetzel, 1956) or working alliance (Greenson, 1967). This is the relatively nonconflictual rational aspects of the relationship between therapist and patient;

2. The anxiety, depression, and suffering caused by the patient's conflicts;

3. The as yet unanalyzed positive transference.

The patient's observing ego, his wish to be rid of his neurotic discomfort, and his wish to transferentially please the therapist combine to facilitate the difficult, painful, and time-consuming labor of transference analysis.

Freud was adamant in viewing the transference "as the ground on which the victory must be won, the final expression of which is lasting recovery from neurosis" (Freud, 1912). If understanding the transference is crucial to resolving psychic conflicts, we need to ask how the transference can most effectively be utilized in working with Vietnam veterans. What special issues might we anticipate? How can we most therapeutically approach them?

Patients bring to the therapeutic process a host of reasonable and unreasonable expectations regarding the therapist as an expert and authority. Vietnam veterans are particularly sensitive to the therapist's role as an authority. They have difficulty differentiating between rational authority and irrational authority. Fromm (1947) sees rational authority as based upon equality of both people, differing only in their skill and knowledge in a particular field. Irrational authority is based on a lack of equality, with differences in each persons value, and with the need for power as the motivating force in the relationship.

TRANSFERENCE AND AUTHORITY

Many Vietnam veterans have great difficulty in dealing with people in positions of authority. These men felt misled by a series of powerful people and institutions. There was, among them, a general feeling of having been deceived by the army and the government. They deplored the lies that the government told about Vietnam. These men often decried the hypocrisy of a war in which officers allowed and encouraged them to rape, brutalize, and sometimes kill South Vietnamese civilians while the army insisted it was fighting to protect the South Vietnamese from evil aggressors. Lifton (1972) refers to soldiers' reports of combat briefings by officers: "I don't know why I'm here, you don't know why you're here. But since we're both here we might as well try to do a good job and do our best to stay alive."

In Vietnam itself there was an unprecedented expression of hostility toward superior officers, who were often seen as the agents of a malevolent authority. The enormity of the soldiers' rage seemed to go beyond the hostility usually born out of the frustrations of army life. The fury of soldiers at the powerful authority embodied in officers may be inferred from the large number of assaults on officers. The killing of officers has been recorded by Levy (1971).

Generally these veterans left the army with feelings of rage and powerlessness. In part this outrage was a response to the absurd and hopeless position of our army in Vietnam. In part it was related to personal feelings toward authority that each soldier brought with him to the war. The intense feelings and fantasies of these men toward authority figures represent an interaction between earlier life experiences and their experiences in Vietnam.

For example, some men who had passive or ineffective fathers consciously or unconsciously hoped that the officers, army, or government would turn out to be the long-hoped-for, all-knowing authority. The authoritarian structure of the army made it easy for these men to give in to the temptation of seeing the army or officer as omnipotent and omniscient and of turning over their sense of responsibility to these authorities.

> Paul, a vet who came from a deeply troubled background, had an alcoholic father and a weak, ineffectual mother. He reported committing a variety of atrocities in Vietnam with little sense at the time that his actions involved any personal decision. Taunting and raping village women was considered standard operating procedure in his army unit. Within this environment Paul was able to enjoy the excitement of forbidden acts with little or no experience of guilt or distress. As long as the officer was seen as all-knowing and all-powerful, the soldier did not have to weigh the morals of the situation.
>
> Near the end of his stay in Vietnam, Paul began to think about what he had done under the auspices of the trusted authority. He felt disappointed. He sensed that he had been betrayed and was filled with enormous anger at the officers and

the army. Not only was it necessary for Paul to keep his deep resentment under cover but he had to be outwardly respectful and follow army orders.

As these issues were discussed, Paul became aware of his guilt over having enjoyed sadistic acts toward women. He was able to understand something about his own susceptibility to the "powerful" officer in terms of his longing to have his father stop drinking and "take charge" of the family. Paul's situation was further complicated by his wish to find not only a strong authority but also a kind, loving, and nurturing one. In this he was most certainly disappointed.

The presence of feelings of betrayal, rage, and impotence in relation to those in authority, the wish to see the authority as omnipotent and omniscient, the passive wish to let the officer take over and give "permission" so that one could act out various fantasies, the longing for the good parent and the disappointment in not finding him are only some of the powerful and complicated dynamics that in various combinations lay beneath the veteran's attitude toward authority.

The army experience served to reinforce or compound difficulties these men had in dealing with people in positions of authority before going to Vietnam. The misuse of power and the abuse of authority were clearly imprinted in their mind during their stay in Vietnam.

On their return to civilian life, many vets were enraged and frustrated at the various government agencies that put them through miles of red tape before giving them benefits that were often seen as inadequate. At the same time, other government agencies freely spent billions on war material. At work, they were overly sensitive to their bosses' telling them what to do. They were angry at the army for having "fucked them over" in countless ways. Sometimes, experiences with army and VA psychiatrists and psychologists added to their cynicism and distrust of authorities.

Therapists are seen as authority figures in a variety of ways. They have an area of expertise, are prosperous members of the establishment, and may have the power to ameliorate anxiety and depression. This dual role of helper and member of the establishment can potentially stir up intense transference reactions in the veteran. If the negative transference becomes too intense we may have a rupture of the therapeutic relationship.

HANDLING THE TRANSFERENCE

Dealing with the distortions, projections, and fantasies in relation to a therapist would undoubtedly be a tremendously difficult and frightening task for many of these men. A powerful working alliance needs to be formed before transference interpretations can be considered.

The working alliance can best be established by "handling the transference" (Horner, 1979) while slowly educating the veteran about the use of transference as a helpful therapeutic aid.

The handling of the transference can be accomplished in the following ways:

1. Restraint from early interpretation;
2. Interpreting by use of extra therapy situations;
3. Accepting the veteran's need to identify with the therapist as a benign authority;
4. Not focusing on unconscious aspects of the negative transference (ie, slips, dreams, etc.). Consciously experienced negative reactions should be dealt with directly to minimize the possibility of their becoming too powerful and disruptive.

AVOIDING EARLY INTERPRETATIONS

Early interpretations of unconscious conflicts, transference to the therapist, and, in group therapy, transference to other group members may raise anxiety to intolerable levels.

> Mark, a drug-addicted veteran, came to only one group meeting. He spoke quite openly about himself and the inner reactions he described struck responsive chords in many of the participants.
>
> The therapist noted that Mark was "dependent" on the army in much the same way he was "dependent" on drugs. He was encouraged to explore other times that he had felt "dependent." Mark found that an interesting idea and said that he would think about it. Mark did not come to the next group meeting in spite of his avowed good feelings about the session. The therapist had taken Mark's openness at face value and pushed for more unconscious material. Mark defended himself by saying that he would "think about it" and by withdrawing from the group.

In the next group meeting there was a sense of disappointment and loss at Mark's absence. One veteran decided to call
Mark. When he reached him, Mark apologized and said he'd
definitely be at the next meeting. When Mark did not arrive at
the next session and it became clear that he was not going to
come, many of the vets responded with feelings of sorrow.
They spoke in ways reminiscent of mourning: "There was so
much I wanted to tell him." "We had so much in common."
"Maybe we failed him, maybe we should have said something
different to him." "I can't believe he really didn't return."

Such an intense reaction to someone whom they had met
only once was undoubtedly rooted in earlier experiences.
Strikingly, the group could express more affect about Mark's
failure to return than they could about losing much closer
friends in Vietnam.

After a great many feelings and thoughts were expressed
about Mark's leaving, the therapist turned to Jim, who had
been particularly moved, and said, "You are obviously very
upset about Mark's leaving the group. It made me think of the
way you felt after Tony stepped on the mine." Jim seemed
close to tears. He responded with "I guess they're pretty heavy
feelings." The therapist agreed that losing someone important is
heavy. Jim began to talk about Tony's death with somewhat
stronger and more immediate affect than he had before.

Slowly and tentatively, over many months, he began to
work on painful memories and feelings that had been guarded
against. In the supportive atmosphere of the group he was able
to go through some mourning.

Some points of technique regarding the therapist's focus emerge
from this example. The therapist was careful not to make the interpretation that sadness over Mark's leaving was exaggerated by earlier
experiences of separation. In this instance the therapist chose not to
designate the surprisingly intense reaction to the loss of Mark as a
displacement. Instead, he simply allowed the immediate experience
to serve as a touchstone to past experiences. The therapist did not,
however, act as if feelings of grief in respect to Mark were perfectly
appropriate to the real situation. He merely underscored the idea
that Jim had experienced similar grief in the past, leaving open the
question of displaced feelings as a possible subject for the future.

In addition, the therapist did not point out that Jim was able to
be more emotional about Mark than about Tony. It was important

not to make Jim feel that he was being criticized for showing too little emotion about Tony's death. Clearly, feelings about Tony were extremely painful and had to be let out slowly. In reality, Mark was not a close friend, and since he was still alive and could still be reached, Jim was able to approach his loss of Tony through Mark. The therapist recognized his over-zealous interpretation of Mark's "dependence" and proceeded more cautiously with Jim.

In order to avoid the possibility of sustaining yet another loss, many veterans steer away from forming close relationships. Often the defensive posture of staying detached adopted during the war keeps the vet from making genuine contact with others long after he has left the war behind (Shatan, 1973).

INTERPRETING VIA EXTRA THERAPY SITUATIONS

Randy feared that he was unfit for anyone's love, given the atrocities he had witnessed and committed. He would constantly recount stories of his own inhumanity. It was as if he were saying, "See how terrible I am; you couldn't possibly like me." In one session Randy reported that he was in love with Gloria, a young woman he had dated for two months. She had just told him that she would like to "cool the relationship." Randy felt he was as open, warm, and caring as anyone could be. He shared his "soul" with Gloria. The therapist asked for an example of how Randy shared his soul: "I tell her things that are the hardest for me to tell anyone. I told her how I stood by and watched three of my buddies rape a South Vietnamese woman and then insert an explosive in her vagina that killed her." After many sessions Randy began to see how his open sharing of horrible details of the Vietnam experience served to test Gloria and simultaneously push her away.

His tendency to test the therapist by perseverating about war atrocities was not mentioned since the veteran may have experienced that as the therapist's wanting to "cool" the relationship with him. It was many months before the therapist could ask Randy how he imagined the therapist felt about the Vietnam stories he was hearing.

IDENTIFICATION WITH THE THERAPIST

Steve was part of a rap group being conducted by Vietnam Veterans Against the War (V.V.A.W.). A very short, thin, 21-year-old man, he was beset by feelings of inadequacy. He

repeatedly told the group he was frightened he would cut somebody up. He carried a push button knife on him and became
more and more obsessed with the idea that he hadn't killed anybody face-to-face in Vietnam. Sure, he was against war and
violence, but most of the men in the group had proven they
weren't chicken. They'd killed men face-to-face in Vietnam.
"All my life I've been a punk. My old man gave me the nick-
name PeeWee. He still thinks I could be knocked over by a good
wind. Even my kid brother is six inches taller than me."

The group pushed him to talk about how he thought he
would feel if he killed someone. He acknowledged that he'd feel
guilty and shitty for cutting up some poor bastard just to prove
himself. The therapist commented that it sounded like he'd feel
like a punk if he didn't knife somebody and a shit if he did.
Either way it sounded like he'd be very unhappy. The group
echoed this "damned if you do, damned if you don't" idea.

Steve turned to the therapist and said he felt like he was
really flipping out. He was really feeling trapped. There was an
outpouring of rage at and fear of his father, a furniture mover
who had once beaten up three guys who tried to mug him.
Steve was overcome with a sense of his own unmanliness. The
therapist intervened by directly questioning the image of manli-
ness perpetrated by the family and the army. The therapist
pointed out the qualities that he admired in Steve as a man: his
sensitivity and gentleness toward various group members, his
actively helping a suicidal soldier who had gone AWOL, his
work at V.V.A.W., his sense of humor, his serious efforts to find
vocational satisfaction. In this case the therapist directly and
deliberately offered his own value system, one that was radically different from that of father, brother, or the ideal soldier.
This view of manhood was relatively new to Steve and helped
him pull himself together.

Steve's wish to become a tough, frightening figure who could
destroy others became a source of intense anxiety during and after
the war. His conflict over aggression was contained before Vietnam,
but in Vietnam acts of violence which were once forbidden became
permissible, socially acceptable, and even praiseworthy. One could
do violence without expecting retaliation. Once external restraints
were removed, Steve felt overwhelmed and confused by his own
hostility. Raw aggression was valued in the family as in the army. He
was opposed to the war on political and moral grounds but had an
urge to kill to prove his courage and masculinity.

The therapist's interventions were directed at Steve's conscious understanding of masculinity. Intellectual controls were offered to help Steve deal with his impulses. The therapist made explicit another view of masculinity. In this situation the therapist underscored aspects of a value system to which Steve, as seen in his V.V.A.W. activities, was already aspiring. The therapist clarified and supported one aspect of Steve's identity while continuing to examine his conflict over it.

NEGATIVE TRANSFERENCE

During the early phases of therapy, transference feelings are best used as a jumping off point to focus on a related problem area outside of the therapy relationship. In instances of clearly experienced negative transference, the therapist should help the veteran acknowledge the feelings before they become too intense. Only after there is a clearly established working alliance can the therapist begin to interpret negative, as well as idealizing, feelings in terms of the veteran's early history.

In one instance, a fairly new patient openly and harshly stated that all the shrinks he had known were "shits" and that he didn't trust them. The therapists had all been seen after his return from Vietnam. He spoke angrily about their lack of helpfulness and their callousness and reported two instances of getting even with them. In one case he broke the windows of the therapist's car. At another time he made a series of obscene telephone calls to the therapist. On hearing these accounts the therapist said that he got the message and considered himself warned. The vet smiled and said sarcastically, "Well, I don't know about you, yet."

When the therapist asked about the specifics of his previous experiences, the vet recounted in considerable detail a series of episodes all of which left him feeling neglected or abandoned.

"This guy I saw in a clinic said, 'Well, we've done all we can; maybe the VA could be of further help to you.' This lady shrink wasn't all bad but she moved to Washington." The vet was not aware of the pattern. The therapist was empathic to some of the vet's experiences. At the same time he focused very pointedly on the veteran's frequently recurring sense of being abandoned.

Eventually the vet was able to talk about other times in his life when he felt that people had given up on him and left him to his own devices. He seemed particularly vulnerable to feelings of neglect.

In this instance feelings about neglect were dealt with partly in terms of the present therapy situation. The therapist made it clear to the vet that he had received a fairly direct communication: If you treat me the way the other shrinks did, I'll get back at you. The therapist, however, did not explore the vet's feelings and fantasies about him. He did not question the vet's statement that he didn't mean this therapist "yet." Here the therapist acknowledged the threat by the vet but did not encourage the vet to investigate why he was threatening him. He did not confront the vet with the paradox of his coming to therapy while thinking all shrinks were terrible.

The therapist, after noting the communication in a clear-cut way, returned to the issue of the vet's past experiences with therapists. By listening to the vet's descriptions of his previous therapy, it became clear that the anger and wish for revenge grew out of the vet's sense that he had repeatedly been abandoned. The therapist heard the vet's anger and expressed his curiosity over its source. The therapist did not interpret the warning to him as a plea of "don't give up on me." Rather, the therapist demonstrated his interest by exploring with the vet his earlier experiences with therapists.

The need for the vet's defensive stand of "don't mess with me or you'll be sorry" was not dealt with vis-a-vis the therapist. Months later it was explored by examining the ways in which the vet's need to be tough covered his fear of being left by important people in his life. As much as possible, the therapist tried *not* to use the therapist-patient relationship as the focal point for therapeutic clarification.

In general, the working alliance is most easily maintained when both the therapist and vet can examine together what is happening outside their relationship. This appears to minimize resistances, defensiveness, embarrassment, and the tendency to leave therapy. At the same time it seems to foster a greater sense of mutual cooperation in working together on the significant and often deeply entrenched problems that preoccupy the veterans.

The therapist, after establishing a solid working alliance, can begin to educate the patient regarding the usefulness of understanding the transference. A first step might include utilizing a transference response as one of a number of examples that highlights a dynamic that has been previously elucidated. If the veteran responds well to this, a questioning of the historical antecedents would be a possible next step. Including the transference response in a more general list of incidents allows the therapist to see how well the veteran can tolerate exploration of the therapist-patient relationship. As a greater tolerance is developed, more pointed questions and later interpretations about the transference can be initiated.

REACTIONS OF THE THERAPIST

The therapist's unconscious reactions to the patient's transference is an important aspect of countertransference: some psychoanalysts in fact, see this reaction as *the* definition of countertransference. We will use the term more broadly. Countertransference refers to the "total emotional reaction of the psychotherapist to the patient in the treatment setting" (Kernberg, 1975).

The literature on psychotherapy puts great stress on therapists' being aware of feelings, fantasies, and attitudes toward their patients. Theoreticians take divergent positions as to how therapists can utilize knowledge of their own emotional reactions to facilitate psychotherapy (Levenson, 1973; Racker, 1968; Singer, 1969). All, however, agree that the more one knows his own responses to a patient, the greater the potential for positive therapeutic results.

In working with Vietnam veterans, therapists need to find a way of confronting material that often is emotionally jolting and difficult to integrate. These men describe harrowing experiences in which they are at times the victims, at other times the perpetrators, of brutal acts. They have seen the bodies of their comrades mutilated by the Vietcong. Frequently they were betrayed by both South Vietnamese civilians and soldiers. Within their own units, nonconformists were often the subject of merciless scapegoating. One junior officer was exposed to intense ridicule for helping a South Vietnamese woman deliver her baby. His fellow officers had found him soft and unmanly. On other occasions veterans label themselves as the agents of evil. It is at such times that therapists often lose their objective footing.

One man spoke of shooting a seven-year-old girl because she tried to steal C rations for her family. A former medic described the thrill of extracting teeth without administering the novocaine he had with him. Listening to such accounts of enacted sadism arouses strong feelings in therapists—feelings that are markedly different from those he experienced when hearing about equally sadistic dreams or fantasies. Again the therapist has to examine the nature and intensity of his reactions and question the effect of his response on the therapeutic task.

The therapist should be aware of the motives that lead him to work with Vietnam vets and should try to anticipate his own reactions to the kind of material that might arise. Therapists working with Vietnam veterans are vulnerable to two distinct technical pitfalls. One danger to therapeutic work arises when the therapist—because of political convictions or personal needs—takes a strong position against the abuses of society. This may lead him away from objective exploration of the patient's experience. This occurs when the therapist becomes overly eager to convey his empathy for the veteran and his understanding of the war situation. There are more and less subtle forms of this unhelpful position. The therapist, for example, who prides himself on being politically aware, may strongly identify with a veteran who feels rage at the social system. He is susceptible to moving in too quickly to explain the veteran's feelings or behavior as reactions to the hypocrisy of our society. He offers support or comfort prematurely. Often this makes it difficult for the veteran to talk about the personally unacceptable aspects of what he had felt and done in Vietnam.

> One veteran spoke of having shot civilians in Vietnam "without the slightest feeling."
> "You shot civilians without feeling anything because the army trained you to respond like an unfeeling robot," the therapist responded. He did not investigate the veteran's lack of affect. On some level the vet knew his actions were not simply a function of army conditioning. He realized that everyone in Vietnam had not responded in the way he had.

In some cases therapists have an urgent need to communicate their sympathy to these men for having been caught in the horrors of Vietnam.

> After hearing one veteran speak compassionately about the destruction United States planes wrought on a South Vietnamese hamlet, the therapist said: "It must have been awful for you to see those people maimed and helpless." The therapist had taken the vet's distress at face value and had subtly reinforced the idea that compassion was the only understandable response to such a situation. The potential for exploring other conscious or unconscious reactions was diminished by the therapist's precipitous intervention.

In both examples the therapists had an intense desire to be empathic and supportive. It led them to act as if they (1) knew how the vet felt, (2) knew why the vet felt and behaved in the way he did, and (3) knew how the vet should have felt.

At times the veterans were aware that some of the emotions strongly associated with Vietnam were similar to feelings they had before the war.

> Tom, a rather quiet man, listened carefully while the therapist criticized the army for turning men into mindless killers. Tom later confessed to a buddy that although everyone else in the group killed because they had been brainwashed, he was excited by the idea of killing "gooks" in Nam. Furthermore, he remembered cutting up animals for kicks when he was an adolescent. Tom felt alienated from the group because he was so aware of his own aggressive impulses. By placing too much emphasis on the army's role in fostering aggression, the therapist failed to help Tom grapple with his destructive wishes.

Conditions of war and internal psychic processes need to be considered in relation to each other. In this situation, the therapist focused too exclusively on the social and political forces impelling the soldier.

Conversely, single-minded preoccupation with intrapsychic dynamics is the source of another therapeutic pitfall. Here therapists tend to view the war situation primarily as a catalyst that exacerbates or brings to the surface already existing psychological problems. Veterans' grievances about the war are automatically treated as a form of resistance to facing inner conflicts. By not acknowledging the tremendous stresses of the war, the therapist can easily underestimate the profound influence of the war experience on the personalities of these men. The veteran's prewar character often underwent important modifications because of Vietnam, and these had to be understood.

> Steve, an articulate, outspoken veteran, became defensive and annoyed with the therapist. "You act like only the shitty parts are real and nothing else counts. You don't know what the Nam was really like." Finally, Steve told the therapist that he was just like his parents who didn't understand the way things were. The therapist pointed out that Steve was blaming the therapist just as he had blamed the army and his parents. He suggested

that Steve's anger at authority figures represented certain feelings he had toward his parents. This transference interpretation was lost on Steve. He saw it as still another attack.

The therapist refused to recognize the fact that in Vietnam the army had often functioned as a disrespectful, manipulative authority. By failing to distinguish Steve's early difficulties with his parents from the reality of his experience in Vietnam the therapist was unable to comprehend the complexity of Steve's reactions.

The therapist can make the first kind of error at one time and the second at another. He can feel particularly identified with a veteran or a situation and err in the direction of being overly sympathetic. On another occasion, he can fail to appreciate the crucial effect of army life or the war on a particular veteran. Here he might insist on the importance of pre-army experiences and ignore the trauma of Vietnam.

For the most part, each therapist tends to err in a particular direction. To the extent that the therapist can recognize his bias, he can increase his capacity to see the interaction between the veteran's pre-Vietnam experience and the effects of Vietnam. He can be responsive to the repercussions of the war on the psychological development of the vet, while remembering that the veteran had a life history before Vietnam that shaped his personality and influenced his perceptions of and reactions to the war. The seemingly obvious necessity of keeping *both* points in mind is neglected more often than one would expect. In part, the emotionally charged quality of the material often leads the therapist to take a defensive unidimensional position so that both he and the veteran might avoid the full impact of the Vietnam experience.

CONCLUSIONS

Therapists working with Vietnam veterans need to move cautiously in dealing with transference reactions early in treatment. Although it may remain unexpressed, the veteran often enters therapy with an underlying sense of cynicism. Transference interpretations may be seen as a misuse of the therapist's authority—a form of intellectual bullying in which the therapist claims to know the veteran's feeling better than he does. Consequently, a dependable working alliance needs to be established before transference interpretations are offered. The working alliance itself is strengthened through careful handling of the transference: avoidance of early transference interpretations, use of extra therapy situations as material for interpretive comments, accepting the veteran's need to identify with the therapist.

The negative transference deserves particular attention. It is often difficult for the veteran to acknowledge the intensity of his hostility or envy toward the therapist—especially in the early phases of treatment. Therefore, the therapist might deal with vague or indirect expressions of anger or distrust by focusing on external situations associated with such feelings. However, when negative feelings are experienced directly and openly the therapist should discuss them in terms of the therapeutic relationship. In this way the therapist does not allow the negative transference to build to a disruptive intensity.

As the veteran develops more trust, the therapist can begin to illustrate the ways that the transference can be used therapeutically. This needs to be done gradually and precedes making of historical reconstructions about the negative and idealizing transference.

The therapist working with Vietnam veterans must be particularly sensitive to his internal reactions when confronting the dehumanizing events these men experienced. The therapist's inner distress over the profoundly disturbing experiences of the veterans may impel him to become either too involved in the external circumstances of the war or too detached from them. The first error arises when the therapist focuses exclusively on social, economic, or political determinants of the veterans condition. He may be eager to communicate his dismay with the social system, to let the veteran know that he understands his suffering. The therapist's overinvolvement with the abuses of society, real as they may be, can interfere with his capacity to explore the veteran's reactions objectively.

The second danger arises when the therapist does not pay adequate attention to the effects of ongoing social pressures. In this case he narrows his scope by minimizing the effects of environmental stress. His preoccupation with early interpersonal phenomena and intrapsychic dynamics leads him to view larger social factors or later traumatic situations as simply intensifying preexisting conflicts. The patient's feeling that he holds a difficult place in society is treated primarily as a resistance. Therapists demonstrate this kind of myopia when they gloss over the psychologically destructive aspects of serving in the army during the Vietnam war.

ACKNOWLEDGMENT

The author wishes to acknowledge the collaborative contributions of Dr. Ruth Shapiro to both the content and style of this paper. Aspects of this chapter have appeared in *Group Therapy 1978*, Wolberg, A., Aronson, M. (Eds.). New York: Statton, 1978, and *Group, Fall 1978*, Vol. 2, 3, New York: Human Sciences Press.

REFERENCES

Freud, S. (1912). The dynamics of transference. *S.E.* 12.
Freud, S. (1917). Introductory lectures on psychoanalysis. *S.E.* 16.
Fromm, E. (1947). *Man for Himself.* New York: Yale University Press.
Greenson, R. (1967). *The Technique and Practice of Psychoanalysis*, Vol. 1. New York: International Universities Press.
Horner, A. (1979). *Object Relations and the Developing Ego in Therapy.* New York: Jason Aronson.
Kernberg, O. (1975). *Borderline Conditions and Pathological Narcissism.* New York: Jason Aronson.
Levenson, E. (1973). *The Fallacy of Understanding.* New York: Basic Books.
Levy, C. (1971). ARVN as faggots. *Transaction*, October 23, 18-27.
Lifton, R. (1972). Home from the war: The psychology of survival. *Atlantic Monthly*, November, 56-72.
Lifton, R. (1973). *Home from the War.* New York: Simon and Schuster.
Racker, H. (1968). *Transference and Countertransference.* London: Hogarth Press.
Saul, L. (1972). *Psychodynamically Based Psychotherapy.* New York: Science House.
Shatan, H. (1973). The grief of soldiers. *American Journal of Orthopsychiatry* 43: 640-653.
Singer, E. (1969). *Key Concepts in Psychotherapy.* New York: Basic Books.
Zetzel, E. (1956). Current concepts of transference. *International Journal of Psychoanalysis* 37: 369-376.

5
Nightmares of the Traumatic Neuroses: Implications for Theory and Treatment

ROBERT BLITZ, PH.D. AND RAMON GREENBERG, M.D.

Nightmares have been a prominent symptom of traumatic war neurosis since it was first described in the literature from World War I (Brown, 1920; Rado, 1942). As a symptom of trauma, the dream imagery of the nightmare can be used to understand the issues that arise from the traumatic experience. The interpretation of these issues and the explanation for the development of the traumatic symptoms are embedded in a theoretical understanding of personality dynamics, and in a theory of dreaming which encompasses the development of the nightmare. This chapter briefly reviews the literature on the personality theories used to explain the traumatic war neurosis and the traumatic nightmare, discusses the implications of recent research on the theory of dreaming, and uses Kohut's theory about the development of the self to provide a more comprehensive orientation for the understanding and treatment of traumatic neurosis.

In general, the term *nightmare* refers to the "bad dream" from which the sleeper awakens feeling frightened and anxious due to mental imagery which usually has some sort of development as in a dream. It is distinguished from the night terror by the lower level of autonomic arousal (Fisher et al, 1970; Kahn et al, 1972) and the more developed dream imagery. Night terrors are sometimes associated with more prolonged disorientation upon awakening and amnesia for the nighttime event. Traumatic nightmares frequently depict content related to real life trauma and are more likely to present images from the experience than to consist of symbolic imagery (van der Kolk et al, 1982). The traumatic nightmare appears to be more like the REM dream nightmare than the night terror, although there is occasional appearance of traumatic nightmares in Stage 2 sleep (Schlossberg and Benjamin, 1978).

The considerable clinical literature concerning the development of the war neurosis has failed to support the position that there is a single premorbid personality type or specific predisposition that results in traumatic war neurosis (TWN) (Fairbairn, 1951; Lidz, 1946; Kardiner, 1959). Kardiner asserts, "Although it is true that a war situation can revive pre-existing syndromes heretofore dormant, it can also create new ones" (1959, p. 245). He defines trauma as an imbalance between the environment and one's adaptive resources. He emphasizes that the traumatic symptoms appear to represent a failure of particular psychological functions and not a "regression" to previous fixation. The strikingly consistent symptom pattern suggests that a particular set of psychological functions has been affected by the trauma although the symptom content is subject to individual elaboration.

Kardiner (1959) described the traumatic nightmare as "the most universal earmark of the traumatic syndrome. These constant dreams of the failure to consummate successful actions are, in fact, the key to the pathology" (p. 249). A typical traumatic nightmare includes images of the dreamer being overrun, ambushed, or frozen in terror and unable to respond while others are being killed. There is a pervasive sense of vulnerability and helplessness. At times, there are images of finding oneself dead. In some cases the traumatic imagery portrays the dreamer as the aggressor. Kardiner writes,

> The altered conception of oneself and the outer world is what lies behind the catastrophic dreams. No action can be completed. Instead, the ego is overwhelmed as it once was. Since the implements for keeping the world at bay (mastery) are now impounded, the world is overwhelming the ego. Hence the hostile world and the impoverished self are two facets of the same pathology. . . . Whether or not the dream may be a wish-fulfillment, it is the best indicator of the structure of the personality. . . . We have the tendency to regard dreams from the

point of view of motivation. But the motivation is contingent on the resources available to carry it out. In other words, the dream gives information about the motivation and of the structure of the personality at the time (p. 253).

The traumatic experience seems to assault one's basic assumptions about oneself in relation to the world, and one's capacity to bear the feelings in response to it. The traumatized person has lost a basic trust in himself and in the world about him and has lost the capacity to self soothe.

The traumatic nightmare and the incident it depicts are emotionally immediate, as they are reported in the therapy (van der Kolk, personal communication). The incidents appear *unintegrated* with or unelaborated by the veteran's current or previous experiences. This lack of integration in the nightmare appears to have parallels in the traumatized person's sense of himself. The veteran frequently reports feeling that he has lost something of himself, that he is not the same person, that things have lost their meaning. Current relationships and accomplishments do not appear to be able to mitigate the sense that something has shattered inside, as if connections with other meaningful memories and present experiences cannot be made.

Other elements of the symptom pattern point to an association of posttraumatic stress disorder (PTSD) with problems in interpersonal functioning (Maskin, 1941; Moses, 1978; Fox, 1974). DSM III (1980) includes as one of the criteria for the diagnosis of PTSD a sense of isolation from others characterized by diminished responsiveness or interest in activities, and a feeling of detachment or constricted affect. The symptoms that result from disruptions of interpersonal connections include impaired self-esteem, a sense of isolation and aloneness, a desire for revenge against the loss, impulsive outbursts, difficulty in feeling close to one's children, and a sense of danger in reinvesting in others (Kolb, 1982; van der Kolk, 1982).

The importance of interpersonal functions is further emphasized by two studies that reported that traumatized persons had a history of problems in early relationships to primary figures, which resulted in difficulty establishing useful, modulated relationships in the service. These relationships were either so close that the death of the other was catastrophic or they relied on previous relationships with parents or a girlfriend and felt hopeless when these were disrupted (Fairbairn, 1952; Lidz, 1946). Although Lidz (1946) argues that these symbiotic relationships were evidence of immature personality structure, van der Kolk (1982) has suggested that for many soldiers this intense investment in a buddy and the idealization of the goals of the immediate group reflect an expected stage of development for the adolescent. Under normal circumstances, these relationships would result in a reworking of issues of differentiation, identity, and ambition. In this model what is traumatic is the premature and violent disruption of the relationships, the loss of idealization of the group, and the destruction of the phase-appropriate sense of omnipotence. Weinberg (1946) reports that units with effective leadership and good group morale had decreased incidence of TWN.

The following review discusses the early literature and then indicates the implications of self-psychology for understanding the traumatic neurosis syndrome and the nightmares associated with it.

TRAUMATIC WAR NEUROSIS: HISTORICAL PERSPECTIVES

Abram Kardiner (1959) writes that the war neuroses are caused by:

a self-preservative crisis due to the danger of destruction. This reaction to impending threat of destruction is the pathological nucleus around which a new style of adaptation can be organized. It is this new organization and the reactions of the subject to it that constitute the syndrome we call the "traumatic neurosis" (p. 246).

He focuses on the specific functions of the personality which are affected by the trauma. These functions are related to the way the person relates to the physical world. He discounts the usefulness of identifying these functions as evidence of a "self-preservative" instinct, suggesting instead that the focus should be on the action systems and the effect on them of the miscarried adaptation to the trauma. The dominant adaptive method used "was akin to repression, the purpose of which was to eliminate the painful environment and to diminish the anxiety created by the curtailment of resources. The neurosis consists of the establishment of a new style of adaptation based upon the truncation of resources" (p. 247). There is a long struggle to maintain meaningful contact with the world which, when it fails, results in reduction in areas of effectiveness and gratification. The world is experienced as a hostile place. "Organized channels of action are broken up, and their place is taken by periodic outbursts of disorganized aggression" (Kardiner, 1959, p. 253).

In focusing on the action systems and their relation to the physical world, Kardiner has removed his conceptualization of the war neuroses from the considerations of instincts, regressions to previous levels of psychosexual development, and unconscious wish fulfillment. From this vantage point he is able to pinpoint the salient parts of the syndrome, the constriction of a broad range of functions, the experience of oneself as not capable of completing actions, and the fragmented, disintegrated qualities of the experience of oneself. He identifies the nightmare as the dream that reveals this state of the organism and its inability to complete a task.

Clinical observation of a number of soldiers with war neurosis led Fairbairn (1952) to conclude that all of the soldiers with this syndrome had earlier overly dependent relationships with a parent. This had blocked the diffusion of the intensity of the need for the primary relationship and had thwarted the development of new relationships with peer groups. He noted that separation anxiety is paramount in the neurotic picture as opposed to desire for secondary gain. He saw in his soldiers a strong need to return home or to reestablish a dependent relationship. He also described a clinical picture of some soldiers for whom reaction formation against their dependence enabled them to appear adjusted to the military. When the situation became stressful and frustrating, the potential for stimulation of the defended against passivity and dependency became disruptive. He found that people who had war neuroses were usually engaged in relationships in which they identified with the other. In this process the individual failed to differentiate himself from the other person, and thus spontaneously identified with those upon whom he depended. This resulted in an inability to tolerate separation from the important object in thought or in deed. Individuation, personality consolidation, and independence are not achieved. This soldier, "finds it too difficult a task to establish himself as a separate personality within the framework of the military organization, subordinate himself to the aims of the military group without any surrender of independence, and maintain stable emotional bonds with the group while remaining differentiated from it" (Fairbairn, 1952, p. 278). Nightmares are viewed as depicting the soldier's experience of persecution by the authorities as a result of the splitting of the "good" home relationships from the intolerable relationships to the "bad" authorities in the army.

In his paper, "Nightmares and the Traumatic War Neurosis," Lidz (1946) observed that nightmares and other symptoms of the traumatic neuroses appeared in patients subsequent to their experiencing the real or threatened loss of an emotionally significant figure. Using the wish fulfilling hypothesis about the nature of dreams and the concept of the death instinct, he proposed that the individual experiences suicidal wishes in response to the loss; these are dystonic and are projected in the dream work and result in nightmares of images that threaten life. He stressed the disruptive early family relationships and the interaction of patients' residual conflicts and immaturity with the combat stress. The family pattern is of absense or insecurity of affection from the parents. This leaves the patient experiencing hostility and guilt toward the parent. Lidz (1946) outlined the dynamics of the nightmare development as follows:

> The soldier's development in an unstable family environment leaves him insecure in his interpersonal relationships and hostile when deprived of affection. He finally achieves a dependent relationship with a single person. When deprived of this bulwark of security when alone in a terrifying setting, he loses his desire to live. The suicidal thoughts are repressed and the danger from within the self is projected in the nightmares as an external threat (p. 40).

Again the theory proposed stresses the importance of the soldier's relationships to others as a primary factor in the predisposition to development of war neurosis and nightmares. Both Fairbairn (1952) and Lidz (1946) suggest that the relationship pattern of persons who have traumatic neuroses and nightmares is related to early dependency issues, possibly at the level of symbiosis.

In a review of the early dynamic theories about the etiology of the TWN, Maskin (1941) pointed to the difficulty Freud and others had in defining the symptoms of TWN as a result of blocking of the libido. His review carefully detailed the two directions that these early theorists took in explaining the war neuroses. One was Freud's conception of instincts which were "beyond the pleasure principle." The "death instinct" and the idea of the repetition compulsion as an attempt at active mastery were suggested as additional factors to explain the development of the traumatic neuroses. Neither was developed in later writings. Another formulation that used libido theory stressed the regression to narcissistic stages of investment of the ego with libido. This reinvestment of libido in the ego was referred to as a regression to an early narcissistic position. The theory stressed the threat to the ego of being overwhelmed with excitation, which resulted when the "stimulus barrier" function of the ego was overwhelmed. Mack (1974) wrote that the traumatic disorders result when the ego experiences a threat to itself, and suggested "these disorders require a reconsideration of the role of self preservation in human motivation and the reintroduction of concepts closely allied to Freud's earlier concept of 'ego instincts'" (p. 219).

In the clinical descriptions from World War II, the traumatized veterans frequently were characterized as narcissistic (referring to the dependency attempts to gain reassurance from authority) and aggressive when their wants were frustrated. The theoretical orientation at that time attributed these symptoms to the discharge of excessive psychic energy and castration anxiety. Theory aside, the descriptions of the clinical syndrome pointed to concerns over body integrity, one's sense of safety in the world, and the capacity to care for oneself.

Other investigators (Sullivan, Kardiner, Horney, and Rado) "are all concerned with the ontogeny in the human personality of techniques for mastering the social, interpersonal and physical world" (Maskin, 1941, p. 112). These workers focused more on the development of the ego and the effect of mastery in motivation and adaptation to the external environment. Kardiner (1959) refers to mastery as the defense against being overwhelmed by external experience.

More recently Fox (1974) found an association between psychiatric difficulties subsequent to combat (including nightmares) and narcissistic injury and rage. Reviewing his clinical experience with 106 Vietnam combat veterans who were referred for psychiatric evaluation after a tour of combat duty with the Marines, he noted the different experience of two types of combat aggression. One type he described as having aggression associated with group effort and following group rules. There is a lack of personal hostility in this type of aggression which was characterized by several patients as similar to that felt in team sports. The second type of aggression was a much more personally felt hostile aggression. He suggested that the transition to this second form of aggression frequently followed the death of a buddy in combat. "Following such a loss, the patient became aware of feelings of murderous rage and wishes for revenge. Even when the subject was studied later in psychotherapy, the predominant theme was one of vengeance rather than of mourning" (p. 808). The intensity of this affective reaction, its persistence after revengeful acts, the accompanying fear of retaliatory action from others, the absence of empathy for the victims, and the emphasis on revenge over grief and mourning all suggested to Fox that the rage is associated with narcissistic injury. He argued that the combat buddy relationship represents a "mirror relationship" as Kohut (1971) describes it. The loss of the buddy then represents a narcissistic injury with the resultant threat to the self which is accompanied by rage and retaliatory action.

Moses (1978) argues for the association of particular types of early object relations and traumatic neurosis in adults. The two psychological functions which he identified as being related to the susceptibility to combat neuroses are self-esteem and a sense of belonging to a primary group in which one has a sense of well-being and freedom. In the comparison of soldiers who developed combat neurosis with soldiers who were wounded, Moses (1978) noted that the former have, "a narcissistic vulnerability based on a frail and insecure sense of self, which is thrown out of kilter by the trauma and turns into a sense of worthlessness, of badness, sometimes extending to the group as a whole (p. 361)." He concluded, "From many different points of view, then, narcissistic factors emerge as playing an important role in the predisposition to combat reactions, in its prevention, in its treatment and, by implication, in all traumatic neuroses of the adult" (Moses, 1978, pp. 361–362).

Van der Kolk (1982) also has suggested that narcissistic issues as revived in adolescence are involved in TWN. As Blos (1979) noted, adolescence is a regression to self-absorption and a reworking of narcissistic issues as the adolescent differentiates from the family group and establishes a new identity in the peer group. This period is characterized by a view of the world as a series of absolutes, the polarities of good versus evil, autonomy versus dependency, action versus passivity, and love versus hate. These polarities are seen to arise from the sense of omnipotence the child has when merged with the mother contrasted with the constant danger of losing her and that sense of well being. Van der Kolk (1982) stated,

> The resolution of adolescence consists of integrating these polarities through the development of self and object constancy. This integration is easily threatened when an adolescent is exposed to trauma which would confirm a world view which is transiently based on a sense of absolute badness and helplessness, and the defense against that: total omnipotence. . . . It was the younger men who had experienced their friend's death, and the concommitant dissolution of the once omnipotent group, as a narcissistic injury and who had persistent nightmares of the traumatic events, in which they regularly relived the state of total helplessness they once experienced on the battlefield (pp. 2–4).

There is the need to regain the idealization necessary to resume the adolescent development. Van der Kolk (1982) described his clinical observations as follows:

> Their relationships to significant others, such as wives or therapists, is characterized by either idealization or withdrawal, rather than by empathy. In groups, initially there tends to be a marked lack of genuine interpersonal differentiation. Rather, the members seem to use each other as mirrors against whom they reflect both the memories of feelings of belonging and omnipotence as experienced in combat, or with whom to relive some of the terror (p. 6).

To summarize, these studies report the following factors as characteristic of persons who have TWN:

1. In the face of combat stress they have the potential to form overly dependent relationships with a peer or with an important figure back home. In the relationship there is a lack of differentiation from the other.
2. A resulting vulnerability to loss which can result in overwhelming feelings of insecurity. This loss can result in chronic hostility and desire for vengeance. This hostility quickly can change to a feeling of threat to themselves from people or their environment.
3. A diminished capacity to regulate self-esteem. They are dependent upon others and the group norms for feelings of self-worth.
4. A susceptibility to concerns about maintaining their psychological intactness and their belief that the world is a safe place.
5. A pervasive depression with felt inability to reinvest in new relationships, initiate gratifying activities, and a sense that something basic about themselves has been altered.
6. Preoccupation with their bodies and health.
7. A vacillation between feelings of utter helplessness and terror, and feelings of omnipotence and yearning for idealized figures.

As we consider these factors, it seems they can be best understood with Kohut's (1971, 1972) descriptions of the personality functions based upon the self. Lidz (1946) and Fairbairn (1951) were explicit in their descriptions of the overly dependent relationships in which the individual fails to differentiate himself from others; this is a major characteristic of the merger-seeking personality (Kohut and Wolf, 1978). Lidz (1946) also wrote of the hostility that prevails when deprived of affection in this group and tied it to insecurity about affection from early family relationships. He identified the loss of a close buddy or loved one from home as frequent precipitants of the war neurosis and the nightmares. This intense reaction to the object loss could arise from the fear of loss of integrity of self because the self was maintained with the aid of the merger relationship with the other. Fairbairn (1951) wrote that there is a failure of individuation and personality consolidation. All these descriptions of the subjects' relationships are markedly parallel to the descriptions that Kohut (1971) provided of the individual with an impaired self who relies excessively on self-objects to function in accordance with his ambition and ideals.

Kardiner's (1959) descriptions of the experience of the world as hostile, the change in self-conception, the inability to focus aggression, and the impairment of psychological structure and adaptive functions all suggest a person struggling with a fragmented self-structure. Kardiner's treatment suggestion focuses on the usefulness of an empathic relationship that helps reintegrate the memories of the trauma and makes the experience bearable and no longer fragmented. Fox (1974), Moses (1978), and van der Kolk (1982) were more explicit in tying the symptoms of the posttraumatic stress disorder directly to narcissistic impairment as seen in object relations.

In general the literature reports numerous factors associated with traumatic neurosis and traumatic nightmares which fit within the framework of narcissistic disorders. These factors seem related to areas of personality function which determine basic aspects of an individual's sense of self in relationship to others and to his external world. These functions are based upon an individual's cohesive self. They form the basis of object relations, self-esteem, experience of continuity in one's life, the experience of an autonomous center for initiative, and the capacity for comforting oneself. The interpersonal dysfunction described is not neurotic distortion of the interaction, but is more like the distortion associated with narcissistic structural deficits. Kohut's (1971, 1977) outline of a theory of the self provides a system for describing and classifying psychopathology in this area. His theory of narcissism and the development of the self within a self-object matrix will be used in conjunction with current theories about the function of dreams to discuss the therapeutic implications of the traumatic nightmare.

Our thesis, then, is that persons with traumatic nightmares have suffered disruptions of the self, experiencing transient loss of self cohesion, difficulty in self-esteem regulation, and loss of a sense of well-being in the face of threatened interruptions in their relationships to important others. They have failed to develop or have traumatically lost their own self functions which would provide a consistent sense of self, maintain their self-esteem, and enable them to soothe themselves as their primary others did at one time.

DREAMS AND NIGHTMARES

Having reviewed the literature on the personality dynamics associated with TWN, we need to consider nightmares as a dream phenomenon. We discuss Freud's theories of dreaming, compare them with material developed from recent sleep research, consider the nightmare as a special case of dreaming, and relate this to the clinical picture of nightmares sufferers that we have presented.

Freud's original dream theory was based upon concepts of drive discharge and wish fulfillment. He postulated that sleep was a state that the person was motivated to preserve. When there was physiological or psychological arousal that threatened to disrupt sleep, the preconscious system substituted mental imagery for the impulse gratifying action of waking life to satisfy the id impulses and preserve the sleeping state. With the elaboration of the theory to include an account of the anxiety dream, Freud (1900) suggested that the dream begins as a "discharge of unconscious impulses." This fits into the model of the mind outlined in the last chapter of *The Interpretation of Dreams* (1900). In this model there are two systems: the unconscious, which represents the instinctual impulses and the preconscious, which is a censoring agency that prevents direct discharge of impulses.

In sleep the impulses that would be motorically expressed or gratified if the individual were awake cannot be directly gratified. According to this theory, the preconscious uses imagery from the day residue to provide fantasied gratification and thus prevents the build up of tension that would awaken the sleeper. Because the repressive barrier of the preconscious is weakened during sleep, there is less censorship of impulses although there is still dream work and secondary revision that disguise the instinctual roots of the dream.

In *Beyond the Pleasure Principle*, Freud (1920) suggested an addition to his view of dreaming. Breger, Hunter, and Lane (1971) summarized it as follows:

Confronted with the evidence that experiences of psychological trauma may lead a person to dream continually about the anxiety-provoking traumatic event, Freud postulated a separate function for dreaming. This function consists of binding the tensions that arise from the trauma; he speaks of it as antedating wish fulfillment. This view of traumatic dreams is embedded in a discussion of the repetition compulsion in which Freud suggests a common underlying principle for certain repetitive neurotic symptoms, traumatic dreams, and the repetitive play of children. All are attempts at mastering, under one's own control, events that one could not deal with originally (p. 10).

This theory is consonant with later theories involving ego function, but for Freud, the wish fulfillment hypothesis remained foremost as a theory of dream function (Breger et al, 1971).

The principle that all dreams and nightmares represent the discharge of unconscious impulses led Jones (1931) to interpret nightmares as sexual dreams arising from Oedipal conflicts. This implies that the persons suffered from neurotic level conflicts. The manifest content of the nightmare, however, appears to reveal more primitive conflicts. Jones himself noted the limitations of an exclusively Oedipal interpretation and suggested that some nightmares may represent issues formed earlier than Oedipal conflicts.

Using drive discharge formulations, the nightmare could thus represent unconscious impulses that were anxiety provoking because they were conflictual or because they represented a traumatic overstimulation that had previously threatened the ego. Freud's suggestion that there is a dream function that antedated the wish fulfilling one, and his suggestions that the traumatic dreams might represent a conflict within the ego, point to a more varied dream function. There remains, however, the implication that the anxiety associated with nightmares results from conflict.

EGO PSYCHOLOGY: DREAM THEORY AND NIGHTMARES

A second contribution to the theory of nightmare development and related personality factors arose from ego psychology. Within the framework of ego psychology, the dream was still seen as an expression of any one of a number of unconscious impulses; however, the nightmare only occurred when the impulse threatened to overwhelm the ego. Mack (1974) described the impulses underlying the nightmare as "the earliest, most profound, and inescapable anxieties to which human beings are subject: those involving destructive aggression, castration, separation and abandonment, devouring and being devoured, and fear regarding loss of identity and fusion with the mother" (p. 16). He has suggested that nightmares represent the arousal of these impulses as a person moves toward more autonomy and separation from primary figures. With this addition to the theory of nightmares, the nightmare sufferer's personality could be described not only in terms of the earlier conflicts that were represented, but also in terms of the individual's capacity to bear the affect or to defend against it. The term "ego strength" is used to describe this capacity.

Briefly, Mack's theory of dreams suggests that the personality factor involved in the development of a nightmare is "ego strength," that is, the capacity to defend against or bear primitive unconscious impulses. These unconscious impulses focus on aggression, maintenance of identity and body integrity, fear of fusion, and object loss either by abandonment, devouring, or separation. For nightmare sufferers these issues, along with a diminished capacity to master the anxiety and impulses, should be prevalent.

Mack's (1965) study of the nightmare at different developmental stages offered an important view of the nightmare as it appears in the developmental sequence. Mack viewed the nightmare as a breakthrough of primitive destructive impulses toward loved ones at a time when the psychological mastery of the impulses is incomplete. The focus of the cause of nightmares is on the threatened disruption of the relationship to an important other. This formulation assumes, however, that hatred and hostility cause the disruption of the relationship to the people who are loved.

Mack noted that the mastery of these impulses increases as the internal representations of others in the dream imagery increases. In a more recent paper reviewing theories about children's dreams, Ablon and Mack (1980) summarized, "A nightmare can reflect mastery and a developmental advance, or indicate areas of vulnerability that lead to the child's being overwhelmed, with resultant impairment of ego functioning or more lasting symptom formation" (p. 200). They anticipate the need to consider the self in relation to nightmares: "There has been little or no research as to how the occurrence of or susceptibility to frequent nightmares applies to the concept of the self, the development of a cohesive self, and impairments or vulnerability in the development of the self" (Ablon and Mack, 1980, p. 201). To pursue this exploration of the relationship of dreaming, nightmares and the self, current research on the function of dreams needs to be considered.

THE FUNCTION OF DREAMS: CURRENT RESEARCH

The results of recent laboratory studies of sleep and dreaming have pointed to an adaptive function for dreams (Webb and Cartwright, 1978; Breger, 1967; Greenberg and Pearlman, 1975a). To be more specific, the studies suggest that dreaming is necessary for the integration of affective experiences so as to maintain or modify defensive and coping strategies. Two types of data have been drawn upon. The first has been demonstrations of the continuity of personality characteristics and affective concerns in waking life and in dreaming. The second has been the results of studies showing that dreaming or REM sleep facilitate adaptation to waking life experiences and tasks.

In a review of dream research Cartwright (Webb and Cartwright, 1978) cites articles by Foulkes that support the conclusion that "children's dreams are realistic representations of their waking life and . . . that when waking life is disturbed due to some personality dysfunction so also are the dreams" (p. 240). Turpin's (1976) investigation of the continuity of ego development between waking and sleeping in children aged 11 to 13 also supports the continuity of functioning between these two states. Cartwright (Webb and Cartwright, 1978) concludes, "All of this literature with respect to longstanding demographic and personality characteristics supports the view that dream characteristics correctly reflect waking emotional concerns and styles" (p. 242).

Breger et al (1971) have demonstrated this connection even more clearly in their monograph on dreams and stress. They found very clear evidence, in the dreams of subjects facing various stressful life situations, of material clearly related to the stress and of efforts to integrate or master the stressful situations. Greenberg and Pearlman (1975b) added to this when they showed the continuity of material from analytic hours with the manifest content of dreams collected in the sleep laboratory the night after the analytic hour. They also found that when the dreams showed evidence of solutions of the problems from the hour, the analytic hour the next day showed evidence of improved coping. They summarized their conclusions as follows:

The manifest dream then provides a vivid subjective view of the patient's current adaptive tasks. . . . Our concept of adaptation is similar to that described by Joffe and Sandler (1968), in which the ego attempts to create new organizations of the ideal state of self in order to preserve a feeling of safety and to avoid the experience of being traumatically overwhelmed. Successful adaptation involves a relinquishing of ideals (wishes) which are no longer appropriate to present reality. That these previous ideal states are not always so easily abandoned contributes to the appearance of infantile wishes and the wish fulfillment aspect of dreaming. We are suggesting that dreams portray the struggle, inherent in the interaction between the wishes of the past and the needs of the present, and reflect the process of integration which appears to take place in REM sleep (p. 447).

A second set of data also points to the role of dreaming or its physiological correlate, REM sleep, for adaptation to waking tasks. This has been extensively reviewed by Pearlman (1982). Briefly, the results of a number of studies of REM sleep deprivation in animals show that REM sleep is necessary for the mastery of complicated tasks but not for simple ones. In a similar way, studies in humans show a role for REM sleep in mastery of complicated, new, or affectively laden situations. We would summarize these studies for the purpose of this discussion as pointing to a function for dreams which involves integration or assimilation of new and important experiences into existing structures or schemata.

We would also suggest that the weight of sleep research studies suggests that the drive discharge theory of dreaming is no longer adequate. Furthermore, it suggests that the manifest dream portrays more than it hides (Greenberg and Pearlman, 1981).

From this perspective we would consider the nightmare a "failed dream," that is, a dream that does not complete the process of integration of present and past experience. Greenberg et al (1970) wrote, "If the new experiences are growth-promoting in nature, ie, correct previous distorted wishes or fears, a modification in ways of dealing with the previously unconscious material may result when the dream brings the new experience into relation to the past" (p. 2). In order to understand nightmares from this theoretical perspective, then, the question is what causes this normal development and flow of the dream to fail. From the above formulation there are three inter-related areas that may affect the successful completion of the dream. The first factor is the psychological make-up of the dreamer. This includes not only the conflictual, symptomatic aspects of his personality, but his character and defensive style. The second factor is the dreamer's relationship to others. If there are facilitating interpersonal interactions available to the dreamer, it is possible that the dream is less likely to fail. Finally, the third factor is the stimulation of the environment. Daily experiences appear to evoke dream imagery differentially depending upon the salience of that experience to the person's concerns (Cartwright, 1979). A particular constellation of experiences might induce a dream failure. The particular personality function suggested by this current review of dream research is related to the person's capacity to integrate experiences and establish a continuity of past and present emotional life.

SELF-PSYCHOLOGY: DREAMS AND NIGHTMARES

As in our discussion of the personalities of nightmare sufferers, we would now suggest that Kohut's descriptions of the function of the self present another perspective. Kohut (1977) suggests that the self also provides the structure for assimilating current experience and maintaining a sense of continuity to one's experience. Both the self and dreams appear to function differentially, depending upon the self-objects or empathic responses available to the individual. As a theoretical speculation, it seems possible that the normal dream process is supported by and supports a cohesive functioning self. The failed dream then can be hypothesized to be related to the dreamer's experience of a threat to his self-cohesion with the accompanying intense anxiety which awakens the dreamer and interrupts the dream function.

Kohut is more specific about this connection. He (1977) noted that some dreams, including children's dreams and nightmares, represent a depiction of the state of the "self" and do not necessarily lend themselves to interpretation as an expression of unconscious impulses. The nightmare frequently depicts a dangerous situation in which the individual is under attack or in danger of losing his or her life. These situations can be interpreted as mental representations of an imperiled self, that is, a self that is potentially fragmenting. This possible association of nightmares and the fragmenting self suggests that persons having frequent nightmares may have fragile self-structures or may have been exposed to catastrophic stress where the possibility of annihilation was so real that the self was shattered.

Traumatic nightmares, then, may result from a disturbance of the psychological functions which allow dreams to function as a means of "making sense of" the day's emotional experiences in light of one's previous experience. Like "self-state" dreams, the content and associations to the dream material reveal attempts to elaborate the experience of a threatened self-state with mental images.

IMPLICATIONS FOR TREATMENT

The changing theories about the personalities of those suffering from TWN and the mechanisms involved in nightmare formation have been paralleled by changing efforts to treat this very serious and painful disorder. We will try to demonstrate how the perspective of self-psychology can help us understand what has been effective in treatment and to formulate a more coherent treatment approach.

As we review some recent reports (Wilmer, 1982; Haley, 1974), we have been struck by the applicability of two major concepts in the treatment of narcissistic disorders. These are the development of either a mirror transference or of an idealizing transference in the course of treatment. Associated with these ideas is the importance of self-object ties and their loss rather than the role of drives and of conflict.

As one reads the case reports in the two reports cited, one can readily see the impact of loss of important self-objects. Most impressive, however, are the descriptions the authors provide of what works in therapy. For example Wilmer (1982) notes the following:

By focusing on the world of dreams, a helpful bond was created. Almost all patients were enormously relieved that at last some professional person was interested in the dreams, not afraid to listen patiently to their nightmares and their combat experiences (p. 47).

Haley (1974) notes a similar need as illustrated in the following excerpts:

The therapists must be able to envision the possibility that under extreme physical and psychic stress in an atmosphere of overt license and encouragement, he/she, too, might very well murder. Without this effort by the therapist, treatment is between the 'good' therapist and the 'bad,' out of control patient (p. 194).

Establishment of the therapeutic alliance for this group of patients *is* the treatment (p. 195).

These reports provide ample evidence of the importance of empathy and the development of idealizing transferences to the therapist or the institution. As a matter of fact, it is probably the loss of idealized self-objects that underlies the frequent observation that Vietnam veterans have been so adversely affected by the sense that their country was bad and got them involved in a bad war.

One of the main problems in treating patients with traumatic neuroses has been their propensity to flee treatment. We would suggest that in some cases this may occur because the condition is seen as a problem of aggression. By contrast a focus on what the patient has experienced, as reflected in his dreams, may help the patient develop a mirror transference in treatment that will allow the eventual integration of the trauma into the patient's experience.

This concept of integration allows us to look at the nightmares and how they can be used in the course of treatment. As mentioned in the theoretical discussion, we view the nightmare as a failed dream in which all one sees is repetition of trauma and evidence of a fragmented self-state. This understanding should focus the therapist on the patient and his state rather than on the possible symbolic meaning of the dream. In effect, the manifest dream is the meaning. If therapy progresses one will find evidence, often in the dreams, of a gradual integration of the traumatic experience and therefore of the self of the patient. Past and present (traumatic) will appear in the dreams. Wilmer, in his report, gives several examples of such an evolution of the nightmares of one of his patients, which seemed to develop as the patient talked about his nightmares and the experiences in Vietnam that they portrayed.

We are suggesting an approach to patients with TWN rather than a specific treatment program. We believe that understanding the condition within the framework we have presented gives a firm theoretical base to this approach. Furthermore, it seems to provide an understanding of what has worked for authors who did not have this theoretical framework but who nonetheless were able to provide the kind of treatment that led to resolution of the traumatic neurosis and nightmares. If one deals with these patients as people who have suffered severe narcissistic injuries because of the loss of sustaining self-objects, either mirroring as in a buddy or idealizing as in a failure of leadership, one can provide a treatment setting in which repair can occur.

ACKNOWLEDGMENT

The authors wish to acknowledge Bessel van der Kolk, MD, for his collaboration in the preparation of this paper.

REFERENCES

Ablon, S., Mack, J. (1980). Children's dreams reconsidered. *The Psychoanalytic Study of the Child* 35: 179-217.

Blos, P. (1979). *The Adolescent Passage.* New York: International Universities Press.

Breger, L. (1967). Function of dreams. *Journal of Abnormal Psychology: Monograph* 72(5) (Part 2): 1-28.

Breger, L., Hunter, I., Lane, R. (1971). *The Effect of Stress on Dreams.* Psychological Issues Monograph, no. 27. New York: International Universities Press.

Brown, W. (1920). The revival of emotional memories and its therapeutic value (I). *British Journal of Psychology* 1: 16-33.

Cartwright, R. (1979). The nature and function of repetitive dreams: a survey and speculation. *Psychiatry* 42: 131-137.

Diagnostic and Statistical Manual of Mental Disorders (DSM III) (3rd ed.). (1980). Washington, DC: American Psychiatric Association.

Fairbairn, W. R. D. (1952). The war neuroses: their nature and significance. *Psychoanalytic Studies of the Personality.* Boston: Rutledge, Kegan, and Paul, Ltd.

Fisher, C., Byrne, J., Edwards, A., Kahn, E. (1970). The nightmare: REM and NREM nightmares. *International Psychiatry Clinics* 7(2): 183-187.

Fox, D. (1974). Narcissistic rage and the problem of combat aggression. *Archives of General Psychiatry* 31: 807-811.

Freud, S. (1900). The interpretation of dreams. *S.E.* 4-5.

Freud, S. (1914). On narcissism: an introduction. *S.E.* 14.

Freud, S. (1920). Beyond the pleasure principle. *S.E.* 18.

Freud, S. (1926). Inhibitions, symptoms, and anxiety. *S.E.* 20.

Greenberg, R. (1980). Is there a good dream? What does it mean? Presented at the 20th Annual Meeting of the Association for the Psychophysiological Study of Sleep, Mexico City.

Greenberg, R., Pearlman, C. (1975a). A psychoanalytic-dream continuum: the source and function of dreams. *The International Review of Psycho-Analysis* 2(Part 4): 441-448.

Greenberg, R., Pearlman, C. (1975b). REM sleep and the analytic process: a psychophysiologic bridge. *The Psychoanalytic Quarterly* 44(3): 392-403.

Greenberg, R, Pearlman, C. (1981). The private language of the dream. In J. Natterson (ed.). *The Dream in Clinical Practice.* New York: J. Aronson.

Greenberg, R., Pearlman, C., Fingar, R., Kantrowitz, J., Kawliche, S. (1970). The effects of dream deprivation: implications for a theory of the psychological function of dreaming. *British Journal of Medical Psychology* 43: 1-11.

Greenberg, R., Pearlman, C., Gampel, D. (1972). War neuroses and the adaptive function of REM sleep. *British Journal of Medical Psychology* 45: 27–33.
Greenberg, R., Pillard, R., Pearlman, C. (1972). The effect of dream (stage REM) deprivation on adaptation to stress. *Psychosomatic Medicine* 34(3): 257–262.
Haley, S. (1974). When the patient reports atrocities. *Archives of General Psychiatry* 30: 191–196.
Hartmann, E., Russ, D., van der Kolk, B., Falke, R., Oldfield, M. (1981). A preliminary study of the personality of the nightmare sufferer: relationship to schizophrenia and creativity? *American Journal of Psychiatry* 138(6): 794–797.
Joffe, W. G., Sandler, J. (1968). Comments on the psychoanalytic psychology of adaptation. *International Journal of Psycho-Analysis* 49: 445–454.
Jones, E. (1931). *On the Nightmare*. London: Hogarth Press Ltd.
Kahn, E., Fisher, C., Edwards, A., Davis, D. (1972). Psychophysiology of night terrors and nightmares. *Proceedings of the 80th Annual Convention, American Psychological Association* (Summary). 7: 407–408.
Kardiner, A. (1959). Traumatic neuroses of war. In S. Arieti (ed.). *American Handbook of Psychiatry*. New York: Basic Books.
Kohut, H. (1971). *The Analysis of the Self*. New York: International Universities Press.
Kohut, H. (1977). *The Restoration of the Self*. New York: International Universities Press.
Kohut, H., Wolf, E. (1978). The disorders of the self and their treatment: An outline. *The International Journal of Psycho-analysis* 59(4): 413–425.
Kolb, L. (1982). Psychoanalysis and conflict: return of the repressed in delayed stress reaction to war. Presented at the American Academy of Psychoanalysis, Toronto.
Lidz, T. (1946). Nightmares and the combat neuroses. *Psychiatry* 9: 37–49.
Mack, J. (1965). Nightmares, conflict, and ego development in childhood. *The International Journal of Psycho-Analysis* 46(4): 403–428.
Mack, J. (1974). *Nightmares and Human Conflict*. Boston: Houghton Mifflin.
Maskin, M. (1971). Psychodynamic aspects of the war neuroses: a survey of the literature. *Psychiatry* 4(1): 97–115.
Moses, R. (1978). Adult psychic trauma: the question of early predisposition and some detailed mechanisms. *International Journal of Psycho-analysis* 59: 353–363.
Pearlman, C. (1982). Sleep structure variation and performance. In W. Webb (ed.). *Biologic Rhythms, Sleep and Performance*. New York: John Wiley and Sons.
Rado, S. (1942). Pathodynamics and treatment of traumatic war neurosis (Traumatophobia). *Psychosomatic Medicine* IV(4): 362–368.
Schlossberg, A., Benjamin, M. (1978). Sleep patterns in three acute combat fatigue cases. *Journal of Clinical Psychiatry* 39:546–548.
Turpin, E. (1976). Correlates of ego-level and agency-communion in stage REM dreams of 11–13 year old children. *Journal of Child Psychology and Psychiatry* 17: 169–180.
van der Kolk, B. (1982). Adolescent vulnerability to post traumatic stress. Presented at the 135th Annual Meeting of the American Psychiatric Association, Toronto.

van der Kolk, B., Blitz, R., Burr, W., Sherry, S., Hartmann, E. (1982). Clinical characteristics of traumatic and lifelong nightmare sufferers. Presented at the 135th Annual Meeting of the American Psychiatric Association, Toronto.

Webb, W., Cartwright, R. (1978). Sleep and dreams. *Annual Review of Psychology* 29: 223-252.

Weinberg, S. K. (1946). The combat neuroses. *American Journal of Sociology* 51: 465-478.

Wilmer, H. (1982). Vietnam and madness: dreams of schizophrenic veterans. *Journal of The American Academy of Psychoanalysis* 10(1): 47-64.

6
Brief Psychotherapy
of the Vietnam Combat Neuroses

JOHN A. MCKINNON, M.D.

Much has been written about the peculiarities of the lost, excruciating American war in Southeast Asia (Bourne, 1970; Lifton, 1973; Haley, 1974; Goodwin, 1980; Blank, 1981), about the psychological sequelae of combat (Swank, 1949; Futterman and Pumpian-Mindlin, 1951; Archibald and Tuddenham, 1965; Horowitz, 1975; Howard, 1975; Defazio, 1978; Kormos, 1978; Shatan, 1978, Wilson, 1980) and of other, nonmilitary trauma (Visotsky, Hamburg et al, 1961; Eitinger, 1964; Des Pres, 1976; Niederland, 1968, 1981). There are clear accounts of crisis-intervention techniques behind the battle lines (Grinker and Spiegel, 1945; Glass, 1947, 1954; Pettera, Johnson and Zimmer, 1969; Colbach and Parrish, 1970; Jones and Johnson, 1975). And there is now an established literature on brief psychotherapy. This chapter, while not an exhaustive review of all these issues, brings together relevant aspects of the literature and adds clinical case material with the aim of making coherent sense of a brief therapeutic approach to selected symptomatic combat veterans.

In the 20th century literature there has been no single "war neurosis" syndrome. Leaving aside frankly psychotic decompensations and enduring personality flaws, which combat may aggravate but does not cause, there remain two broad distinctive categories:

"war neurosis" (Ferenczi, 1921) and "posttraumatic stress disorder" (DSM III). The first, which preoccupied Freud and his colleagues (Freud et al, 1921), was made manifest in gross motor symptoms: paralysis, tremor, or spectacular disruptions of gait. These functional symptoms were understood (Ferenczi, 1921; Freud, 1919, 1920a, 1920b, 1922) to result from a rigidly effective repression that banished from awareness a soldier's quite sane, but nonheroic motives as well as memory of the precipitating trauma. The onset of symptoms tended to coincide, more or less, with the traumatic event.

The second syndrome (posttraumatic stress disorder) has been the preoccupation of psychiatrists writing of emotional casualties since World War II. Its more diffuse dysfunction is captured by terms such as *battle fatigue.* Descriptions list a welter of symptoms and signs, including disturbances of sleep and dreaming, mood, arousal, cognition, motivation, motor and autonomic functioning (Swank, 1949). In one early conceptualization (Grinker and Spiegel, 1945), it appeared to be a reactive disorder of the autonomic nervous system: "excessive or deficient sympathetic activity." More recently, Horowitz (1974, 1976) has provided a coherent, synthetic, psychoanalytic conceptualization of a "general stress response," a reactive syndrome common both to military and nonmilitary experiences of stress.

One exemplar of this stress response is uncomplicated grief, the normal reaction to object loss (Parkes, 1970). Bereavement normally sets into motion a biphasic, pendular, working through whose extremes are: (1) an experience of dulled forgetting (my term)—an emotional numbing associated with avoidance of conscious memories or thoughts to do with the traumatic event, alternating with (2) an experience of intrusive remembering (again, my term) a distracting assault of images, ideas and dysphoric affects often accompanied by rivetting anxiety. Various latent self-images are reactivated in disturbing juxtaposition with previously stable and ego-syntonic self-images and role relationships (Horowitz, Wilner et al, 1980), and in this active process the event and its implications become assimilated; enduring concepts of self and the world accommodate to the painful new facts of life.

A completion is reached, marked on the one hand by an abatement of anxiety and affective arousal in reaction to any memory of loss, and on the other, by an end to the reflexive warding-away of memory and emotion. The pendulum comes to rest. The person finished with grieving is no longer bombarded by images of his lost love at the chance reminder of a song or an empty chair. And yet he can remember what he's lost when he wants to; he finds himself again open to his feelings and to new attachments. No longer does he readily experience himself in regressive, unexpected and unwanted ways, eg, as abandoned and helplessly longing, as shamefully defective, or as guiltily at fault.

As in the case of grief (Freud, 1917), the pathology of the general stress response is not in its occurrence, but in its paralysis, its breakdown, and failure to reach a timely completion. A rigidly reflexive clamping-down upon remembering may render indecisive the intrusive reiterations of the stress response, prolonging its pointless oscillations like a needle stuck in the groove of a scratched record: the *chronic* stress response syndrome. Or else the dread of memory may remain so imperative as to prevent remembering from occurring at all for weeks, months or even decades. A constricted, phobically avoidant, or simply a relatively numb hiatus of 'forgetting' may persist. Much later, however, this muddy stagnant pond may be eruptively disturbed by the surfacing leviathan: the *delayed* stress response syndrome.

Those able on their own to put Vietnam combat stress behind them have presumably done so. They have reached their own completion. Vietnam veterans presenting now with stress response symptoms are suffering chronic or delayed variants of the syndrome.

Whether or not a particular combat experience is traumatic, ie, whether or not it provokes symptoms, must depend in part upon prior experience and character structure, ego-strength, and defensive style. Through no fault of their own, men differ in what we may call resilience. The same event turns out to be more traumatic, less readily assimilable, for one man than another. And this is true whether the response is nil, or a normal self-limited recovery, or one of the pathological forms. But equally beyond doubt, now, the enormity of the bolus of trauma has much to do with a person's capacity to digest it and go on. Some experiences (eg, Nazi concentration camp imprisonment) (Eitinger, 1964) prove impossible for anyone to swallow and remain stuck in the throat, an enduring discontinuity for a lifetime. As was said after the experience of World War II, "Everyone has his breaking point" (Grinker and Spiegel, 1945).

Both the classic war neuroses and the general stress response are symptomatic reactions to trauma. Despite the surface disparity between them, they share fundamental elements which have a crucial bearing upon the task of treatment. The traumatized patient is "suffering from reminiscences" (Breuer and Freud, 1893-95). He is shackled ("fixated") to a past which "alienates [him] from both present and future" (Freud, 1922). Underlying both syndromes is a motivated struggle between an urgent wish to forget and a persistent, implacable "compulsion to repeat" in the interest of mastery (Freud, 1920b). This compulsion is manifest in a central, shared symptom, the repetitive nightmare, which "astonished" Freud and compelled him to postulate this insistent drive toward mastery. It is, he said, an urge distinct from ("more primitive, more elementary, more instinctual" and "beyond") the pleasure principle, "which it overrides."

But these two posttraumatic syndromes also are different. A paralyzed limb does not reduce to an anxiety attack. A central distinction seems to lie in the enduring, repressive obliteration of both the traumatic event and its etiologic connection with the motor symptoms of war neurosis. Repression seems the prerequisite to a symbolically elaborated, derivative "reminiscence" in the guise of conversion symptoms (Ferenczi, 1921). A combat veteran with stress response symptoms also contends with repression, but does not have a global amnesia. Rather, his memory of the most painful events may be punctured with holes, details he has forgotten or implications he has ignored or misconstrued. These are crucial to reconstruct in therapy, because they usually dredge up in train those dreaded, repressed self-images (and associated experiences of shame, guilt, rage, fear or grief) which are the basis for the indecisive sticking of the integrative process.

It may be supposed that the interpretation of a war neurosis symptom (eg, a paralyzed limb) and the recovery of banished memory and repressed motivation would leave such a patient subsequently in the throes of a stress response syndrome. For having remembered, he remains (like the stress response patient) with the equivalent task of repeating the traumatic event in thought, word and feeling until he has worked through to completion. For this reason, and because dissociative, conversion symptoms are apparently relatively rare sequelae of Vietnam combat (Blank, 1980), the discussion of treatment that follows is centered upon the combat stress response syndromes.

THE THERAPEUTIC TASK

The task in the treatment of either syndrome is difficult, but simply stated. It is to free the hampered pendular swings of the normal stress response, to foster a measured associative remembering, and to reach a point of completion. I rush to add that this task does not reduce to a cathartic lancing of an emotional 'boil.'

Case A

A 37-year-old single Marine veteran was the only son of a stern, laconic ex-Marine, who held "inspections" once the patient's chores were completed and "always failed me at least once." His religious mother raised him in her faith. He did well enough in school, was an athlete if not a scholar, and he enjoyed many friends. His idols included the martyred President, who shared his faith and sense of duty, the Marines of World War II, and John Wayne. Shortly after John Kennedy's assassination he enlisted in the Marine Corps. His parents proudly attended his graduation from boot camp. He went directly to Vietnam in 1965, and saw much action. When he returned from his first tour he was disappointed not to be able to talk with his father, who "never asked me about Vietnam," for he was sick at heart at what he had seen and done. But his father had never talked about his own combat experience, and seemed not interested to hear about the patient's. He reenlisted and volunteered for a second tour, which he completed in 1968.

When he returned again and was posted to a stateside camp he "decked" a noncommissioned officer who ordered him to police a sidewalk; he was quickly discharged. Shortly afterwards he had an argument at home in which he pulled a combat knife on his parents, who then called the police. He fled, not to return until the time of his father's final deterioration and coma in a Veterans Administration hospital. He could not bring himself to attend the funeral. He drifted from one job to another over the next decade, losing one after another after altercations with the boss over matters of discipline. Afraid of crowds he avoided subways and sat in restaurants with his back to a wall. He jumped if approached from behind. He found himself looking for people breaking a rule (eg, smoking in a theatre where it was not permitted), and would tell them either to "stop or come outside." He worked as a guard in a store, filled with fantasies of some criminal trying to rob it "so that I could blow him away!" He was soon fired; the manager found him "too intense."

He presented to an Outreach Center, joined a rap group, but became disgusted when the others refused to discuss 'guilt.' He came to the VA outpatient clinic worried sick about his recent violence, his nightmares, and his compulsive confrontations with law-breakers. He thought his behavior was "crazy." He had a loaded pistol at home, and he had contemplated suicide, although he did not think he was in acute danger.

During his first interview he became visibly agitated when speaking about his father, about his mother's recent illness, about his jobs and his bosses, but most particularly when speaking about combat in Vietnam. He broke down and cried bitter tears about the mayhem. "I thought we were there to save those people from communism," he said angrily, "but in the first village we came to guys just started killing everybody who ran out. We were running down women and old men and emptying clips into them! It was so *wrong!*" But the worst of it was, he confessed, he soon came to like the killing. Admitting to this, he became visibly pale and agitated.

When he missed his next appointment, I called him. He told me he was "overwhelmed," that he was "tired of crying," and that he could not come back in now. A letter brought a reply in which he wrote of "surfing alone" on a stormy beach when young. He had been "overwhelmed by a wave," and had almost drowned. He ended: "I want to talk with you again, because I think you might help me, but I just can't talk now about anything!" I believe he has left the city, as he proposed he might do. I hope this is all. I have written, but have received no further communication. His telephone has been disconnected.

This case serves to make vivid a therapeutic failure. As Blank (1975) has pointed out, missing the opportunity to help a panicky combat vet get a grip on himself (in whatever way necessary) may be an opportunity lost for good. This was not a man who needed a catharsis, and to let him become overwhelmed was insufficiently cautious (assuming this could have been avoided). Those reassuring efforts I made to shift the subject, to help him intellectualize, to discuss the options of medication and hospitalization and the steps we could take to unload his gun and rid him of it, were insufficient to this fundamental task: to manage his anxiety.

For the management of anxiety is the fundamental problem here, as it is, perhaps, in any therapy. With combat veterans, whose inhibitions in the field of violent action have been deliberately undermined in military training and whose visions of their own capacity for mayhem are anything but fantasies, the treatment is neither "anxiety-provoking," solely, nor solely "anxiety-suppressing" (these terms are from Sifneos' excellent papers, eg, 1967; see Horowitz, 1973, 1974, 1976, and 1979), but rather each in its proper season. As in dermatology: "If it's wet, you *dry* it, and if it's dry, you *wet* it." Patients who present or become numb and avoidant will need prodding to come back to "remembering," so that they can work through their experience. But it is best to presume (particularly when the vet is a relative stranger) that his defensive perimeter is mined with potentially explosive anxiety and dysphoric affect.

BRIEF PSYCHOTHERAPY

Not wanting to be left sounding like Marie Antoinette, some modern psychoanalysts (eg, Malan, 1963, 1976; Balint et al, 1972; Sifneos, 1967, 1972; Wolberg, 1965; Mann, 1969, 1973; Horowitz, 1976; Davanloo, 1978) have studied the cake of "full" psychoanalysis to discover what, if anything, could be sacrificed as frosting and what shorter recipe or quicker yeast might bake a less costly, and yet wholesome, loaf. Brief psychotherapy turns out to be anything but a new idea, and has roots in the work of Freud, Ferenczi, Rank and Alexander (for a review of this history, see Straker, 1977; Marmor, 1979). But those papers directed toward the treatment of Vietnam vets tend to emphasize problems in proper diagnosis (eg, Van Putten and Emory, 1973; Blank, 1975; DeFazio, 1978), or peculiarities of the war and its combat (eg, Goodwin, 1980), or barriers to empathy and other countertransference problems (eg, Egendorf, 1970; Haley, 1974, 1978; DeFazio, 1978). There is little specific guidance and there are few case reports specifically to do with brief treatment of Vietnam combat veterans. This is to say, the direct relevance of suggestions and admonitions offered in the mainstream of brief treatment writings cannot be taken for granted.

With this cautionary note, the following discussions of patient selection and technique are offered, supplemented with suggestions from my own experience, from which I will present (disguised) case material.

PATIENT SELECTION

The point in selection is to discover whether the patient has the capacity for doing the work of psychotherapy. This being so, the criteria offered for the selection of candidates for brief treatment have tended to coincide with criteria for classic psychoanalytic therapy (Marmor, 1979). "The critical issue," Marmor writes, "is not diagnosis so much as the possession of certain personality attributes, plus the existence of a focal conflict and a high degree of motivation." These "personality attributes" or evidence for them, include: (1) ego strength; (2) at least one meaningful, ie, trusting, relationship in the past; (3) a capacity to interact with the therapist in a constructive way, ie, some hint of a potential positive transference; (4) the capacity to think psychologically, as manifest in responsiveness to test clarifications, confrontations, or interpretations; and (5) the ability to experience feelings.

It must be remembered, however, that "the ability to experience feelings" may be dulled by the very pathology in question. Moreover, a cross-section of combat veterans includes many who are neither well-educated nor naturally glib about their own psychology. This being so, and taking into account a broad (VA) responsibility for veterans, whose lack of psychological-mindedness did not preserve them from posttraumatic symptoms, and in the absence of clear-cut empirical evidence to exclude them a priori, we have tended to err on the liberal side in patient selection. Some veterans can learn to work in psychotherapy, even if they do not appear apt, while of course others cannot. No doubt our unwillingness to take these criteria too narrowly to heart has had much to do with periodic treatment disappointments, but on the other hand, significant improvement sometimes crowns an improbable beginning.

These criteria should have some give to them, from our point of view. But we have to assess with considerable care the two other traditional selection criteria: (6) motivation for change; and (7) the presence of an identifiable focus.

Motivation can be tricky to assess. Explicit enthusiasm for treatment and impatience with symptomatology are hopeful signs, as is a significant degree of obvious pain, frustration with disruptions of work, interpersonal and sexual relations, and an absence of ulterior motives. To the extent that motivation for change comes from external sources, eg, from wives, bosses, courts, and friends, the prognosis must be to that extent guarded. Pending claims for service-connected disability compensation must be carefully evaluated. Frequently claims are filed simultaneously with presentation for treatment for the simple reason that troubled visits to Vietnam Vets Outreach store-fronts may result in a filed claim and a referral for treatment. A pending claim is not, in itself, a barrier to treatment. But the disability evaluation and the treatment must be kept separate. For no one can be expected to be entirely frank if he thinks it is going to cost him money. I make it quite clear I am willing to give my opinion as to diagnosis, but equally clear that I am unwilling to participate in a charade of unwanted "treatment."

A *focal* problem is a critical criterion for brief treatment. Naturally, if a major combat trauma is discovered to be at the heart of a patient's pain, this trauma will constitute one aspect of the focus. And if posttraumatic stress disorder, or combat neurosis, is the correct formulation, then such a historical focus will be present. In addition, however, the formulation of focus needs to include a grasp of the meaning of the trauma, the conflictual issue which makes of his experience a tar-baby. This need not be a search for pre-war pathology by any means; rather, this aspect of the focus constitutes a recognition that events, particularly traumatic ones, have very personal meanings.

THE WORK-UP FOR A BRIEF THERAPY

The evaluative stage should be brief, if a brief treatment is contemplated. For an extended, leisurely work-up is not only out of proportion, but tends to subvert the enterprise with an implicit promise of timelessness. On the other hand, there is no excuse for an inadequate history, nor for failing to reach a specific dynamic formulation. I use a "two session rule" of thumb and force myself to come to written terms with an inevitably elliptical set of facts. I divide this evaluation from the treatment with an explanation of my findings, a proposal for treatment, if indicated, and an explanation of what I will expect from him and what he can expect from me. We agree to a time limit, if I choose to set one, and discuss and agree upon a focus. I explain my expectation that he will say out loud whatever comes to his mind, tell him why, and answer any questions which seem straightforward. Then I propose we "start now."

Brevity in evaluation conveys the correct implicit message:"We do *not* have forever! But it makes exhaustive exploration impossible, occasionally leads to selection errors, and occasionally leaves spectacular gaps in the history, as Case B demonstrates.

Case B

A 31-year-old ex-Marine, still single, educated part-way through high-school, a caucasian from an Italian, Catholic, Pittsburgh family, presented first in 1980 referred from a surgical clinic, where he was followed for residual pain and disability from combat gunshot wounds to his left hip, right knee and left chest. A bullet near his heart and spine had been left as a "sleeping dog," better undisturbed.

When first referred he complained entirely about knee and hip pain, which interfered with his sexual relations with his girlfriend, who was in apparent consequence on the point of leaving him. He had no prior psychiatric history. In the course of a triage interview he became convinced his problems were nonpsychiatric and that the surgeons had been trying to get rid of him because of his repeated requests for help with his pain. He refused further interviews.

Some months later he presented again, and I did the evaluation. Seven months before he had been injured in a motorcycle accident, which had exacerbated his pain. The surgeons prescribed analgesics. But a month before his encounter with our triage worker, he had been fired from a plumbing apprenticeship because (1) his pain medications had interfered with his concentration: he had flunked a key exam; and (2) when they learned additionally about his disability and pain, which made the medications necessary, the school authorities had decided he was unfit to be a plumber in the first place. He had been "terminated" from the program. When he went back to his surgeons, he felt they wished not to be involved. A school physician who had been required to examine him said he was physically unfit for such strenuous work. Angrily, he was busy filing grievances with various agencies; he contemplated a lawsuit, and found himself imagining violent revenge.

What brought him this time to the Mental Hygiene Clinic, however, was a resurgence of his combat nightmares; in his dreams he was variously getting "overrun" or was trapped in a bunker, likely to be blown up by a tossed grenade. He awoke from these dreams in a disheveled bed soaked with his sweat to the mattress. He slept with a shotgun in bed, near to his hand, as he had in the field in Vietnam; and he lay awake for hours afterward filled with dreadful fantasies of someone coming in through the door or window. If he slept at all, he woke at the slightest sound. There were no daytime flashbacks, no intrusive images of combat, but he was "going crazy" with fantasies of killing the training program foreman, who "wouldn't give me a chance." The school authorities seemed like "Germans," who "just took orders," and who deserved, he thought at moments, to be killed. These fantasies and the rage that went with them, preoccupied him, made him oddly "aloof" from his girlfriend, whom he cared about abstractly but did not live with nor contemplate marrying. She complained about the disruption of their sexual life which his pain caused; he was simply unwilling to move with his former enthusiasm. There was no mechanical disfunction.

He was the second of seven children; his sisters and brothers were married with children of their own and lived near his family's home in Pittsburgh. His father was a firm, stoic, intelligent and hardworking steelworker, a man without significant vices. His mother was "angelic," an overworked, gentle and warm housewife who was "probably in the kitchen right now!" His aunts and uncles lived close by and occupied positions in the police and fire departments or in building trades. In school he had been bright, but an average performer, with many friends. He played football on the high school team, drank beer out of the trunks of friends' cars, liked loud parties, and got into minor truancy difficulties with the nuns. He had had a longtime sweetheart, a girl whose family was closely tied to his own, and he imagined readily that "except for the war" he would have settled into a "box house" with her, and by now "we'd have four kids and I'd work at the mill." This did not happen.

Instead, after a minor disciplinary action at school, he left home in his senior year to enlist in the US Marine Corps. It was 1966; he was filled with patriotic fervor, wanting to be "John Wayne." His friends admired the uniform; his girl promised to wait for him, and he went off to bootcamp, where he did well. He volunteered for Vietnam, where he imagined "we had a job that had to be done." In 1967 he was sent to I Corps near the DMZ, assigned to a Combined Action Platoon in support of local militia, and for months moved along Highway 1 from one village to another. Each night two patrols went "out" and one remained "back" in the village in reserve. They set up ambushes, waited to spring them, and saw much action.

But, by late 1967, they had become disillusioned in various ways. Moreover, they were vastly outnumbered at night by enemy troops moving south in preparation for what would be the TET offensive. Sometimes they would go out at night to "hide," which meant to set up other than in the place to which their officer had pointed on the map. On such a night his patrol set up at the fork in a road, and their position was literally stumbled over by a much larger unit of enemy soldiers. One soldier "walked right into my hole!" In the ensuing firefight which lasted only seconds, he was wounded, three of his patrol were killed, and a number of NVA corpses were strewn around in the dark. When the "back" patrol came out of the village to support them, it was ambushed and badly mauled. Artillary flares, which were supposed to light up the paddies where the enemy had taken cover, went awry; instead they "lit us up like Yankee Stadium." There was a delay getting help by Med-evac helicopter, enough time for the medic to crawl over under fire to examine him and tell him, "they both are still there!" He was covered with his own blood and that of a "hole-buddy" who had been killed; it felt like "someone had thrown mud on me." The Huey arrived, and he was rushed over open ground on a poncho "like a turd on a blanket" and "popped" into the helicopter, which already was lifting away.

He was evacuated to a hospital for immediate surgery, got probed for bullets and bandaged, and soon was back in the United States, where he endured five more surgical procedures over the next year.

Hundreds of other men were there as well, many of them screaming
in pain and dying. His family visited frequently, but his girlfriend
never did. "I think she heard my nuts had been shot off," he suggested. He denied feeling angry about this, and rather only a "kind
of numb sad feeling." When fit a year later he was assigned to a
"nothing unit" in the US and then discharged. He ended up in
California, worked on a ranch and "sort of drifted" after a fall
from a horse brought a resurgence of his pain and made riding
impossible. He came to San Francisco to take a plumbing apprenticeship a year prior to his presentation for treatment. At the time of
his "termination" from the apprenticeship he had done much of
a year's work in good standing, except for flunking the final written
exam.

   He was a cleanshaven, tidy, good-looking Latinate young man
with a sense of humor apparent in cynical cracks about "bureau-
crats" and "idiots" in the military and in the VA, and he had a
ready, friendly smile. He limped slightly, sat trying not to move his
hips, occasionally slapped at his wounded knee, but otherwise did
not make his pain obvious. He wore informal levis and cowboy
boots. He was courteous enough with me, called me "Doctor" and
later "John," and evidenced no hostility, even when he was enraged
about the "idiot doctor" at the school, who had suggested he was
too disabled to do plumbing. He spoke of his wounding readily, but
with a detachment that left little room for anguish or anxiety; there
was a lingering wish to justify his behavior there as part of his duty,
but no other evidence of guilt. There were few complaints about his
wounds, and virtually all his conscious anger was directed at the program authorities who had fired him from his apprenticeship. He felt
no grief about his wounded and killed acquaintances in the platoon,
for many of them had been "new guys" whose names he could no
longer remember. The notion that he might feel guilt over surviving
struck him as "interesting," but aroused no feeling. There was no
hint of psychosis, nor of paranoia, nor was he suicidal, then or in
the past. But he was much troubled by his homicidal fantasies, although not worried about acting upon them. They were "making me
crazy," he complained, riling him up and intruding upon his concentration on anything else.

   I was not to know of this history's gaping hole until some weeks
later, when the work of reiterating the details of his post-Vietnam
adjustment provoked a full-blown, anxious "remembering."

TECHNICAL CONSIDERATIONS

Making it Brief

Freud seems to have been the first to set an explicit termination date to move a stalled analysis, but Mann (1969, 1973) has elegantly made the general case for a deadline in brief treatment, which makes separation the central issue. I doubt it makes a difference just how many sessions are planned, although various authorities have preferences. No doubt it makes good sense to set such a deadline from the outset in treating patients for whom the focal issue is separation; certainly this is often true of combat veterans.

But it may not always make sense. An arbitrary number of sessions may be just that, ie, arbitrary, and bear no relation to either an earlier or a later, more natural ending point. Any long treatment, however indeterminate at the outset, will be punctuated by "commas," which are marked by a tentative, if partial, resolution of some issue which has preoccupied a period of the work and by latent talk of termination. Such commas may be turned into "periods" by a skillful therapist. But such a flexible approach requires the therapist to be alert for the proper ending; he must himself be willing to let go. Setting an arbitrary number of sessions at the outset relieves the therapist from facing the imperfect result which is inevitable. Without this arbitrary limit, he must be ready to let the patient go "unfinished, sent before [his] time . . . scarce half made up." But on the other hand, predelimited therapies can, on occasion, drift on past a focal resolution and an end to symptoms.

Focus

"Everything is grist for the mill," so long as there are no constraints on time or energy to run the mill. As soon as there are, however, some matters must be made priorities (even if by default). Finding a focus and sticking to it constitute the most radical parameter in brief treatment, apart from the limitation upon time itself, and require what is termed "activity" on the therapist's part.

Symptoms that appear to result from combat imply a focus upon the combat experience itself. But invariably (and without implying the patient was "sick" before his experience) there will be one or more "core" conflictual issues which the trauma reactivates. This core conflict may be inferred from the precipitating event, from repetitions in the history, and from the veteran's experience of dysphoric affects around which reactivated "latent self-images and role relationships" tend to surface. Material in therapy hours can be viewed from the therapist's point of view, then, as moving toward or fleeing from these traumatic events and the core, latent conflicts which are "activated" in train. The therapist's tactics at any given stage must be determined by means of a reading of the patient's level of anxiety.

Case B (Continued) The formulation with which I began this treatment was a little vague. I was aware of his enduring rage at authoritative men who had let him down, and also of his disappointment about them. This was the red affective thread that ran through his conscious anger at the government, which had "used" him, at the training authorities who had "terminated" him, at the VA physicians who seemed to want to be rid of him, and hypothetically, at his father who at some point had let him down.

Second, there were the soldiers who had damaged him, almost "terminated" him; he had been hurt, sexually impaired and left in chronic pain. He had been made a "turd on a blanket," a man assigned to a "nothing" unit. And he does not entirely accept the medic's reassurance that "they're both still there."

Third, his high-school sweetheart abandoned him, married someone else, when (as he would have it) she heard his "balls had been shot off;" his present girlfriend was on the point of leaving him because (as he would have it) he was not sexually functional. It was my hypothesis that he had, accordingly, experienced his "outgunned" platoon's discovery and firefight and his severe injury in part as the echo of an oedipal (fantasied) defeat, which now had cost him both his "balls," and his woman. His ejection from the training program, too, was experienced as vindictive and cruel. The foreman was telling him he was not man enough to be a plumber. Instead of a father's kind help in his development, he got retaliation. He got pushed out.

Finally, somewhere in Vietnam or just afterward, "John Wayne" had been entirely lost. His adjustment since the war suggested no coherent, satisfying image of manhood to take the place of this ideal.

Of course there were other issues as well: his legalistic struggles over who had said what and which regulations had been traduced; his grief over those "who got it worse than I did," which made it difficult for him to complain about his own fate; his envy of real and figurative "siblings" who had got ahead of him while he had gone to war; and his concern and doubt about whether his violent participation had been, in the end, moral.

But I proposed we focus upon his "termination" from the plumbing training program and the murderous rage he thought out of proportion and "crazy." I told him I thought he had Vietnam "still up [his] craw," and that we would discover just what connection it had once we got to work. He agreed, seemed calmly interested in these ideas, and we began work which I suggested would take "about three months." As well as going over the details of his firing from the training program, I suggested he tell me again in detail about his experience in Vietnam and about his coming home.

The Barometer of Anxiety (I)

Keeping the surface and latent aspects of the focus in mind, the therapist must keep track of the patient's anxiety, helping him to flee for respite when he grows panicky, and firmly herding him back toward the loaded focal issue when he wanders too far. During respites a certain amount of "chatting" is permissible, but must be brought to an end when it has served its purpose; without active prodding, these flights can straggle aimlessly from the focus.

In this situation, something must be done to bring the patient back toward his anxiety-provoking focus. Sometimes this "something" happens to be an external, fortuitous event, some reminder (common predicate) of the traumatic experience. In the case of Patient B, the motorcycle accident and his flunking an exam and getting "terminated" were such triggers, and when he presented, he was already symptomatic. But there are active steps the therapist may take, including (1) pressing for additional historical detail, (2) interpretation of defensive avoidance, (3) suggesting the patient imagine the event in visual images, if he tends not to (Horowitz, 1973), or (4) shifting from a present event or affect to the past by means of a common thread connecting them. This technique can be illustrated with a vignette from another patient's treatment (Case C):

Patient: "I've just been numb, and I couldn't care less about anything. I just feel dead half the time. I should be in a bag."

Therapist: "That's how you described yourself when you walked out of Khe Sanh: 'In a bag.' Then you changed the subject."

Patient: (silence).

Therapist: "You look reminded of something."
Patient: "Yeah. I saw Eddie "in a bag" you know. His boots
were sticking out (crying now). I just looked at them, you know?
And I just felt nothing! I always feel bad about that. I mean, he
was with me through all that shit. And then when he got wasted,
I didn't feel anything. You know? . . ."

In Case B, I had imagined the patient's getting shot would turn
out to be the moment he dreaded to remember. But this was not the
case. It was the reiteration of his homecoming.

Case B (Continued) In the first few sessions we concentrated
upon (1) the details of his wounding, (2) his homecoming and recovery, (3) his family history, and (4) details of his training course in
plumbing and its "termination." There were external reminders, for
he was having to give formal affidavits in the course of his appeals.
Moreover, hostages were taken in Iran, and there was talk of reinstituting the draft, which aroused his angry protest. His nightmares
grew worse, his retreat from his girlfriend more complete, and he
grew more irritable with those around him. Then he became panicky,
and began to feel out of control.

The Barometer of Anxiety (II)

It is not tolerable anxiety, but panic, which requires action. No
productive work occurs when a patient is terrified, and the patient's
most rigid defenses are called into play. The risk of suicide increases,
as does the potential for violence, and of course (see Case A earlier)
there is the very real risk the patient may come to think his disease
preferable to the cure.

The aim of intervention is clear enough: it is to help the patient
defend himself, help him do what he naturally wants to do, ie, to
flee his memories. He needs to be helped to calm himself. Sometimes
simply a deft change of subject to more neutral material will suffice.
For example:

Patient: "If I had just moved quicker! (crying bitterly) I
could have got that little girl out of the way. If I had seen her!
Oh, god (starting to get up), I've got to go."
Therapist: "Why don't you stop now and go back a step.
Before you came to the road. Please sit down. I want to know
why you were going out on that patrol. What was its point?"

Patient (sitting down): "It was just routine. Nothing special about it, I don't think. We had day patrols and night patrols. I always preferred the day patrols, because at night you couldn't see a goddamned thing."

Therapist: "You were alert, but not expecting much of anything in particular."

Patient: "Right."

Therapist: "OK, go on."

The patient's characteristic defenses (eg, intellectualization, denial, phobic avoidance) may be encouraged until he is calm enough to go on. Explicit exhortation to stop thinking and talking about it now, or to calm down, can help. Horowitz (1973) suggests taking over ego functions from a patient who has been immobilized by anxiety (eg, planning how he'll manage problems, helping him test reality, helping him to reduce external stimulation and demands), and suggests providing a model of calm which the patient can use as a source of identification. When these means will not suffice (eg, Case A), medication may be indicated (Blank, 1975; Hogben and Cornfield, 1981). Some "activity" on the therapist's part is not only unavoidable, it is—in the interest of keeping properly to the focus and modulating anxiety within tolerable bounds—desirable.

Case B (Continued) Between session five and six the patient called, sounding unusually tense and desperate, and insisted he had to see me immediately. When he arrived, he looked stricken, out of breath, excited. Not sitting down, he unbuttoned his cuffs, rolled up his sleeves and showed me eight fresh needle tracks running up a prominent vien. "I'm doing it again!" he exclaimed. I told him to sit down and calm himself. Then he sat on the edge of his chair and told me in a rush he had "left out" part of his history because of shame and worry over what I would conclude. He had become addicted to morphine during his long stay in the military hospital; there "they use it like water," because so many men have so much pain. When he left the service and joined the "nothing unit" he had gone to street drugs, injecting himself, and when he returned home to Pittsburgh and moved in with his family, he kept his habit a secret. In the course of months, however, one of his brothers learned about his habit and blurted it out at the dinner table, from which his father rose, putting down his fork, and walked out. The next day after his father left for work, his mother presented him with an airline ticket and his father's ultimatum: he was to get out of Pittsburgh before sundown and not to come back until his addiction was cured. His mother took him to the airport, and he left for California, where he found a residential drug treatment program. He worked on a ranch and "rode horses." He successfully rid himself of opiates, became a member of the staff of the program, and stayed for some years.

Two weeks before this blurted confession he had taken money from a friend, who now had discovered the loss and asked him about it with friendly concern. The patient was filled with remorse and shame, reported that in the past 24 hours he had put his shotgun barrel into his mouth two or three times, and that he feared he might pull the trigger.

I suggested we take the steps we had to to protect him, get him calmed down so that he could think and put matters into perspective, and to this end, I immediately arranged a hospital bed, which he accepted gratefully. Mindful of his father's reaction, I added that this admission would put him nearer to my office and make it possible for us to work together more frequently. He would not have to go it alone. He looked visibly relieved, and arranged to have his friend remove his shotgun and not return it until he (the patient) and I agreed it was safe for him to have it again.

Working Through

The central task which active holding to a focus is solely intended to accomplish is the patient's reexperiencing and reconsidering his trauma, to which he has become "fixated." There may be some relief in catharsis, but working through involves a tracing of associations and an exploration of the implications of the event. This "remembering" should reveal echoes in the more remote past with which the traumatic experiences reverberates and demonstrates the "latent self-image(s)" around which the patient's present dysphoria emerges. The focus of treatment almost invariably becomes much more precise in the process.

In this case, the abrupt confession of his shameful habit and his suicidal panic reiterated for this man an experience of shameful revelation before his father. Just as the military discharged him once it had "used" and damaged him, his father turned his back upon his disgraced, defective son. His mother joined his father in banishing him from home, and he was left alone to fend for himself, to find his own cure. And of course such a revelation and rejection had occurred just before his beginning treatment, too, when he was fired from his training program after his failed exam revealed him to be a drug-taker with a disability, a man unworthy to continue. Although not clearly revealed in his treatment, the suspicion must remain that these adult oedipal repetitions echo in some fundamental way a childhood experience or fantasy.

Case B (Completed) During a five-week stay on the inpatient ward the patient visited my office twice a week on a regular schedule. I shared responsibility for his care with the ward staff and with a kind, calm resident, who also spent hours talking and planning with him. Reminders of war and combat injury, inevitable in a Veterans Hospital, stirred up his memories and aroused intense anxiety. The Iranian hostage crisis filled the news, and there was talk of reinstituting the draft. These external proddings kept him in the "remembering" phase, in large part, but his basic needs were met, his days structured, and he had other support from patients and staff. He went off opiates "cold turkey," had little trouble doing so, and may have taken comfort in his consequent suffering. But his nightmares disturbed his sleep, in fact made him afraid of going to bed, and sedation was carefully offered. He got help sorting out his VA benefits, including his eligibility for additional schooling. In brief, the full-blown "remembering" phase of his delayed combat stress response now expressed itself within the protected walls of the hospital. The psychotherapy remained "hot."

Part of this work involved increasingly explicit, joint attention to the level of his anxiety. Early in his hospitalization, a documentary of the war appeared on television, catching him by surprise with introductory filmclips of combat, including sounds of small arms fire, machine-gun bursts and mortars. He reported he tried to "turn away from it, just not to look and get the hell out of there," but not in time. His night filled with images of fighting, the memory of a rocket-attack upon a village, which left the village women and children torn apart and strewn, bleeding and screaming, and of course, the virtually accidental encounter which resulted in his wounds and enduring pain. A certain amount of this material was worked over simply as detailed remembering. That is, he told what happened, and in my explicit wish to know all about it, an initially impressionistic, florid description became detailed. For example, I wondered how it could be so that after months in the field with some of the men in his patrol, he could so completely have forgotten their names?

Patient: "I don't know exactly. Some were just 'fucking new guys,' and I avoided them. But there was this one guy, Jesus, what was his name? Frank? I think it was Frank something. He was the guy who got it in the guts when they opened up. See, after the first firing ended, there were three or four gooks lying on the road, and this guy, Frank or whoever, and some of the others, went out there to kick them over. Then some of the gooks in the paddy over the road opened up, and one guy got it in the knees, but Frank took a whole burst in the guts. It got his spine, you know, and . . . I was just thinking I did see him afterwards. It was in Japan, I think. I saw him up on one of those racks they put guys on who have paralysis, you know? Like a grilled chicken. Man, I hadn't thought of that for a while. Somebody, maybe a doctor or maybe an aide, went by my bed and said, 'That dude's Romeo days are over,' or something like that."

Therapist: "You mean he couldn't get it up."

Patient: "That's what I took it to mean. He might as well have got 'em shot off! I felt sort of lucky, I think."

Therapist: "Glad yours were still in working order."

Patient: (laughing) "Glad they were still THERE!"

Therapist: "No wonder you didn't want to remember his name!"

Patient: (somberly) "Yeah, I felt real bad about him."

Therapist: "Yeah, I understand, but glad it wasn't you."

Patient: "That sounds really shitty, but yeah. I'm glad it wasn't me."

In addition to this remembering out loud what he wanted to forget there were themes which emerged in various ways over and over again. For example, his "crazy-making" rage at the foreman who had fired him came under scrutiny. His strenuous efforts had been directed solely toward reinstatement. Little thought had been given to whether this made any sense.

Therapist: "Can we ignore whether the 'prick' foreman should have done what he did more politely, and whether the doctor obeyed the proper rules, or treated you with courtesy? I don't mean these aren't important. But can we set that aside for a minute?"

Patient: "I guess."

Therapist: "Because I wanted to ask you frankly whether it makes any sense for somebody who endures as much pain as you do to try to be a plumber? Or for that matter, to do any work that strenuous?"

Patient: "I was doing a good job, except for the test, doc, and they wouldn't even have known I was hurt, except for the exam, and because I then told 'em I was taking the codeine. They wouldn't have ever known!"

Therapist: "Sure, but you're avoiding my point. I don't doubt your courage, if that's what it is, or that you could do the work. I'm asking whether it makes sense for you to be training to do something that hurts you to do it! Standing up, carrying heavy pipe, hunkering down to do a seal—it *hurts*, right?"

Patient: (looking down, slapping at knee).

Therapist: "You'd just as soon not admit it. You'd rather I kept my big mouth shut about that?"

Patient: "Yeah, it hurts." (silence)

Therapist: "Something special about plumbing? Do you have to be a plumber?"

Patient: "Oh, I don't know. It's a guy's kind of job, and I like that about it. I like heavy work. And I like fixing things, you know, and cutting the joints and being real careful, specially with the inside work, 'cuz some of it's under pressure, and if you fuck up, you ruin the whole shebang."

Therapist: "You like that, having to be careful, because it's important."

Patient: "Yeah. Careful, and clean. It's good if you work clean."

Therapist: (joking) "You make it sound like surgery."

Patient: "That's funny you say that, because I was thinking that too. You know I told my father once, when I was little, that I was going to work in the mill with him, or else be a surgeon, like this doctor on tv.

Therapist: "You were trying to do both!"

Patient: "What?"

Therapist: "Plumbing. It's a man's job, like your dad's. But it's kind of like surgery, too, don't you think? You get to fix things like your orthopedist: cutting, sawing, making "joints."

When he left the hospital he enrolled in a training program in computer technology, having given up the notion of reinstatement. But this was only the practical matter of "getting back in." There was, of course, more to this wish for "reinstatement," and he accepted my suggestion that he wanted—even more than to get back to plumbing—to get back into his parents' good graces, to undo the war and his injury and his addiction and be restored to his old self, to be again a guy "sure to marry the girl and live in the box house with the kids and the cocker spaniel." Some of his rage and sense of injustice had to do, I said, with his conviction an "injustice" had been done.

After all, he had "done a good job for a year." He had earned something, he believed, and only an injustice could be keeping him from it. This helped him let go of plumbing, in the end, since it was not a substitute for the restitution he really wanted.

Subtly, the story he had told at the outset changed, at least in tone. A theme of forgiveness recurred. He expressed an empathy for the villains in his life, and his enmity and anger began to fade. It had turned out that the foreman and the physician in the training program had had a point, even if their method seemed disrespectful. The "gooks" began to be "young guys," who "probably just wanted a box house and a cocker spaniel and some kids, too." They became less flat, less abstract, less malevolent, and more human. He imagined himself in their place fighting off an invader, a thought which made him the more resentful of American leaders, who had sent him over to kill and had made him a "sucker." More important, however, was his remembering that his father's brother had died of an overdose of illicit drugs. This made his father's stern repudiation comprehensible, certainly, and after all, his father had sent him away in large part to force him to get help.

Our final sessions ended on a nostalgic note. He began to complain of the "wasted" years. He faced the prospect of his computer training with a quiet, optimistic determination. He would have little money to live on, but enough; much hard work, but the prospect of a trade sufficient to support a family, if he could find the right girl. He continued to have occasional nightmares, but did not fear sleep; he was less often bothered by them. Intrusive fantasies of violent revenge had stopped, although he never felt other than that he had been treated shabbily. He reported he felt "more like myself" and did not need to sleep with a gun. When he left the hospital we were near the three month period we had roughly set, and we had no difficulty agreeing to stop. I left the door open for a return someday, should he want to take up unfinished business, but he doubted he would do so (and has not).

I saw him once more, six months later. He was going over to see his orthopedic surgeons. He was not on analgesics and was sleeping without the gun. His nightmares had become rare, not much of a bother, and he was not angry.

Neither did he ask to begin therapy again. He had gotten back in touch with his family in Pittsburgh and hoped to be home for a visit at Christmas. He said he had "just stopped by to see you."

RECIPROCAL IMAGES OF MASCULINITY
IN THE FIELD OF VIOLENT ACTION

American soldiers in Vietnam usually entered service and fought during late adolescence, when appropriate developmental tasks involve the consolidation of identity and the establishment of a firm capacity for intimacy (Erikson, 1950). At 19, these young men were at the point of leaving home to find social and economic roles for themselves. Combat disrupted just these adjustments. Men presenting now in their mid-30s can often be preoccupied with moral issues more familiar in the mouths of college students fifteen years ago. Some of these veterans have become "stuck" around the tasks of the 20s; they complain of feeling "left behind," as indeed, some have been. For some, it is in just this sense that they have become "fixated" to a past that deprives them of the present and future.

War raises for a young man the masculine issue of decisive competence (versus restraint) in the field of violent action. John Wayne's name surfaces so regularly that I have been driven to consider what aspirations he embodied, what young men facing combat hoped to discover to be true about themselves? In summary, John Wayne suggests a strong, brave and moral man, who never "draws first," nor backs away from a fight; he invariably wins with decisive, violent action, which is always justified by the moral circumstances. He opposes bullies, defends women and children; he is a potent, kind lover and a loyal friend. Finally, he is rarely in doubt what right action constitutes; the bad guys always wear black hats (or pajamas).

This American ideal is worth considering. For identity consolidates around such identifications, or partial identifications; its coherence results in part from an active repudiation of other, despised part-identifications, other unwanted experiences of self. Traumatic events dredge up in train those repudiated, unwanted aspects of self (Horowitz et al, 1981).

If bereavement brings to the surface certain typical constellations of ideation and affect (eg, an ashamed sense of defectiveness) combat does, too. But it tends to reactivate concerns about a man's proper behavior in the field of violent action. The Vietnam war tended to dash young mens' hopes to discover themselves to be John Wayne, and raised deep questions about America's moral stance. Disappointment with self and with America constitutes a central theme: the discovery of the dark, repressed, underside of the

American ideal of heroic masculinity. In common with every other war ever fought, probably, the men who fight and return must struggle with a loss of innocence, doubt about their fellow men, and about themselves. Many troubled vets worry about sadism (Case A), about being bullies instead of moral white-hats; they may not have felt themselves or their country to be protectors of the family, but rather its destroyer, the killers of women and children; or else they felt themselves to have been saps, "losers" caught up helplessly, "used" and then discarded, impotent to protect themselves; they hate to feel like "suckers."

Thus, it may not be solely the traumatic particulars of combat which are precariously warded-off, but also their excruciating implications, which clash so confusingly, so bitterly, with a young man's ideals. In Case B it was not simply getting wounded, but being hurt and then rejected by his parents as "bad" and "defective;" he feared he had become a "turd on a blanket," a castrated "nothing." In Case A the patient was more preoccupied with the suicide-provoking knowledge that he could like killing people, that he was a sadistic criminal who deserved to be shot down like a mad dog. These issues are particularly moral in the way young men tend to be concerned with ethics; for they continue to struggle, and are fixated around these moral issues, unable to consolidate an identity out of ethical confusion in which their experience, and their coming home, left them. Many of these men had their identity consolidation derailed by their combat experience; they continue into their mid-30s trying to get back on track, to recover the momentum, the sense of themselves moving into a confident, proud future, which they feel they have lost.

OUTCOME

However long or brief, psychotherapy does not erase life's scars; it will not wipe out the memory of battle, traumatic injury or the spectacle of war's victims. These are not images a man ever entirely forgets. But it is also true that *without* therapy, the symptoms of an uncompleted stress response can last for decades and constrict a soldier's life. This fact makes a psychotherapeutic effort, however brief, well worthwhile.

REFERENCES

American Psychiatric Association. (1980). *Diagnostic and Statistical Manual of Mental Disorders* (DSM III). Third Edition.

Archibald, H. E., Tuddenham, R. D. (1965). Persistent Stress Reaction after Combat: A Twenty Year Follow-up. *Archives of General Psychiatry* 12: 475-481.

Balint, M., Ornstein, P. H., Balint, E. (1972). *Focal Psychotherapy*. Philadelphia: J. B. Lippincott Co.

Blank, A. S. (1975). A Guide to Evaluation and Treatment of Vietnam Returnee Patients. Unpublished.

Blank, A. S. (1980). The Unconscious Flashback to the War in Vietnam Veterans: Clinical Mystery, Legal Defense and Community Problem. Presented to the American Psychological Association, Montreal, September 1-5, 1980.

Blank, A. S. (1981). Stresses of War: The Example of Vietnam. In: *The Handbook of Stress*. L. Goldberger and S. Bresnitz (Ed.). New York: The Free Press, 1981.

Bourne, P. G. (1970a). Military Psychiatry and the Vietnam Experience. *American Journal of Psychiatry* 127(4): 481-487.

Bourne, P. G. (1970b). *Men, Stress and Vietnam*. Boston: Little Brown.

Breuer, S., Freud, S. (1893-95). *Studies in Hysteria*. S. E. Vol. 2.

Colbach, E. M., Parrish, M. D. (1970). Army Mental Health Activities in Vietnam: 1965-1970. *Bulletin of Menninger Clinic* 34(6): 333-342.

Davanloo, H. (1978). *Principles and Techniques in Short-Term Dynamic Psychotherapy*. New York: Spectrum.

Defazio, V. J. (1978). Dynamic Perspectives on the Nature and Effects of Combat Stress. In: Figley, C. R. (Ed.). *Stress Disorders Among Vietnam Veterans*. New York: Brunner/Mazel.

Des Pres, T. (1976). *The Survivor: An Anatomy of Life in the Death Camps*. New York: Oxford University Press.

Egendorf, A. (1978). Psychotherapy with Vietnam Veterans: Observations and Suggestions. In: Figley, C. R. (Ed.). *Stress Disorders Among Vietnam Veterans*. New York: Brunner/Mazel.

Eitinger, L. (1964). *Concentration Camp Survivors in Norway and Israel*. London: Allen and Urwin.

Erikson, E. H. (1950). *Childhood and Society*. New York: Norton.

Ferenczi, S. (1921). Two Types of War Neurosis. In: J. I. Suttie (Trans.). *Further Contribution to the Theory and Technique of Psychoanalysis*. New York: Basic Books.

Freud, S. (1917). Mourning and Melancholia. Standard Edition. J. Strachey (Ed.). *The Complete Psychological Work of Sigmund Freud*, Vol. 14. London: Hogarth Press.

Freud, S. (1919). Introduction to *Psychoanalysis and the War Neurosis*. S. E. Vol. 17.

Freud, S. (1920a). Memorandum on the Electrical Treatment of War Neurotics. S. E. Vol. 17.

Freud, S. (1920b). *Beyond the Pleasure Principle*. J. Strachey (Trans). New York: Bantam Books.

Freud, S. (1922). *Introductory Lectures on Psychoanalysis.* Joan Riviere (Trans). London: George Allan and Urwin.

Freud, S., Ferenczi, S., Abraham, K., Simmal, E., Jones, E. (1921). *Psychoanalysis and the War Neuroses.* New York and London: International Psychoanalytical Press.

Futterman, S., Pumpian—Mindlin, E. (1951). Traumatic War Neuroses Five Years Later. *American Journal of Psychiatry* III (12): 401–408.

Glass, A. J. (1947). Effectiveness of Forward Treatment. *Bulletin of US Army Medicine* 7: 1034–1041.

Glass, A. J. (1954). Psychotherapy in the Combat Zone. *American Journal of Psychiatry* 110: 725–731.

Goodwin, J. (1980). The Etiology of Combat-Related Post-Traumatic Stress Disorders. In: T. Williams (Ed.). *Post-Traumatic Stress Disorders of the Vietnam Veteran.* Cincinnati: Disabled American Veterans.

Grinker, R. R., Spiegel, J. P. (1945). *Men Under Stress.* Philadelphia: Blakiston.

Haley, S. A. (1974). When The Patient Reports Atrocities. *Archives of General Psychiatry* 30(2): 191–196.

Haley, S. A. (1978). Treatment Implications of Post-Combat Stress Response Syndromes for Mental Health Professionals. In: Charles R. Figley (Ed.). *Stress Disorders Among Vietnam Veterans.* New York: Brunner/Mazel.

Hogben, G. L., Cornfield, R. B. (1981). Treatment of Traumatic War Neurosis with Phenylzine. *Archives of General Psychiatry* 38(4): 440–445.

Horowitz, M. J. (1973). Phase Oriented Treatment of Stress Response Syndromes. *American Journal of Psychotherapy* 27: 506–515.

Horowitz, M. J. (1974). Stress Response Syndromes. *Archives of General Psychiatry* 31(12): 768–781.

Horowitz, M. J. (1975). A Prediction of Delayed Stress Response Syndromes in Vietnam Veterans. *Journal of Social Issues* 31(4): 67–81.

Horowitz, M. J. (1976). *Stress Response Syndrome.* New York: Jason Aronson.

Horowitz, M. J., Kaltreider, N. B. (1979). Brief Therapy of the Stress Response Syndrome. *Psychiatric Clinics of North America* (2): 365–377.

Horowitz, M. J., Wilner, N., Marmer, C., Krupnick, J. (1980). Pathological Grief and the Activation of Latent Self-Images. *American Journal of Psychiatry* 137(10): 1157–1162.

Howard, S. (1976). The Vietnam Warrior: His Experience, and Implications for Psychotherapy. *American Journal of Psychotherapy* 30(1): 121–135.

Malan, D. H. (1963). *A Study of Brief Psychotherapy.* Springfield, Illinois. Charles C. Thomas.

Malan, D. H. (1976). *The Frontier of Brief Psychotherapy.* New York: Plenum Press.

Jones, F. D., Johnsen, A. W. (1975). Medical and Psychiatric Treatment Policy and Practice in Vietnam. *Journal of Social Issues* 31(4): 49–65.

Kormos, H. R. (1978). The Nature of Combat Stress. In: Figley, C. R. (Ed.). *Stress Disorders Among Vietnam Veterans.* New York: Brunner/Mazel.

Lifton, R. F. (1973). *Home From The War.* New York: Simon and Schuster.

Mann, J. (1969). The Specific Limitation of Time in Psychotherapy. *Seminars in Psychiatry* 1: 375.

Mann, J. (1973). *Time-Limited Psychotherapy.* Cambridge: Harvard University Press.

Marmor, J. (1979). Short-term Dynamic Psychotherapy. *American Journal of Psychiatry* 136(2): 149-155.

Niederland, W. G. (1968). Clinical Observations on the "Survivor Syndrome," *International Journal of Psychoanalysis* 49: 313-315.

Niederland, W. G. (1981). The Survivor Syndrome: Further Observation and Dimensions. *Journal of the American Psychiatric Association* 29(2): 413-425.

Parkes, C. M. (1973). *Bereavement.* New York: International Universities Press.

Pettera, R. L., Johnson, B. M., Zimmer, R. (1969). Psychiatric Management of Combat Reactions with Emphasis on a Reaction Unique to Vietnam. *Military Medicine* (9): 673-678.

Shatan, C. F. (1978). Stress Disorders Among Vietnam Veterans: The Emotional Content of Combat Continues. In: Figley, C. R. (Ed.). *Stress Disorders Among Vietnam Veterans.* New York: Brunner/Mazel.

Sifneos, P. E. (1967). Two Different Kinds of Psychotherapy of Short Duration. *American Journal of Psychiatry* 123: 1069-1074.

Sifneos, P. E. (1972). *Short-Term Psychotherapy and Emotional Crisis.* Cambridge: Harvard University Press.

Straker, M. (1977). A Review of Short-Term Psychotherapy. *Diseases of the Nervous System* 38(10): 813-816.

Swank, R. L. (1949). Combat Exhaustion. *Journal of Nervous and Mental Diseases* 109(6): 475-508.

VanPutten, T., Emory, W. H. (1973). Traumatic Neuroses in Vietnam Refugees. *Archives of General Psychiatry* 29(11): 695-698.

Viotsky, H. M., Hamburg, D. A., Goss, M. E., Lebovitz, B. (1961). Coping Behavior Under Extreme Stress. *Archives of General Psychiatry* 5(11): 27--52.

Wilson, J. P. (1980). Conflict, Stress and Growth: Effects of War on Psycho-Social Development. In: Figley, C. R., Leventman, S. (Eds.). *Strangers at Home: Vietnam Veterans Since The War.* New York: Praeger Special Studies.

Wolberg, L. R. (1965). *Short-term Psychotherapy.* New York: Grune and Stratton.

7
The Role of Psychodynamic Group Therapy in the Treatment of the Combat Veteran

ERWIN RANDOLPH PARSON, PH.D.

OVERVIEW OF THE USE OF GROUPS
IN THE TREATMENT OF COMBAT VETERANS

The literature on group therapy continues to flourish and to grow at an unprecedented rate. Numerous techniques abound, and fall under the general rubric of group psychotherapy: Gestalt, bio-energetics, psychosynthesis, encounter, sensitivity training, trans-actional analysis, fantasy-imagery, theatre of encounter, rolfing, group games, family, couple, and many others. These techniques and maneuvers have been applied to a number of patient populations to include inpatients, outpatients, addicted individuals, delinquents, mixed ethnicity groups, the handicapped, marital pairs, as well as other group membership classifications. However, there is a curious and conspicuous barrenness in the group literature on the group treatment approach to combat veterans and other persons having suffered a catastrophic life event or pattern of events.

This seeming lack of interest in or appreciation for the importance of the unique clinical and investigative problems posed by such survivors is perhaps due to two competing traditional perspectives on the psychological reactions of survivors to stressful experiences.

One of these views places the onus of responsibility for stress reactions on the survivor himself, while the other attempts to explain stress reactions in terms of the specific properties of the event itself. The first view is called the *predisposition* hypothesis or perspective, which holds that any persons succumbing to a stressful event by a manifestation of symptoms, was so predisposed by characterological vulnerabilities and defects existing before the stressful event. This view has been especially prominent in contexts in which the traumatic event was judged as mild. The second view is referred to as the *conditions of the event* perspective, and maintains that reactions to stress is related to factors intrinsic to the event itself. This point of view was held especially when the inciting event or events were highly intense and catastrophic. Smith (1981) discusses these perspectives in a monumental review of the psychological literature on reactions to combat from the Civil War through the Vietnam War, spanning a period of 120 years (from 1860 to 1980). In addition to these two traditional views on stress reactions to trauma, he presents a third. Whereas the first two views focus on the issue of causality, the third perspective, called the *process* perspective, emphasizes the importance of understanding and exploring the reactions themselves as a continuous process. For when stress reactions in human beings are understood from this perspective, the clinician and research investigator is able to address a number of issues as these relate to the ever-changing vicissitudes of the normal, expectable recovery process (involving cyclical periods of denial and numbing reactions, pseudo-normality, and intrusive images, thoughts, and affects) as well as the abnormal and disordered patterns of adaptation.

This seeming diversionary account on the traditional views held regarding psychological reactions to stress is important in giving the reader some useful explanation for the reasons the literature on the group treatment of combat veterans and other survivors of trauma is virtually nonexistent, despite the fact that reactions to catastrophic events is not new (Cavenar and Nash, 1976). With very few exceptions, clinicians and researchers who hold to the predisposition perspective, tend to understand stress-related reactions such as nightmares, flashback to the event, high levels of anxiety, insomnia and other sleep disturbances, panic, numbing, etc. as they understand any other neurotic manifestation; namely, as pathology stemming from problematic, maladaptive patterns of learning with their origins rooted in the reinforcements of childhood experiences. It is thus not very difficult to understand how this focus and orientation would limit interest and exploration of stress-related pathology as a clinical entity in its own right. Specific survivor populations (for example, combat veterans, or survivors of concentration camps, natural catastrophes, fires, car accidents, etc.) have therefore been grouped together along with other populations of persons suffering from neurotic or characterological conflicts. There is no wonder, then, that the literature on the treatment of combat and other survivors is so sparse. This chapter presents the view that stress-related mental conditions can be conceptualized along different lines, and so requiring a different kind of treatment planning than more traditional approaches.

As indicated earlier, in contrast to the voluminous number of papers and symposia over the past several decades on the relative efficacy of group treatment with various types of patients, very little has been published on the group treatment of survivors of combat or catastrophic events. In fact, Krystal's (1968) book, *Massive Psychic Trauma*, on the conceptualization of clinical issues and treatment of survivors of Nazi concentration death camps, makes only one overly terse statement on the usefulness of the group approach to treating the mental and interpersonal woes of these persons. He states, "Group therapy may be of special value in handling the aftereffects of social mistreatment. This area, however, still remains to be explored" (p. 2). Grinker and Spiegel (1945), in their book *Men Under Stress*, reported on the treatment of war neuroses in American bomber pilots in the North Africa Campaign. They discussed two approaches: the administration of drugs, especially narcosynthesis with sodium pentothal, and individual or group therapy. Regarding the use of group therapy with these stressed pilots, Grinker and Spiegel state:

Dealing with groups has a positive value in that the group more nearly approximates the state of the human being in his natural surroundings, as a gregarious animal seeking a satisfactory niche in his social setting. His inhibitions and repressions are motivated by the mores of the group, and his difficulties in adjustment and failures to express his emotional troubles are partly the results of his ability to conform to what he thinks the group demands. Place this person in a small group that is friendly toward him, composed of fellow sufferers, and eventually he will be able to express his aggressive tendencies, his hates, his loves, and his wishes without an accompanying sense of guilt. By working out his problems in a small group he should, theoretically, be able to face the larger group, that is, his world, in an easier manner.

These authors believed that group therapy was a useful therapeutic modality in its own right; however, they felt that group treatment, in general, had significant limitations that could only be overcome by individual psychotherapy. This view differs from more modern perspectives on group approaches to treatment which maintain that deep unconscious anxieties and character disorders can be analyzed in groups (Kissen, 1976).

The military has used group treatment for many years. However, the group modality was utilized, not because groups were conceived as useful in treating combat related pathology in the soldier, but rather because of expediency in offering treatment to a large number of persons in the absence of a sufficient number of trained mental health professionals. Rome (1944) discusses the various advantages of the group approach in military settings. He lists nine critical factors that facilitate the healing process in groups:

1. The similarity of symptoms relieves the therapeutic burden of any one individual.

2. Tensions based on feeling unique are dissipated.

3. Stigma is ameliorated.

4. The doctor-patient relationship is eased.

5. Emotional release is controlled.

6. A too penetrating analysis is controlled.

7. Individual sessions may be added, if indicated.

8. A 24 hour schedule avoids undirected lulls.

9. Monotony is avoided.

Though Grinker and Spiegel (1945) agree with Rome's list of critical factors, they maintain that factors 4, 5, and 6 are critical issues in any treatment, and so believe the group approach is limited by its inability to (1) develop useful transference reactions (via the doctor-patient relationship); (2) free emotional expression; and (3) offer a penetrating analysis of neurotic and character pathology, due to reliance on the conscious maneuvers of coercion, persuasion, suppression, and goal-setting in dealing with problematic thoughts, feelings, and actions. They thus concluded that group therapy should be reserved for limited therapeutic goals: "If all that is desired is merely an outward appearance of unstable normality, group therapy can achieve this goal." They continue, "For patients who are mildly ill, group therapy suffices. . . ." Additionally, Grinker and Spiegel believed that "not much time is saved" since the patient with deep anxieties spontaneously seeks out an individual experience (p. 87). This biased view on the utility of group therapy had been reported previously in 1940 by Wender, whose extensive paper, "Group

Psychotherapy—A Study of Its Application," had insisted "that individual therapy must be carried on in private interviews during the course of group therapy" (Grinker and Spiegel, 1945, p. 387) in order to bolster the overall efficacy of the group experience. This may be yet another reason for the relative absence of published reports on the group psychotherapy with survivors of trauma-inducing events or pattern of events.

From the discussion so far, it is possible to isolate two traditional perspectives on the role of group therapy in adequately handling stress reaction derived from a catastrophic inciting experience. The first perspective holds that group therapy is a treatment of choice—a treatment modality in its own right—for persons who have shared in a life-event and desire to make useful integrations of their catastrophic experiences. Rome's view above discusses the utility of group therapy as distinct from other modalities for combat soldiers who suffered a variety of psychiatric reactions following their war engagements. The latter perspective views group therapy only in terms of the adjunctive role it can play in the total treatment plan of the survivor; and its overall value is conceived as minimal. These two views relate to an ongoing controversy that has existed for several decades.

The most progressive conception of the group modality of treatment is perhaps one which considers the utility of groups in a flexible manner, that they are amenable to addressing a broad spectrum of changing patient needs. Groups as a whole have an organic property of their own that moves naturally through a series of developmental phases toward maturity (Bennis and Shepard, 1976), in which group members go through these phases together. For certain patient populations such as survivors of a traumatization such as war, it is this author's experience that patient needs are often best met by highly specialized groups, designed to meet specific immediate psychological or psychosocial needs, then progressing to another group designed to further increase insight, growth, and maturation. This manner of viewing groups eliminates the biased perspective that "rap" groups are useless or inferior to other kinds of group experiences. Thus, rather than fostering Walker's (1981) viewpoint that "rap" groups are no longer useful in the treatment of Vietnam combat veterans, the point of view here is that "rap" groups have an important place in the overall and comprehensive treatment of most Vietnam veterans who have for years—perhaps for over a decade—felt alienated from culture and who have been unable to formulate for themselves a consistent and personally useful philosophy of their own suffering, losses, and about the onus of responsibility for their personal actions in Vietnam. "Rap" groups, as a therapeutic modality will be discussed in a later section of this chapter.

Historically, the "rap" group concept evolved out of the need of Vietnam veterans to find *meaning* in their Vietnam and post-Vietnam experience, and from a desire to deal with the psychological symptoms they suffered. As reported by Shapiro (1978), the early rap groups were organized by a small group of Vietnam veteran political dissidents in 1971 belonging to the veterans organization called the Vietnam Veterans Against the War (VVAW). This organization had contacted mental health professionals to assist them with a number of readjustment problems that they had been unable to adequately deal with alone. Lifton (1973), Shapiro (1978), and Shatan (1973) have discussed their experiences as therapist-participants in the early self-help "rap" groups organized in 1970 and continuing until 1974 in New York City. These group experiences for these veterans departed in significant ways from traditional systems of group treatment. For example, the veterans insisted that the groups be conducted on their "own turf—in their own familiar setting, away from the formality of a therapist's office or mental health agency facilities. The veterans wanted the group experience to remain in their control; the therapists were referred to as "the professionals," while the vets were referred to as "the veterans." Basically, the group "experience focused our [the seven therapists who met regularly] attention on the question of how to encourage psychological growth in a group of men who felt simultaneously alienated from society and committed to social change (Shapiro, 1978, p. 157). From the therapist's perspective, the groups were organized and conducted with significant modification of prevailing techniques in group work. The rap group sessions were conducted in VVAW offices which were often crowded, noisy, often sitting on crates, boxes, etc. The VVAW veterans set many of the rules: they decided that any veteran could attend the rap group who desired to do so, and they preferred no hard line on member attendance. Thus, some veterans would attend the group once, and then disappear for several days, weeks, or even months. Group hours would last up to four hours; and by the end of the first year two rap groups were operating on a once-per-week basis. In all, several hundred veterans and some 20 therapists participated in the rap groups, individual therapy, or the theme-centered workshops that grew out of the rap sessions (Shapiro, 1978, p. 159).

In terms of the therapist-veteran relationship, a number of factors prevailed that distinguished this experience from traditional group therapy. For example, therapists became political allies, which, although resulting in intimate contact with the veterans, nonetheless might have prevented the therapist-veteran relationship from mutual exploration of hostile feelings toward the therapist. The therapist's role as an authority person was minimized in this rap group structure, and though powerful rageful feelings were expressed toward bosses, military officers, and toward the "system," very seldom was any negative feelings directed toward the therapist as authority figures. The exploration of transference feelings which could conceivably have helped the men to deal better with their Vietnam and post-Vietnam experience was only tangentially attended to by the therapists. As Shapiro notes, certain critical questions arose regarding whether or not transference feelings toward the therapist could be fruitfully explored directly without raising the level of anxiety related to repressed and split-off troublesome memories, affects, and cognitions in the veteran group members. Raising levels of anxiety could conceivably result in acting-out by leaving the group, or in some other manifestation such as destructive behavior transactions in the group. The therapists felt as though they had to make a choice between keeping the veterans in the group by maintaining a "supportive"*modus operandi*, or risking the men leaving the group out of fear related to transferential affects, distortions, projections, and denial.

In their good judgment, the therapists realized that in order to explore transference phenomena the veteran would need a relatively well-integrated ego, adequate motivation, purpose, and commitment. Since these essential factors were not possessed by the veterans, it would have been disastrous had transference feelings been explored with these men. As I have discussed elsewhere (Parson, 1982), the analysis of transference in the psychological context of arrested ego development is bound to prove ineffective or even harmful to the veteran. This is because an ego weakened by flashbacks and other intrusive trauma-related symptoms is lacking in the necessary integrative and synthetic capabilities to usefully "decode" the symbolic nature of transference feelings, and then to integrate this into ongoing personality structure. By its very nature, transference involves distortions; and a weak, primitive ego is unable to recognize and align the distorted transferential perceptions with the reality aspects of the therapist's here-and-now qualities.

The therapists in the early rap groups were, for the most part, psychoanalysts, psychoanalytically-oriented psychotherapists, and other dynamically-bent professionals. It seems remarkable that professionals of these orientations could put aside their ordinary mode of treatment functioning and intervening and make the necessary adaptation to the needs of these men. Many other therapists of like bent would decry the "looseness" of the group structure and the general conduct and interventive procedures that characterized the rap groups. But it is precisely this very type of structure that has given this type of group experience its unique identity. I refer to the rap group approach which, for the most part, avoids transference exploration as the "oblique technical approach," as opposed to the "frontal technical approach," in which transference phenomena are allowed to unfold and becomes a central ingredient in the therapeutic effort. The oblique technical approach in rap groups addresses the need of the veteran to come to terms with his war experiences and postwar realities, but on his own terms, in his own time. The oblique technical approach, like the frontal technical approach is "technical" because its use is strategic, purposive, and intentional. Thus, the employing of the oblique approach of rap groups is not haphazard, but is deliberate and designed as aspects of useful technique with these veterans.

For Lifton (1973), three principles seemed important in describing the nature of these rap groups: *affinity*, *presence*, and *self-generation*. By "affinity" he meant the coming together of persons having shared a special and common sociopsychohistorical experience and are available to each other for mutual exploration, contact, and discovery. "Presence" refers to *being there*—a mutual availability to the other among participants of the rap groups, while "self-generation" reflects the members' need to change, achieve insight and self-knowledge as they assume responsibility for their own processes and lives.

Working with higher functioning Vietnam combat veterans at the Queens Hospital Center in New York, Parson (1980) reports on the essential ingredients of experiential group psychotherapy with these combatants. He explains, "Experiential group therapy encourages the veteran to recollect and make public (within the group) his *there-and-then* experiences of the Vietnam war. For its underlying principles recognize the veteran's psychological need to return to the land 'where it all happened,' indeed, to where it all began, in working through the war. However, the *central* focus is on *experience-at-the-moment* as this transpires in the *here-and-now*" (p. 6). Experiential group therapy, he maintains, leads to *personal meaningfulness* (Beukenkamp, 1966). The attainment of personal meaning is a critical and very necessary by-product of rap group experiences (Smith, 1980).

Brende (in press) reports on a 12-session, "educational-thera-peutic" group experience with alcohol and drug-abusing Vietnam veterans, who also suffered from a variety of posttraumatic stress symptoms. Group development themes included (1) breaking through emotional detachment and meaninglessness; (2) images and experi-ences of death, dehumanization, victimization, and *killer-victim* identification; (3) encountering the loss of self; and (4) the beginning of the grief and reparation process.

Walker and Nash (1981), charging that "no systematic approach to group treatment of those men [Vietnam veterans] has been proposed," set out to outline a number of treatment issues they have found to be central in any therapeutic venture with these war com-batants suffering from posttraumatic stress disorder. They insist that their groups are *not* "rap" groups, but are therapy groups, though they have failed to demonstrate the specific features that distinguish the "rap" group from their proposed group therapy model. By implication, a very important distinguishing feature might be the development and maintenance of clear demarcation between therapist and group members. We shall see later that this biased view against rap groups is technically unwarranted, since rap groups do have a place in the total scheme of overall treatment-planning for the Vietnam war combatant, as will be demonstrated in this chapter.

In a rather comprehensive treatment regime for Israeli soldiers after the Yom Kippur War of 1973. Moses et al (1976) discuss the overall goal and structure of the therapeutic community. The over-all goals of the treatment was to prevent or minimize regressive forces in the soldier by fostering a milieu that identified and incor-porated the soldier's strengths and positive resources in its on-going operations. The treatment unit had all the features of a social system or a therapeutic community, and relied on a systematic daily routine and physical activities for each soldier. Staff emotional reactions concerning their work with the soldiers, their feelings about the war and about working on the particular unit, were allowed free expres-sion as an aspect of the comprehensive treatment for these patients. Group psychotherapy was a vital and intrinsic part of the program. Loyalty and group cohesion began early in the groups, and provided a useful forum for a number of important explorations of war and post-war realities and reactions.

Cognitive, behavioral, and social learning techniques have also been reported as approaches to the treatment of Vietnam veterans. For example, Scaturo (1980), using a cognitive-emotional model, discussed a number of issues pertaining to the selection of clients, the development of group cohesiveness, the cognitive component of

war trauma and its treatment through the group modality. The therapeutic function of the *reattribution* process was discussed as a key
element in the cognitive aspects of war actions to which the combatant responds with guilt and self-blame. This process is geared to assist
the veteran in the group setting to arrive at a greater acceptance of
external attribution ("other or situational blame"), while personal
acceptance of *internal attribution* ("self-blame") is discouraged.
Marafiote (1980) also used cognitive procedures and techniques in
working with stress-disordered Vietnam veterans in groups. She
emphasized behavioral consequences, and attempted to make the
group attractive by communicating to the veteran that he was not
alone: by informal interaction a half hour before group, by the use of
refreshments, and by a buddy system to include the exchange of telephone numbers. Additionally, target behaviors were selected and an
individualized treatment plan involving goals and objectives were
instituted. The final section of the paper presented a selection of
techniques and procedures that the author had found useful in the
group treatment of Vietnam combat veterans, but only in the first
phase of a proposed multiphasic developmental group process as will
be presented in this chapter. Marafiote recommends the following
techniques and procedures she has found useful in groups of Vietnam
veterans: cognitive restructuring, rehearsal, thought stopping, home-
work assignments, modeling, assertiveness training, charts and graphs,
fee refunds, and bibliotherapy.

Stress disorders in noncombat contexts have also been presented
in the literature. For example, Fogelman and Savran (1980) have
discussed their experiences as group leaders in support groups of
children of Holocaust survivors. These second generation group
members had suffered a number of psychosocial problems directly
related to having survivor parents with a traumatic past. Central
problems explored by these authors in these *feeling* groups were
difficulties in communicating with parents about their traumatic
experiences; problems in coping with their own rage, shame, guilt,
and scarred feelings; and the conflicts around separating from their
parents psychologically and living independent, guilt-free individuated
adult lives. Psychotic posttraumatic stress disorder, as a nosological
entity and its treatment through the group modality was the subject
of a paper by Bloch and Bloch (1976). The central goals of the treatment with these psychotically traumatized patients were support and
increasing coping capacities in the survivor, who had suffered a
variety of traumatic life-events to include industrial accidents, which
resulted in a concussion and other injuries in one patient; the loss of

four fingers of one hand, in another patient; severe disabling back injury in still another patient; etc. The authors discuss the broad spectrum of human reactions to loss and trauma: anger, depressions, suicidal ideations and actions; acting-out; regression; helplessness; murderous aggressiveness in fantasies of retaliation; paranoid panic; feeling singled out by fate; and viewing the outer world as cold, rejecting, and blameworthy for their misfortune.

MULTIPLE-GROUP DEVELOPMENTAL TREATMENT MODEL WITH VIETNAM VETERANS: FROM "RAP" GROUP TO PSYCHOANALYTIC GROUP PSYCHOTHERAPY

Special Needs and Problems of Vietnam Veterans

There is an abundance of literature now coming on the scene that have specified the unique problems and issues related to the Vietnam war combatant. For example, Figley (1978), in his magnus opus, *Stress Disorders Among Vietnam Veterans*, has presented a wide array of special psychosocial problems in these persons, to include their reactions to death and dying; drug-use as self-medication; aggression and violence; impoverished marital relations and general problems with intimacy; shame and guilt; nightmares; and other stress-determined symptoms. Niff (1976) spoke of the "flashback" syndrome, while Shatan (1972, 1973) has alerted us to the pervasiveness of "impacted" grief among Vietnam veterans. Haley (1974) has eloquently outlined the problems faced by the therapist when the patient veteran reports on the gruesome acts done in the war zone, namely, atrocities. She offers a fresh perspective on inner suffering these men go through in their daily lives as they seek some solace from their internal haunting persecutory superego related to having committed acts of violence on another human being, far beyond "the call of duty." In the area of parenting, Haley (1975) discussed the special issues that emerge in the veteran's interaction with his child, and how having either in fantasy or in actuality been involved in killing a child in Vietnam, adversely affects the nature of the veteran's parenting competence. Friedman (1981) reports on the remarkable underlying physiological mechanisms and correlates of the *Post-Vietnam Syndrome* in Vietnam veterans, especially as these relate to sleep disturbances, and disorder of the circadian rhythm.

Parson (1983) has catalogued a number of clinical symptoms found in the Vietnam veteran: the "pan-suspicious attitude," affectively-induced pain syndromes, generalized bodily tension states, the "walking time bomb anxiety," chronic grief states, survivor-related guilt, atrocity-related guilt, accidental death-related guilt, profound and pervasive sense of personal vulnerability, "Agent Orange anxiety," memory and concentration deficits, and narcissistically-determined isolation and narcissistic injury (Parson, 1982). DeFazio (1978) has offered a classification of stress pathology: (1) classical symptoms of traumatic neurosis—"bad dreams," irritability, aggression, memory problems and amnesias, and psychosomatic disorders; (2) exaggerated character pathology—character neurosis, borderline personality, and narcissistic personality disorder; (3) dissociated symptoms. A comprehensive discussion of the various dimensions of regressive phenomena in Vietnam veterans is presented by Brende (1983) which includes identity splitting, pathological identifications with the aggressor, identity diffusion, and a pathological fusion of both "executioner" and "victim" identifications referred to as the "killer-victim identification."

The "gook-identification" in minority Vietnam veterans is also a clinical phenomenon described by Parson (1982), in which soldiers, while in Vietnam, identified with the squalor, demeaned status, poverty, and general wretchedness of the Vietnamese nationals. He found this phenomena primarily in black and other minority Vietnam veterans, but also in white veterans as well.

The National Council of Churches statistics reported by Eisenhart (1977) reveal a number of striking statistics on the Vietnam war combatant: before 1971, as many as 45,806 soldiers were killed in Vietnam. This figure is contrasted to the large number of veterans who died since their return from the war (49,000), according to this report. As reported by Brende (in press) on the Presidential Review of 1979, violent and antisocial behavior has resulted in 29,000 Vietnam veterans in federal prisons, 87,000 are awaiting trial, 250,000 are on probation, and 37,500 are on parole. The U.S. Bureau of Census found that 70 percent of incarcerated veterans had honorable discharges. Walker (1981) states that a large number of veterans are problem drinkers, have marital difficulties, and committed suicide over the post-war years. It is estimated that up to 800,000 veterans are in need of psychiatric assistance with their mental woes; and social scientists believe that this figure will escalate up to 1.5 million in the near future (Figley, 1978; Wilson, 1977).

Etiologic factors contributing to the tremendous problems of Vietnam veterans just mentioned stem from the nature of the war itself, as well as from the hostile, blaming, and rejecting repatriation experience which this author has referred to as the "dysreception of Vietnam veterans"—to denote the painful and troublesome nature of these veterans' reentry into the United States.

It is this author's belief that the social support and structure needed to "contain" the harrowing intrapsychic "aftermath" of war within the veteran has essentially been undermined by the lack of acceptance and respect shown by the American people for the Vietnam war combatant's sacrifices. In the absence of the essential "holding" function of "Mother-America," the maturational environment needed to quell the veteran's inner tide of affective chaos, persecutory superego feelings and projections, annihilation anxiety, and fear of the return of powerful "split-off" dissociated aspects of the self, cannot occur. The tremendous "impingements" (in Winnicott's sense) originating in the environment have essentially interfered with the "going on being" (Winnicott, 1962) of the Vietnam veteran, and these impingements have produced non-adaptive reactions, especially self-protective isolation—away from the world of people. Impingements from the environment, in the case of the Vietnam veteran, were in the form of what this author has referred to as the "anti-hero syndrome." The *anti-hero syndrome* is an American phenomenon characterized by cold, blaming, and hostile displacements and projections upon the Vietnam war combatant. In response to such impingements "The sense of self is lost . . . and is only regained by a return to isolation" (Winnicott, 1958, p. 222).

"Object Relation," as a theory of personality development and functioning, "refers to specific intrapsychic structures, to an aspect of ego organization, and not to external interpersonal relationships. However, these intrapsychic structures, the mental representation of self ("self-representations") and other ("object-representation"), do become manifest in interpersonal situations" (Horner, 1979, p. 3). For a large number of Vietnam veterans their stress reactions and disorders have precipitated a passionate and constant threat of self-dissolution and fragmentation, with attendant regressive mental and interpersonal functioning. The damage sustained in the veteran's object relations is manifest in primitive, devitalized mental representations of self and others. Low self-esteem and emotional detachment from others represent a *core* set of posttraumatic symptoms, whose origins for many veterans began during the basic training experience. Shatan (1974) writes of the sense of alienation in many of these persons: "Alienation and detachment from feelings and people are a natural outcome of the repression of compassion and inhibition of sensitivity. Some GIs often speak of undergoing 'emotional death' as if *frozen into stone-like gargoyles* . . . or withdrawing from their emotions as if *retreating into mental foxholes*" (p. 10, my italics). To bring the veteran out of these "mental foxholes," and rehumanize the "cold granite" isolation which surrounds the veteran, the treatment approach must be geared to promote a *re-linking experience* (to the world of people), through the gradual accretion of new psychic structure in a "good-enough," containing environment that facilitates maturation, trust, unrequited devotion, and *nonimpingement.*

Such a therapeutic environment would allow the veteran to grow at his own pace, while providing a social structure that can "contain" the disquieting fantasies, memories, and ideations of war experiences (Schwartz, Chapter 9). Moreover, the treatment setting would take on the characteristics of a microcosm (or miniature "Mother-America") in which sanctions are given for war actions, and the opportunity for seeking and finding a personal philosophy (that would infuse the veteran's war and postwar experiences with *meaningfulness*), and working through developmental deficits.

Rationale for a Multiple-Group Model (M-GM)

The multiple-group developmental model proposed in this chapter features a group approach which addresses the progressive and changing spectrum of psychic, interpersonal, and social needs of the veteran over time. As the veteran moves toward renewal, toward maturation, and integration of the trauma into his/her identity system, a flexible and adaptable treatment plan is essential—one that considers this *changing spectrum of needs.*

In reference to Vietnam veterans and many other survivors of psychic trauma, a single-group treatment approach may not be sufficient in meeting the immediate and post-immediate (or long-term) requirements for a complete (as possible) structural (ego) renewal in the survivor. In group treatment contexts, this writer's experience suggests that it is sometimes necessary to formulate a treatment plan for some veterans that utilizes two or three distinct group types whose purpose, organization, and function are geared to accomplish specific goals in the overall readjustment treatment process. For example, for treatment goals that focus on the alleviation of acute stress symptomatology only, a one-group peer-centered supportive treatment experience is often sufficient in effecting rapid symptomatic relief (Yalom, 1970). This group-type, however, is not effective in bringing about important structural "healing" or development to any significant degree. This is to say, that the adverse and "structure-altering" effects of the traumatic experience and attendant developmental (psychic) suspension (Parson, 1982c) cannot be reversed or frontally addressed by the supportive group (that is, single-group) format alone. If, on the other hand, treatment goals are to repair underlying structural impairment and effect long-lasting characterological change by altering the existing pathological psychic formation related to war trauma, then a treatment approach which analyzes pathologic defenses within the group context in the treatment of choice. Experience with Vietnam veterans reveal that significant underlying structural deficits born of traumatic insult, do often persist far beyond the initial relief period of acute symptomatology. This writer is in full agreement with Shatan (1977) when he asserts that studies of concentration camp and combat survivors had taught us that psychic structure might not be as immutable as we used to think. What this means is that under the impact of severe trauma, the individual's habitual modes relating to self and world, regulating the expression of the drives and their derivatives, and the general harmonization of inner needs with the imposing demands of the external world, may become structurally altered. Such a structural alteration in the personality often results in *uncharacteristic* modes of coping for the veteran (survivor). The veteran's character structure is thus expected to falter "in its maintenance of psychosomatic homeostasis . . . patterned self regulation of esteem . . . stabilization of the ego identity, and the automatization of threshold and stimulus barrier levels, both shifting in accordance with the intensity of internal stimuli (Blos, 1968). Moreover, adversely affected by the traumatic experience are the ego's regulatory functions over the fluctuation of emotional processes.

The rationale or the use of multiple-groups in working through the "structural imbalance" (Cohen, 1980), fragmentation and schizoidal isolation of the self, and the narcissistically injured psyche of the Vietnam veteran (1982b) is presented in the following:

1. Support groups (single-group) are useful in allaying high level anxiety and restoring hope, courage, and meaning in the life of the survivor. These groups have been used successfully with survivors of miscarriages (Friedman and Cohen, 1980); hostages taken in prison (Wolk, 1981); and with the combat Vietnam veteran (Smith, 1980). However, since we know from longitudinal studies that post-war

trauma symptoms persist over time, and may become exacerbated by increasing age of the veteran (Archibald and Tuddenham, 1965), the need arises for a more comprehensive system of longer-term treatment that would go beyond the mere alleviation of acute symptoms, to the strengthening of defenses and to the maturation of the ego. Psychoanalytically-oriented psychotherapy would be the treatment of choice at a later time during the developmental course of the treatment experience, since this approach affects deeper psychic structures and trauma-altered personality systems that are in need of a reactivation of developmental arrest (Mednick, 1981).

2. In order that support groups offer maximum benefit to the veteran (or other survivor), the groups must be homogeneously composed along three dimensions—combat (ie, all combat veterans), diagnosis ("posttraumatic stress disorder"), and a strong motivation for growth and readiness to talk about their war experiences in Vietnam. The inherent dilemma in such group compositions is that it is precisely because of this homogeneity that the very necessary pre-curative element of *cohesion* is achieved, but too rapidly and often persists in the group process for too long a time, thus reducing individual differentiation and growth in group members. This is to say that even though cohesion is a critical factor in group treatment (Yalom, 1970; Tropp, 1976), it is also true that "a group may become too cohesive, so cohesive that it becomes incapable of adjusting to the environment. . . . In such a group there is a great uniformity of norms. Everyone has the same frame of reference, and these determine to a serious extent the group's expectations about what is going to happen next. They therefore routinize the behavior of members toward one another and toward the environment" (Klein, 1956, p. 124). For the veteran, who, since repatriation has been unable to feel comfort, harmony, and "fellow-feeling" with others, it is not difficult to understand how these veterans would together form a solid cohesive "group mass" that would be virtually impervious to any process or procedure that would interfere with the "coziness" of group's integratedness. This author uses the term "primary group cohesion" to distinguish this process from maturationally more advanced forms of cohesion that occurs during the later stages of group life ("secondary group cohesion"). During primary group cohesiveness, group members are indistinguishable from the other, and there is intense fear of separateness and individuation. Any attempt to dissolve the cohesion usually results in profound anxiety and threat of dissolution of the self. Since individuation is the goal of group treatment, persistent group

"we-ness" is a resistance to growth and separateness. The multiple-group developmental model proposed in this chapter uses an instrumental approach in which primary group cohesion, as a group defensive process, is worked through by adding two or three new members whose psychological development and insight are congruent with the direction the group process is to take; namely, individuation. The inclusion of these new members begins a new group, and a new shift in dynamic process within the group occurs. The new members should be Vietnam era veterans (not combat veterans). The diversity provided by the era veterans will provide a truer microcosm of the real world. The third group, the psychoanalytically-oriented group, is composed of combat veterans, Vietnam era veterans, and non-veterans. Each of the three group-types will be discussed in more detail later in this chapter.

Multiple-groups are not widely applied in the group literature, except when alluded to in the context of pre-group preparation and screening for cognitive-informational (eg, Rabin, 1970) and cognitive-experiential (eg, Piper et al, 1979) group psychotherapy. The most prevalent form of group therapy is the single group which have been noted to move progressively from one phase of development to another throughout the life of the group. Many authors have discussed the various group developmental shifts that occur "naturally" during the course of the single group. For example, Kissen (1976) holds that group development progresses from early "anxiety-dependency" to a later "reintegration" phase. Bennis and Shepard (1956) view group development as moving through a two-phase process of "dependence" to "interdependence," with a number of subphases pertaining to a broad array of dynamic issues that evolve during the life of the group. Bibbard et al (1974) have isolated three models of group development, especially in reference to analytic group therapy: (1) linear-progressive, (2) life-cycle, and (3) pendular. In the first model, the group moves during the initial phases to a conflict stage, then to resolution, to the development of cohesiveness (referred to as "secondary group cohesion" by the present writer), and finally to the attainment of the group's task. The second model emphasizes termination or the death of the group, while the third model highlights the various recurrent dynamic themes during the course of the group's life. Kellerman (1979) has attempted to integrate these models into a linear-regressive model, which demonstrates that the group progresses toward the expression of conflict and then toward the resolution of a variety of psychosexual level-specific conflicts. Unlike the linear-progressive model which emphasizes the group development along a singular, unidimensional line, from immature functioning to matured forms of integration, the linear-regressive model espouses the view that group development moves regressively (in its progression toward maturity) in accomplishing its task.

In contrast to the single-group whose developmental shifts occur *naturally*, the multiple-group approach (M-GM), as discussed in this chapter, features a developmental scheme which is aided both by the natural emergence of group process and by externally-imposed manipulation (or instrumentation) in order to address the developmental needs of group members over time. The generic, general group process of the M-GM is what this writer refers to as the "developmental-regressive" model (D-RM). This means that the underlying process inspires a regressive dynamic in group members, beginning in the first-phase support "rap" group and culminating in the psychoanalytic group in which deeper dynamic and conflict issues can be analyzed and resolved.

First-Phase Peer-Centered Support Group: The "Rap" Group with Vietnam Veterans

In essence, the function of the "rap" group is to provide support to the veteran's characterological defenses until he is able to tolerate the regressive requirements of psychotherapy. This is to say, that the "rap" group avoids all active encouragement to regression, but instead attempts to stabilize the veteran's internal world. In such a group, the therapist is integrated into the group, and maintains "low visibility" in his interventions. Moreover, the leader shares his feelings and experiences with the same intensity of affect and openness that is expected of any other group member. Essentially, the demarcation between therapist or leader is virtually nonexistent. Technical consideration here would point to the need for this basic "ghost presence" of the leader, not as some "spineless" or avoidant posture, but as a very necessary prerequisite to repairing what had been damaged, and restoring that which had been disintegrated. This does not mean that the group leader does not intervene during the "rap" group process. In the beginning of the "rap" group, the central core dynamic issues revolve around *phallocentric* psychosexual concerns such as masculine identity. Even though the surface theme of the "rap" group appears to reflect the veterans' feelings of anguish, terror, anxieties, and anger regarding their war experiences—both in and after Vietnam—underlying themes of power, dominance and authority relations abound. A typical indication of these dynamics during the first phase of group treatment of Vietnam veterans is the group's focus on the United States Government, the Veterans Administration, and other agencies and persons of demonstrable power, influence, wealth, and phallic narcissism. The powerful feelings that accompany these issues are deflected away from the leader or therapist to an external power symbol, especially if the group leader is a Vietnam veteran. Power play and "power gaming" is an important aspect of this phase of the group's development. The back and forth questioning among group members during early periods of the group's life, regarding where they were, what they did, and with which unit they served in Vietnam serves two purposes. One, it serves to lay the very necessary foundation for trust, inter-personal comfortableness, and dependence; two, it serves to lay the foundation for role differentiation (or the "who's who" of the group). This back and forth sharing and mutual exploration of in-theater unit assignments (or "Who were you with?" "Where were you over there?" etc.) also results in superior-inferior self-assessments among group members. Those members who served in Vietnam during the 1968 TET counteroffensive and in other well-known perilous enemy engagements, emerge as the most prestigious group members, while those in support units are viewed as having made less significant sacrifices in the war. However, unlike most other types of non-Vietnam veteran groups, in which tight subcliques form based on members' past experiences, in "rap" groups with veterans there is a natural tendency to move toward group cohesion, toward *dependency* rather than confrontation. Each group member attempts to spare others in the group from their resentments, anger, hatreds, and general feelings of antipathy, since the common sentiment is that "We all share common anxieties, frustrations; we were all in Vietnam. All we have is ourselves. It's us against them—the ungrate-ful world." The outpouring of strong emotions is encouraged, and the group's cohesive support system offers the members a safe, non-judgemental, and sanctioning atmosphere of sensitivity and mutual respect in which such emotions can be expressed with minimal impingements.

As mentioned earlier, group cohesion, a vital therapeutic element, is attained very rapidly in "rap" groups. This achievement is aided by the common suffering experienced by these combatants, as well as the shared anger and resentment toward society, family, and friends. The mutual sharing of "war stories" involving danger, intrigue, and suffering proves a tremendous facilitator of mutual bonding among group members. Thus, non-Vietnam combat group members become group isolates very quickly. "Group cohesion" refers to "the total field of forces which act on members to remain in the group" (Festinger et al, 1950, p. 164); and its presence in the group motivates members to "value the group more highly and will defend it against internal and external threats; voluntary attendance, participation, mutual help, and defense of the group standards are all greater than in the groups with less esprit de corps" (Yalom 1970, p. 37). High cohesiveness in the group has been positively correlated with self-disclosure (Kirshmer et al, 1978).

The cohesion that occurs in first-phase groups is referred to here as *primary group cohesion.* In this type of cohesion, group members have come to experience each other's problems and concerns as their own, and come to understand their own problems through hearing, feeling, and experiencing others' difficulties *as their own.* During primary cohesion tension among group members is low, and self-boundaries of individual members become unstable, permeable, and uncertain. Also existing in this group developmental phase is an admixture of varying degrees of "true self" and "false self" organization (Winnicott, 1960). The "false self" functions to hide the "true self" by complying with the external environment. Thus, it is the compliant "false self" organization that appears to be a salient factor in the relatively rapid attainment of group cohesion with Vietnam veterans. As a group, Vietnam veterans have had to hide their "true self" (the self of spontaneous action, creativity, and regulated *primary process*), while extending to the world a compliant self (the self that generates ideas, feelings, and actions congruent with the image society has attributed or projected onto the veteran).

This group phase, additionally, is characterized by a group-as-a-whole phenomenon in which the group is experienced by members as a parental object or image—one that provides a "good-enough," facilitating environment. In this environment, the self and its structures can develop and mature. Only a group experience that is able to contain powerful projections, defensive "splitting," annihilation anxiety, and other primitive defenses, can reactivate the arrested or suspended development of these group members (Parson, 1983). It is generally not unusual for any social matrix such as a "rap" group to which is attributed critical growth-promoting events to be experienced by group members as possessing life-giving maternal qualities. Hence, the group has been attributed the qualities or characteristics of nurturant, loving, supportive, caring, and protective. The group as parental figure is supported by authors such as Money-Kyrle (1950) whose observation of group process has lead him to maintain that the group represents three fundamental parental figures: (1) the "good parents," *particularly the mother*, representing the norms and ideals of the group; (2) the "bad parents" in the role of persecutors against whom the group values have to be defended; and (3) the "good parents," *especially the father*, who as his role as the mother's defender reappears as the group leader. For Grotjahn (1972) "as a general rule, the group is a truly good and strong mother, not only in fantasies of transference, but also in the reality of the group process" (p. 318).

In terms of the processes involved in the *maturational-developmental* progression from the "rap" group phase of group primary cohesion, which when prolonged becomes antitherapeutic (Slavson, 1964), to more matured and later phases of the group's development, van Dalfsen's (1966) concept of the "concentric circles" appear to have relevance here. He views the progression of human life as moving from an inner, small circle in the beginning of life toward outer larger circles. He thus writes,

> . . . human life as such expands in concentric circles, the smallest circle being that of the mother and newborn child. It is the task of the mother to direct the attention of the growing child toward the wide circle of father and siblings, while later on the growing adolescent learns to encompass the school, the village or town, the nation and ultimately humanity as a whole (p. 656).

When applied to first-phase groups with Vietnam veterans, van Dalfsen's notion of concentric circles locates the "rap" group, as a maternal object, at the first, innermost, and smallest circle. Within our multiple-group context, phase II and other later group types structure the group's development from relatively immature, homogeneously composed, trauma-centered dynamic themes to personal growth, independence, mature interaction with people, and a greater desire and capacity to make contact with, understand and appreciate the various cultural agencies (ie, the home, school, church, governmental agencies, etc.) of the external world. Like any other population of symptomatic individuals who desire mastery over stress and conflict, Vietnam veterans need a first-phase group experience ("rap" group) *before* he or she is psychically ready to "take on" the various dimensions of a world he has perceived as unnurturing, unempathic, and hostile.

It is this writer's experience that the group-as-a-whole is often experienced as a *maternal object*, while the leader is perceived within the dynamic processes of the group as the *paternal object.* Since the core underlying emotional theme in first-phase groups with symptomatic Vietnam veterans revolves around phallic concerns of aggressive displays, guns, rifles, knives, war actions, toughness, masculinity, etc., it is critical that attendant feelings are kept at manageable levels, as positive affect coloring is actively maintained in the group climate. Creating and maintaining a positive affective coloring to the group's emotional life lay at the basis of the technical recommendation that the leader maintain a consistent participative, nonauthoritarian treatment posture ("ghost presence"). It has been found over and over again with Vietnam veterans that the overzealous, over-anxious, over-directive group learder is destined to fail in his/her responsibility to move the group along toward maturity and the attainment of the group's task. This group leader type often plunges the group head-on into rage-dominated conflictual feelings, reducing the succorant and refuge qualities of the group-as-mother. With combat veterans, the directive, "forced presence" of the leader (rather than "ghost presence") would tend to provoke the unleashing in the group's process the very aggressive and potentially destructive drives and feelings within group members that have given them such tremendous problems in relating to self and others since Vietnam. And because analysis of aggression is best reserved for a later phase in the group development, it is a technical error to actively explore aggression-dominated dissociated symptoms during this phase.

In addition to the group dynamic processes discussed above, a series of immediate first-phase group goals may be identified.

1. Manage acute symptomatology related to "automatic incursive mental phenomena" (intrusive ideation, memory, and affects).

2. Manage acute symptomatology related to massive denial, psychic numbing, and schizoidal isolation.

3. Increase psychological control over the subjective sense of being "explodable" ("walking time-bomb anxiety").

4. Learn to tolerate getting close to others (or dissolving the "counter-tender tendency").

5. Begin the process of working through guilt, "death imprint," grief states, and depression.

6. Offer sanction for personal actions in the war zone, (group-as-microcosm).

7. Enhancement and maintenance of good self-esteem regulation.

8. Begin the process of stabilizing the veteran's self-concept.

9. Development and maintenance of trust in people (or bridging the "schiziod gap" between self and others).

10. Organize a personal philosophy of the turmoil and politico-social chaos of the 1960s, and the finding of personal meaning to the war.

11. Manage "Agent Orange anxiety."

12. Begin the process of self-identity consolidation and self-repair.

13. Reaffirmation of self as belonging to a universe of human beings.

14. Modulation and increased management of rage, violence, paranoid irritability, and phobias, addictions, thrills, and risk-taking behaviors (Lipkin et al, 1982).

15. Restoration of the veteran's connectedness to and desire for "life processes such as marriage, career, and social and political institutions" (Lipkin et al, 1982, p. 911).

16. Beginning of the capacity to tolerate being touched and affected by another's emotional anguish and pain, as well as by others' joy.

17. The beginning of new psychic structure through the avail-ability of "transmuting internalizations" (Kohut, 1977) generated in the group-as-a-whole (or group-as-maternal-one).

18. Lay a solid preparatory foundation for succeeding develop-mantal group phases.

As described elsewhere, in the context of technical consider-ations in the individual treatment of the Vietnam veteran, this writer (Parson, 1983) has outlined a number of first-phase treatment techniques. A number of these have been found useful in group approaches as well; for example, cognitive restructuring and reattri-bution (of blame); relaxation (progressive) and other stress-reduction techniques; bibliotherapy; and as intensive program of educational procedures which aims to assist the veteran in understanding his symptoms. Brende (in press) reports on a special therapeutic approach with self-medicating (drug-use) Vietnam veterans in a group format. Called the "educational-therapeutic" technique, this approach integrated a variety of cognitive and behavioral, as well as experimental components in restoring function, increasing self-esteem, and instilling hope in these veterans. The first phase of Brende's approach utilized a systematic review of the symptoms of posttraumatic stress disorder and explained related factors and issues to the veterans along with pertinent reading assignments. This writer has also used weekly written summaries that chronicled the group session as described by Yalom et al (1975), and later by Lowenstein and Morris (1979) in their "Newsletter" concept.

Selection Criteria for First-Phase "Rap" Group Membership. The multiple-group model limits participating group members to men who were *in* Vietnam, whether in heavy, light, or in no active combat. The introduction of noncombat veterans ("era" veterans) is reserved until the second phase of the group developmental multiple-group process.

On the Issue of Diagnosis. It is critical to have determined the absence of sociopathic character-disordered members. Such members adversely affect the group process, precipitously increasing group tensions, paranoid preoccupations, and instigating paranoid rage reactions in group members. Basically, the sensitivity of veteran group members often "exposes" the sociopathic "agenda" which is perceived as manipulative, controlling, and insulting to group members (to many, reminiscent of the manipulation and trickery wrought upon them by the American society, government agencies, and military leaders). The significantly paranoid veteran must also be screened from group participation. These veterans often "infect" the group with increasing levels of the *pan-suspicious attitude* (Parson, 1980), resulting in a variety of anti-cohesive maneuvers, acting out, fear, anxiety, and other affects and behaviors that may lead to the untimely demise of the group. The paranoid veteran's general group functioning often proves antithetical to the establishment of trust— a critical achievement in any therapeutic work with Vietnam veterans.

Though some psychotic-level posttraumatic stress pathology can be adequately dealt with in the "rap" group, care must be taken not to include the veteran with schizophrenic disturbances. The inherent thought disorder, regressed state of being, replete with hallucinatory and delusional symptoms will adversely affect the group process, distilling unneutralized aggression into the group climate. The schizophrenic veteran interferes with the group's move toward cohesiveness, growth and maturity. In addition to the harmful effects to the group's process, the veteran with schizophrenic disturbance is himself unable to utilize the group experience due to impoverished reality-testing and impaired capacity for ego-integrated mental operations. Psychological distortion observed in such persons relates to the concommitant over-involvement with the internal world of psychotic processes and the virtual exclusion of significant involvement with others due to a reduction in libidinal investment. For this person, moreover, "the objective world has broken down . . . that the world seems 'empty,' 'meaningless,' 'monotonous' . . . he reflects in all this the withdrawal of his libido" (Fenichel, 1945, p. 417) from others. Veteran group members who, for some time following their repatriation, have feared "going crazy" or "being crazy" due to the incomprehensible nature of their readjustment psychic and interpersonal difficulties, may experience the presence of the schizophrenic veteran group member as a threat to his striving toward ego integrity and general well-being.

The first-phase group with Vietnam veterans, as mentioned earlier, must be homogeneously-composed, along the lines of diagnosis and combat status. The uniform diagnosis of "Posttraumatic Stress Disorder" (DSM III, American Psychiatric Association, 1980), albeit mixed with character disorder traits, is to be sought. And all group members are to be veterans who served in Vietnam (not merely in Southeast Asia). Another critical selection criterion is the motivational factor. The unmotivated group member is deleterious to the group, and should not be allowed membership in the "rap" group. The most workable and effective group size is 6 to 8 group members. For the first few months of the first-phase group, the group is open to whomever desires to join and share his or her feelings and experiences about their participation in the war. However, the group is to become closed as soon as a stable number of participants who are motivated to change (not just symptom relief) can be selected as *core* group members of the "rap" group.

Essential Qualities of the "Rap" Group Leader. Ideally, the group leader would be a combat veteran, with a Vietnam era veteran or a non-veteran co-leader who is very knowledgeable, sensitive, and experienced in working with Vietnam veterans. A large majority of Vietnam veterans believe that it is not possible for anyone to ever fully comprehend his or her problems unless the professional was in Vietnam (in heavy combat or not). Though in reality this assumption may not be true, from the subjective world of the veteran group member, this "conviction" has great merit. For ultimately, it is the veteran's own subjective experience of his life and his external environment that must be seriously taken into account if useful intervention is to occur.

From this writer's experience as a mental health professional and as a combat veteran of Vietnam who has had extensive involvement in the readjustment woes of Vietnam war veterans (both as therapist and supervisor of veteran cases), there arises the personal conviction that the group leader need not be a combat veteran or even an "era" veteran (a veteran who served during the Vietnam era, but not in

Vietnam). What is needed is a leader who is sensitive, empathic, and knowledgeable, and who is able to use these qualities in a constructive manner with the Vietnam veteran. Such a leader must consistently be in touch with countertransference feelings, and be ready and willing to utilize these feelings to enhance the therapeutic work. The therapist is to present and maintain himself or herself as someone with whom it is possible to have a relationship—one that is sustaining, containing, and growth-enhancing. The group leader with Vietnam veterans must have the capacity, moreover, to remain constant; he or she will be required to tolerate intense feelings, particularly "raw," unneutralized aggression. Each group member needs to know that the group leader will be there for him or her when members feel most vulnerable.

Since the establishment of *trust* is a critical achievement in any psychotherapeutic venture with the veteran, the group leader must seek to maintain an *openness to experience*, candor, and honesty. For the veteran's "natural" *pan-suspicious attitude* (or hypervigilant functioning) can decipher, on the affective level, certain thoughts, feelings, and actions of the leader that may be dishonest, perfunctory, or insincere. A leader that communicates dishonestly his feelings and group experience will prove a catalyst for increased paranoid flavoring of the group process, which will, essentially, cause some group members into self-protective narcissistic retreat. From this writer's experience, it doesn't matter whether the leader is a Vietnam veteran or not—group members demand honesty from the group leader, as they expect honesty and candor from each member of the group as well. The leader must also believe in the therapeutic power of the group culture to effect meaningful and lasting changes in the life of the group member, and escort him through the various phases of the group work.

The group leader, additionally, is called upon to possess the capacity to adapt to the changing spectrum of needs of the group members, and the intuitive and technical knowledge essential in guiding the group process from one developmental milestone to the next. Of great importance to the success of group work with Vietnam veterans is the leader's willingness and capacity to share his own spontaneous feelings, reactions, thoughts, and experiences as these transpire both within and outside the group setting that bear relationship to critical group process elements. This writer thus agrees with Yalom (1970) when he states "that the therapist who judiciously uses his person increases the therapeutic power of the group by encouraging the development [of a variety of group-born skills]. He gains considerable role flexibility and maneuverability and may, without concerning himself about role spoilage, directly attend to group maintenance and to the shaping of the group norms. By decentralizing his position in the group, he hastens the development of group autonomy and cohesiveness" (p. 102).

In the first-phase "rap" support group, the leader's effectiveness is predicated upon his ability to establish and maintain the group and its boundaries; to shape the group's norms; to utilize special knowledge available on stress pathology in Vietnam veterans in order to comprehend and efficaciously manage the group process; and adopting the "ghost presence." By "ghost presence" is meant the leader's ability to maintain a "nonimpinging," nonintrusive interactive style. Many therapists will object with the "ghost presence" posture since they believe that all symptomatic Vietnam veterans suffer from intractible characterological deficits and problems. These therapists thus adopt an unrelenting authority-dominant confrontational approach, as if confrontational "bombardments" against the character structure of the veteran will eventuate in useful therapeutic regression then to personality development. From this writer's experience such thinking and technique may be useful in later phases of the group's development, but not in the first phase. This is because the basic instability of ego functions in the group member during the first phase is not yet sufficiently integrated in order to withstand and integrate the therapeutic "assault" of persistent confrontation. The authoritarian, confrontational therapist is often experienced by combat veterans as insensitive and angry. This stirs up, rather than supports, the veteran group members' own hostile impulses and "violent" projections, which may lead to a premature and stormy "revolt against the leader." Though it has been well-established that "revolt against the leader" dynamics have adaptive and growth-promoting properties (Kissen, 1976), with Vietnam combat veterans in groups such dynamics usually end in the early demise of the group. The group is destroyed because the intense aggression inherent in the "revolt" is too reminiscent of the unleashing of aggression against others in Vietnam and the veteran's basic fear of being killed or of killing someone. Apparently, the critical issue here revolves around the recognition and security of boundaries, which, for the most part during the first-phase group, still remain undifferentiated and insecure, so that group members experience each other as though the other was themselves. During this emotional revolt against the leader, group members also experience the leader in an undifferentiated manner. This perception results in group members' experiencing the therapist's aggression-dominated confrontations as an active, volitional attempt to humiliate and destroy them. The evolution of these dynamics should be managed to prevent their premature manifestation in the group process.

In general, when the group leader is a combat veteran a different set of group dynamics emerge that contrast in important ways with those dynamics operating when the group leader is a nonveteran or noncombat veteran. If the leader is a combat veteran, "primal horde" sentiments are minimal and the group moves toward cohesion (primary) rather rapidly, with a relative absence of demarcation between leader and group. This observation differs from groups with other populations of persons in that the primal horde revolt against the leader occurs mostly when the group leader is nondirective (Kissen, 1976). Just the opposite happens when the group members are combat veterans, as described earlier. In contrast, when the group leader is a noncombat veteran or nonveteran, the group process moves toward cohesion much slower, and the leader is perceived as separate from the group (providing the group is homogeneously composed of combat veterans), and is subjected to a number of *testing encounters* by the group members. Whereas in the combat veteran-led group the sentiment among group members is "he and us are one," in the noncombat or nonveteran-led group the feeling underlying the group process is "he versus us." Infused with angry projections against the leader, the group regresses along the lines of primal horde behavior. Providing the leader and group survives this period of group development, progress may now be made toward cohesion, and then to later phases of group development and maturity. Though primal horde insurrection takes place early—during the formative period of the group—with the nondirective, noncombat leader as it does with the authoritarian leader, the insurrection or revolt is much less intense and disruptive to the group in the former.

Second Phase Group: The "Rap" Psychotherapy Group with Vietnam Veterans

Primary group cohesion during the "rap" group phase, which extends well over the first year, is the result of a series of common perceptions, shared problems, and shared "victimization." For "rap" group members, these common perceptions originate in the common experience of mutual participation in the Vietnam war, and now sharing a number of symptomatic responses to the war experience. Because group members feel that only a combat veteran can understand them, there is a "fantasied familiarity" (Day, 1976) among members. The implicit assertion here that underlies the group process is, "We are Vietnam vets, have had the same experience in the bush, have all been put down by our society, and now we share the same mental and social problems. We feel anxious and overwhelmed by our symptoms and hostile feelings and by our obsession with power, guns, rifles, and the like." As Collins and Guetzkow (1964) stated, "Under the condition of a common fate, the individuals will develop interpersonal attraction" (p. 142).

As time progresses and group tensions mount in response to the changing dynamics of the group during cohesion, the changing socio-political climate, and the awareness among group members of their increasing age, a profound sense of restlessness predominates the group. Additionally, underlying this first-phase tension is a budding awareness of the shared group "myth," and its variance with the real world and with group members' true feelings. Much of the group myth in the "rap" group phase has to do with the shared perception that Vietnam veterans are either better, worse, or special human beings when compared with others at large. As this *developmental crisis* gradually emerges, the ground work for the *second-phase group* would have begun.

The second-phase group is formed by the systematic and careful introduction of two or three Vietnam era veterans whose diagnoses and personal psychological development and integration are congruent with the progressive needs of the group. What might these special group needs be? Having alleviated acute and some chronic symptomatology, established trust, secured sanction, and increased self-esteem during the first peer-centered support "rap" group phase, continuing group needs involve the "hatching process" or an *expansion beyond the symbiotic orbit* (Mahler et al, 1975). This is to say that the needs of the group, in order to further its development, require opportunities for members to differentiate or individuate from each other and from the group. The "coziness" of the first-phase group by this time has become a resistance to further growth and self-awareness. The groupness and "we-ness" must now give way to differentiated outwardly perceptual activity. Thus, the added group members (Vietnam era veterans) must be free of acute symptomatology, and be relatively healthy psychologically in order to be useful catalysts for the group.

The rationale for the second-phase group formation just described is that the addition of these specific group members (men who served during the Vietnam era, but whom did not go to Vietnam) will provide a critical heterogeneity of the group's cognitive-affective interpersonal matrix. The added range of internalized object relations, ranging among members from the most primitive to the most integrated and differentiated, lays the foundation for "new" affective materials from which "transmuting internalizations" (Kohut, 1977) can be derived. Through these internalizations new psychic structure develops in individual members, which make it possible to accomplish the group's task of mutual self-exploration and self-confrontation without undue anxiety. The second-phase group emphasizes the here-and-now of relationships, not symptoms; and the intense sharing of war stories and mutual experiences in Vietnam of the first-phase group now recedes to the background. During this phase, intense and extended group discussion of the war is regarded as a resistance and must be put to therapeutic scrutiny.

The introduction of the new veterans ("the catalyzing group agents") into the second-phase group is by no means an inconsequential event. Though group members (of the first-phase group) are alerted much earlier of this occurrence, members, for the most part, react strongly to the "unwanted foreigners." At this time it becomes appropriate for the group leader to gradually emerge to the stature within the group as "the Leader" (with a capital "L"). As the leader, now demarcated from the group he manages the group experience in a different manner than he did in the first-phase group. The integration of the new members into the heretofore homogeneous all-combat veteran group is a crucial challange of this group phase, and offers tremendous therapeutic benefits. These advantages are two-fold: (1) the new members provide a broader range of human problems, personality systems, needs, attributes, talents, etc. than was present during the first-phase group experience; and (2) the new members act as catalysts to propelling the group process from a basic provincial, "autistic," symbiotic dynamic to the beginning of individuation and separateness that could not be achieved by all-combat veteran group alone.

The advent of the *catalyzing group agents* and the changed posture of the leader stirs up a variety of vertical and horizontal parental and sibling feelings of anger and resentment. These feelings relate to the group members' perception of having been rejected, and displaced by the new members. And the proverbial "revolt against the leader" begins or intensifies. It should be noted that the "revolt against the leader" or the so-called "primal horde" phenomenon occurs in most groups, whether they be structured or unstructured, reality-oriented or dynamic, laboratory or therapeutic, or "leader-centered," or "group-centered" (Kissen, 1976). For the Vietnam veteran group members this revolt has a special significance. For some members it represents a "getting even" with a rejecting and narcissistic paternal autocracy (or an emotional explosive rebellion against the United States Government and its various agencies including the Veterans Administration). For still other group members the revolt represents a manifestation of a most feared and abhorred fantasy: the reactivation of "split-off" memories and affects related to past killings in Vietnam, along with the attendant excitement and revulsion. Examples of outwardly rebellious behavior are observed in a number challenging group queries: "Why do we need new members, anyway?" "They weren't over there, what do they know about Vietnam? You've got to be there man to know what's going on;" "You (leader) are going to destroy this group. In fact, you already have. It's a shame." These sentiments are usually reflective of the group dynamics of "You (leader) and Us." The newcomers are usually intimidated by the group (older members) and soon identify with them, joining them against the leader. Newcomers also are angry with the leader for subjecting them to a "hornet's nest;" and together with older members join in the rebellion against the leader. As a full-blown *developmental crisis*, the "primal horde" phenomenon brings group members together, closer than they had ever been before. This crisis results in a critical shift in dynamics from "pleasure principle" indulgence and symbiosis to "reality principle" objectivity and interdependence (Appelbaum, 1963), from a "basic assumption" group to a "work" group (Bion, 1959). Many believe that unless this *symbiotic killing* of the group leader (as in the "revolt") takes place in the group's process the attainment of true interpersonal relatedness and a sense of freedom and autonomy among group members would not be possible.

During the second-phase group the old group sense of mutual harmony and universal acceptance and love is recognized for what it is—a patent unreality born of group irrational processes. Moreover, the myth of mutual universal victimization by the world is given up, and now emerges a group sense of shared responsibility for the group experiences and each member for his contribution to the process. It is by no means easy for a group which had been enmeshed in a group cohesion characterized by the mutual self-view of victims, to give up this view of self and world. It requires a herculian capacity on the part of the leader for managing difficult group therapeutic processes. Whereas the first-phase group was characterized by *high structure* despite the leader's "ghost presence," the second-phase group fosters a relatively less structured group environment, focusing on the here-and-now interactive dynamics and feelings expressed and unexpressed in the group setting. The second-phase is *leader-centered*, in that his or her group role is clearly defined and demarcated, in contrast to the first-phase period in which no such demarcation was established. This leader-centered (as opposed to *group-centered* approach) is a critical occurrence in the group experience, for many of the power-dominated, phallic drive concerns with domination, submission, with "being ripped off" by the Government, as well as the group members' fear of being punished by authority persons for their war actions, can only be worked through as these feelings and related concerns are projected onto the group leader and the group works toward resolution and integration of these critical issues. For the Vietnam veteran, treatment is never complete unless therapeutic provisions can be made that would address powerful issues related to phallic or power relations with self and others. The veteran, therefore, must be given the opportunity to work through authority problems with others by understanding the roots of his distorted perceptions of the leader. Whether Vietnam veteran or not, the leader will be tested as he has never been tested by group members before. Angry group members will accuse the leader of "selling out" to society, of being just like the Veterans Administration, of using the same tactics of deception used against them by the United States Government who "sold us down the river." These and other such "assaults" upon the leader are quite integrating and healing to group members, and they present a tremendous challenge, much discomfort, and testing to the leader. It is essential that the group leader be firmly anchored psychologically. The goals of this group phase attempt to:

1. Enlarge the group's resources in terms of novelty, originality, uniqueness, and distinctiveness by the introduction of new members into the group's environment. Diversification of intrapersonal psychodynamics and enrichment of interpersonal learning is to be accomplished in this phase. This relates to the observation that "the more heterogeneous the membership, the more accurate does the group become, for each member, a microcosm of the rest of his interpersonal experiences" (Bennis and Shepard, 1956, p. 416).

2. Deepening of trust.

3. Expanding members' self and interpersonal awareness of their feelings, thoughts and behavior and how these impact upon others, as well as how others affect them internally.

4. Beginning of direct exploration of the "false self" organization (Winnicott, 1960) and its various interpersonal manifestations within the group.

5. Establishment and maintenance of true and heightened peer interaction.

6. Stimulate growth from "mirror-reflected," symbiotic over-identification to matured forms of interpersonal relating.

7. Establish the foundation for the therapeutic work of the third-phase group (the psychoanalytically-oriented group).

Selection Criteria for Second-Phase Group Membership. The members that form the second-phase group are selected for the good of the group. Thus, rather than asking, "Is the group *good for this veteran?*" the leader asks instead, "Is the prospective veteran member good for the group?" This approach is essential to selection, though not widely discussed in the group literature. Improper introduction of particular patients into a group can deteriorate the group process, instigating acting-out, heightened resistances, and other forms of regressive dynamic activity that thwarts the on-going developmental movement of the group (Kellerman, 1979). Whereas the first-phase "rap" group is composed of *all* combat veterans exclusively, the second-phase group is made up of Vietnam era veterans to include a woman veteran, whenever possible. A woman Vietnam veteran who can tolerate the anxieties, anger, resentment, and male-chauvinistic posture within a male-dominated group environment, could conceivably help facilitate her own growth while providing an atmosphere in which developmentally useful internalizations for the group could occur. These internalizations usually assist the male veteran to become more familiar with the "female side" of himself, thereby learning to become more comfortable with tenderness and interpersonal warmth, with both men and women. To be able to feel and share tenderness, sensitivity, or "just plain feeling soft" as one veteran put it, represent a major psychological achievement for many symptomatic Vietnam veterans. Many combat members have for many years adopted a trained inability to feel (Egendorf, 1978) that this writer refers to as the *counter-tender tendency*, which actually began during basic military training and became more pronounced during combat and postcombat experiences. While in Vietnam many soldiers were still struggling with developmental adolescent issues revolving around self identity and sexuality in general. Thrown head-on into an environment in which women were conceived as inferior, treacherous, dangerous, unfeeling, and untrustworthy during this relatively vulnerable developmental epoch, these persons have become arrested in their conception of women. Additionally, young American troops (enlisted men) often felt despised and rejected by

American women who preferred officers to enlisted men. Feelings and perceptions generated and crystallized by these experiences with women in Vietnam persist today in many veterans of that conflict. But these feelings and perceptions remain distortions, and will continue to persist unless an appropriate therapeutic forum in which these issues could be explored, confronted, and worked through, can be established. The second-phase group experience is such an appropriate forum. Women who were in the military and in Vietnam also have perceptions that place men in a negative category of personal experience. They often view men as uncaring, abusive, contemptuous of women, and basically "anti-woman." For both sexes, many of these mutual distortions have gone virtually unchallenged and therefore unexplored and so remains unenlightened.

In general, the second-phase group selection process focuses on persons who are "diagnostically facilitative" to the group; that is, persons whose needs and psychodynamics are basically congruent with the developmental needs of the group-as-whole. Thus, severe forms of psychopathology are to be excluded in this selection process. New members are to fall within the "higher-level" borderline (Kernberg, 1975), neurotic, mild characterological disorder categories, with a predominance of "higher-level" defenses (Laughlin, 1979). First- and second-phase group inclusion of ethnic, gender, diagnostic, and psychodynamics diversity provides the group's environment with a true microcosmic representation of the real world. Additionally, the nontheater veteran ("era") will have a useful opportunity to work out his or her guilt feelings about not having served in Vietnam, and, perhaps, for the first time be able to put into a personally meaningful perspective the national and personal confusions of the war era.

In line with the proposed "developmental-regressive" model mentioned earlier in which first-phase group dynamics were located within the phallic stage of psychosexual development, the second-phase group has a predominance of "anal stage" concerns (particularly during the revolt against the leader period) about the leader's ability and willingness to punish. But these concerns and conflicts are soon resolved with good and competent leadership. The group then moves on (during the second phase) to a subphase of *interdependence* (among members). This interdependence among group members is a new level of interacting, and for many Vietnam veterans this event marks the advent of the "restoration of broken linkages" between self and culture, and an attempt at reparation of the "derailment of the dialogue" (Mahler et al, 1975, p. 94) between the veteran and society at large. Unlike during the first-phase "rap" group experience in which members were tied to each other in a boundaryless, identity-diffuse manner, the second-phase group represents a move toward preoccupation with individual identity and shared responsibility. This phase, also, marks an important milestone in the attainment of ego autonomy in group members. "Ego autonomy" is a concept developed by Heinz Hartmann (1950) and elaborated upon in a number of papers by David Rapaport (1958). It refers to an aspect of ego strength in which the ego exercises its voluntary control and regulation over external as well as external stimuli. The group member who achieves ego autonomy will manifest increased personal independency from the group's norm; and, in Winnicott's sense, can now allow more of the "true self" to emerge.

But the interdependency of the second-phase group is not free of conflict. The conflict that develops, however, is of a different nature. It is a conflict among members, born not of a symbiotic merger as in the first-phase group ("I don't like this about you, but we are all despised veterans."), but of a recognition of emerging ego boundaries and individual identity ("I understand what you feel, but I feel this way.") among fellow group members. Thus the first-phase group sentiment, "We are all Vietnam vets, despised and hated by all, filled with anxiety and stress, we are all we have," to "We are Vietnam era vets, perhaps despised by some, but not by all, and we cope with differing degrees of success with our anxiety, we can count on others." Perhaps stated in a rather exaggerated manner, this writer likens the Vietnam veteran's rediscovery of human contact and interest as the toddler's "love affair with the world" (Greenacre, 1957), and represents an important maturational shift in the veteran's struggle toward self readjustment.

Essential Qualities of the Leader in the Second-Phase Group. The leader's second-phase leadership posture is pivotal. For this phase of the group's development requires the leader to "shift technical gears" from being an "integrated" member of the group (the undifferentiated "ghost presence"), to a more active therapeutic stance in which he *asserts himself as leader.* This assertive position will "set up" the group leader as an object of group transference reactions. This means that the group members are to be allowed to perceive him as an "infallible" expert problem-solver—a magical one who can make all things right. The new leader posture differs from phase one, then, in that he is no longer "one of the guys" but has emerged as the leader upon whom the group's projections can be directed.

The group leader must also have the ability to tolerate projected group aggression, as well as be able to understand and facilitate positive and nurturant emotions and their appropriate expressions among group members. Moreover, the leader is to allow the group's process to converge upon him, and to manage the group dynamics by the technical use of clarification, confrontation, and empathic reflection. It is during this phase of the group treatment that the leader has the most therapeutic leverage in exploring and clarifying institutional transference feelings toward the Veterans Administration (Parson, 1981), and toward the Government as a whole. Chronically complaining veteran group members need to achieve insight into their motivations and feelings that do not align themselves with reality. The leader, then, is a beacon of orientation to reality.

Third-Phase Group: The Psychoanalytically-Oriented Group with Vietnam Veterans

The third-phase group is initiated when the developmental goals of the first two group phases have been achieved. The advent of the third group is predicated upon the more or less full recovery from stress-related traumatic symptoms such as flashbacks, nightmares, and general autonomic hyperresponsivity. The assumption is that sufficient psychic structure would have developed in each group member during the first- and second-phase group experiences. Such development of new psychic structure would conceivably assist group members in withstanding and tolerating the new regressive "pull" inherent in the analytically-oriented group experience.

The goals of the third-phase group intend to:

1. Achieve characterological change by continuing and deepening the affective and experiential group processes of the previous group phase, and by the systematic exploration of unconscious mental life and character defenses and resistances, *within* the individual group member and interactively *among* members.

2. Enhance self-insight and awareness begun during the second-phase group.

3. The working through of remaining personality deficits related to person-specific dynamic meanings of the war experience for the veteran group member (Hendin et al, 1981).

Selection Criteria for Third-Phase Group Membership. The composition of the third-phase group aims to achieve a still more diversified personality dynamic type. It is recommended that new members' dynamics and needs systems facilitate the group process rather than hinder it by the inclusion of severely depressed, low-level borderline, or psychotic group members. Group members' diagnoses for this group phase (third) should fall generally within the neurotic to high-level borderline to narcissistic range of pathology. Higher-level veterans with posttraumatic stress disorder symptoms can also be included as new members in this group, provided he or she had had the opportunity to deal adequately with the Vietnam experience and related stress symptomatology, as well as have attained a reasonable degree of psychological-mindedness (or psychological sophistication). This group formation is not for the veteran who is either beginning or failed to have addressed his reactions and possibly disorders stemming from the war involvement, though his or her symptoms may seem mild and few. This writer's experience suggests that the introduction of non-veterans (prospective members with no military experience), women, and ethnically diverse persons (whenever possible) into the group provides a rich working group environment. This kind of group formation facilitates the exploration and working through of war-linked dynamics; women and sexuality (for men, and men and sexuality for women group members); as well as ethnic prejudice within the group.

Essential Qualities of the Leader in the Third-Phase Group. During this phase the leader is to have the ability to engage members in interactively intensive group work. He or she is thus expected to understand the nature of character resistance, ego defenses, and the therapeutic use of dreams in the group to enhance the analytic group process. The leader is expected, moreover, to have a relatively integrated ego, and be capable of engaging his own feelings in the group work and use these feelings toward the constructive ends of promoting growth among group members. Formal training and supervision are important prerequisites in conducting a therapeutically useful third-phase analytic group. To meet the individual and group needs, the leader will also be expected to understand the subtle metacommunicational signals and to intervene from the vantage points of both *individual-within-the-group* and the *group-as-a-whole*.

Kissen (1976) discusses a number of qualities of the analytic group leader and the challenges and issues that arise in the work. He writes:

The task . . . is indeed mind boggling. One must attempt somehow to synthesize, through a variety of intervention strategies, many complex and partially overlapping data sources and therapeutic demands. One should not fall too easily into a stylistic interpretive format that neglects particular domains of therapeutic knowledge in favor of others. All levels of inquiry (ie, intrapsychic, interpersonal, group dynamic, sociocultural, etc.) must somehow be incorporated into an overall intervention strategy during the source of the group psychoanalytic experience (p. 342).

The ability of the leader to shift flexibly between intervening on the intrapsychic level to processes converging upon the group matrix is invaluable in analytic groups.

It is important to note that leadership in the multiple-group model proposed in this chapter makes extraordinary demands on the group's leader. Throughout the three group-types (the first-phase, second-phase, and third-phase), the leader is expected to remain constant, though exercising great flexibility and adaptational capacities as the group moves developmentally from the first-phase "rap" group through the second-phase "rap" psychotherapy group to the third-phase analytic group. Elaborating on the psychic capabilities essential for good group leadership, Kissen (1976) states:

The leader must be acutely aware of the impact of a particular style of intervention (ie, intrapsychic, interpersonal, group dynamic, etc.) on the largely circular feedback and validation processes received in return from the group members. The ideal group leader, according to Kernberg, utilizes a solid ego synthetic capacity and firm sense of ego identity both to select a particular constant (or even shifting) style of intervention and to tolerate the dissonance and conflict created by the complex variety of hierarchically structured intervention strategies available. The leader's ego strength should also be associated with a freedom from undue countertransference distortions such as the need to be a "charismatic" figure and obtain narcissistic gratifications from interaction with the group members (p. 341).

The analytic group leader is to be able to provide the group with "containing" and "facilitating" functions in being a "good-enough mothering" one (Winnicott, 1960), and to assist group members in regulating closeness and distance among themselves. He, moreover, is to be attentive to the various transferences and interactions between and among group members; attuned to intrapsychic as well as to interpersonal dynamic operations; understand and utilize cross-countertransferences (between leader and co-leader); and the subtle metacommunicational nuances that pregnate in the group's multipersonal matrix.

Early during the formative period of the third-phase group, certain specific group ideas, emotional, and motivational expressions eventuate in conflict. The group process, like in the first phase group, may proceed toward cohesion, but this cohesion is defensive or resistive. What might third-phase group cohesion defend against? Often the underlying feelings and concerns revolve around "covert" group anxiety and conflict over perceived sense of separateness generated by the multiple and diverse personalities, gender and ethnic differences. Cohesion, at this juncture, must be transformed into differentiation, which leads to conflict, then to resolution. This resolution of the group's conflict stage is essential, and leads to a form of cohesion. Unlike other phase-specific group cohesion of earlier group phases, this latter cohesion is a higher-level cohesion, in a developmental sense. Whereas the cohesion of the previous group phases was based on the "false self" organization, this latter form of cohesion is based on the emergence of the "true self" organization. As Wong (1981) notes, "the maintenance of the 'false self' may help in the formation of group cohesion because the individual wishes to comply with the desires of the group leader and the group norms" (p. 319). This kind of cohesion, according to Slavson (1964), is antitherapeutic. Third-phase cohesion (secondary) may lead to group member individuation and psychic and interpersonal growth.

The major generic underlying conflicts of the third-phase group are "oral" conflicts, in contrast to the oedipal-competitive dynamics related to guilt and power of the first-phase group, and the "anal" dynamics influence of the second-phase group experience. This "dematuring" (Kellerman, 1979) principle and process involves structural regression of the group process toward maturity by "laying bare" the relatively more primitive levels of the psyche, and make them available to be influenced by the third-phase analytic group work. That is, the third-phase focuses on primitive modes of psychological defense with the intent of effecting maturational trends within the group and individual personality. This point of view of group development postulates that oedipal derivatives emerge before oral ones during the course of the group's development (Kellerman, 1979). Third-phase oral issues and feelings that are worked through for group members are feelings of vulnerability, deep desire to be understood by others, compassion, empathy, sympathy, affection, and the fear of being rejected. Additionally, in the third-phase group, all other psychosexual stage derivative conflicts converge to be worked through, to include oedipal-competitive urges and guilt; idealization of the leader, the military, emblems and insignias, and the Government; anal-concerns over duty and punishment, and oral conflicts.

Integration of the Multiple-Group Tri-Phasic Model

The position advanced and elaborated in this chapter thus far is that the psychic and social needs of the Vietnam war veteran can best be met by a system of group treatment that utilizes multiple groups, each group experience addressing more or less specific progressive needs of the veteran over time. This writer agrees with Paul Senft when he stated that the term "adjustment" is based on a fallacy. He believes that "one cannot 'adjust' a personal subject to a reality which is still to be structured by him, if it is ever to confront as 'objective' environment" (Senft, 1966, p. 285). The multiple group model is based on the observation and belief that the Vietnam veteran must be charged with the responsibility of structuring his own reality, for it is only then that true adjustment or readjustment can occur.

Description of "Rap" Group Members

1. Joe D. is a black 36-year-old man who served as an infantryman in Vietnam. At age 19 he saw heavy combat that seemed to radically alter him internally. He had had frequent engagements with the enemy, and had experienced the loss of buddies on two separate occasions. Joe is unmarried, but would like to be married some day. His problems with women seemed to revolve around inappropriate expressions of rage, and the basic problem he had experienced since Vietnam of not feeling close to anyone.

Joe grew up as the eldest of three boys. He relates that he had always wanted to be his father's favorite, but was constantly disappointed by his father's rejection. His youngest brothers were the favorites, especially the younger of the two. Joe had thus always envied his younger brothers.

Clinical symptoms presented were delayed onset to include sleep disturbance, hyperactivity of autonomic system, rage reactions, isolation, numbing and denial, constricted affect, survivor guilt, nightmares, depression, and flashback experiences. The trigger event for his current posttraumatic stress reactions was his losing his job held for five years, and the dissolution of an eight-year relationship with his girlfriend after a heated argument.

Joe's diagnosis: DSM III—I. Posttraumatic Stress Disorder; II. Borderline Personality Disorder, with numbing and paranoid features.

2. Art J. is a combat veteran of Italian heritage. Like Joe he had seen much war action, and left with a number of psychic scars related to his survival of a search-and-destroy mission that wiped out almost half of his unit. He recollects with vivid clarity the memories and intense emotions of that day.

Art grew up as the eldest of two boys and two girls. His father was strict, rigid, punitive, and overly demanding of him, especially to perform in a manner "a real man can and should." His father offered no praise for things he did well, but heaped criticism upon criticism upon him. Art believed his mother did not like him, and felt used by her in that she demanded that he care for his younger siblings and was held responsible for everything they did. Art recollects his anger and resentment at being misunderstood by his parents, and being made to feel "bad" about himself if he failed to meet his siblings' wishes. As he approached adolescence he began to experience duty as submission and passivity. He would actively avoid situations that induced passivity in him. He has always had difficulties in relating to women—before, during , and after Vietnam, and was able to relate to male authority figures only in an intensely ambivalent manner as he had with his own father.

Art's clinical symptoms at the time of the initial interview were repetitive nightmares, flashbacks to the war, insomnia, and rage reactions. The contents of his nightmares were crying children and adults killed by his unit, and his crippling anxiety and fear of his being attacked by the Viet Cong. Moreover, Art had witnessed a number of his buddies killed in a barrage of heavy enemy machine gun fire. Art's symptoms began five years after Vietnam, and persists to the present. He had been unable to hold a job, because, as he puts it, "no job was good enough for me."

Art's diagnosis: DSM III—I. Posttraumatic Stress Disorder; II. Borderline Personality Disorder, with impulsive, intrusive, and paranoid features.

3. Danny L. is a 34-year-old Hispanic combat veteran who served in the Navy's riverboat patrol. His boat would transport troops from one point to another in the Mekong Delta. He was 18

years old at the time. His boat was fired upon constantly and was almost sunk on four occasions by the Viet Cong. One day, Danny and men from his unit were caught in an ambush which left eight civilians dead, including two or three children. After this event, he became bewildered, filled with guilt and despair. He began to drink: he drank to be able to sleep and to forget the grisly sight of the dead bodies.

Danny grew up in an orphanage. He felt abandoned by his mother and father who could not and did not want to care for him. He got into fights frequently as a young child and adolescent. His parents were alcoholics and hard drug abusers for years. His presenting problems involved an alcoholic problem he had been treated for at a local Veterans Administration Medical Center; impulsivity; rage reactions; general "ego weakness" (Kernberg, 1979); intrusive ideation and affects; isolation and aloneness; numbing of the self and "Agent Orange" anxiety (Parson, 1982, 1983).

Danny's diagnosis: DSM III—I. Posttraumatic Stress Disorder; II. Borderline Personality Disorder, with impulsive and explosive features.

4. Tom H. entered the service at age 18, and a year later was sent to fight in Vietnam in the infantry unit. He fought in the TET Counteroffensive of 1968, and saw intense combat for prolonged periods of time in the jungles of South Vietnam. Within a year after he returned from 'Nam he got married to a long-time sweetheart. He was angry over how Vietnam veterans were maltreated by the American society, and he spent much of his time and money working to enhance the quality of life for Vietnam veterans. Tom was obsessed with work; and veteran activities absorbed his life and its energies. These activities often led to discord and conflict, which was, among others, a presenting problem at the initial interview. Tom is 34 years old.

Tom's early developmental history was a stormy one, complicated by the dissolution of his parents' marriage at age six. He had always felt abandoned and rejected by his father whom he subsequently saw once a year until age 16, at which time his father completely disappeared from his life. Tom grew up a bitter child, blaming his mother, his father, and himself for his "rotten lot" in life. Much of his anger was directed toward himself for being "such a terrible kid," because "If I weren't so terrible dad wouldn't have left us and we wouldn't be this poor." Tom felt stuck taking care of his mother and younger brother, but felt he had to because "no one else would."

Tom's diagnosis: DSM III—I. Posttraumatic Stress Disorder; II. Borderline Personality Disorder, with depressive, impulsive, and explosive features.

5. John T., a 35-year-old white Jewish war veteran, was a heavy combat infantryman in Vietnam, who saw considerable combat. He was well decorated for heroism and valor. He was divorced from his wife of five years; they have a four-year-old son. John had tremendous readjustment psychological problems over the years since his return home in 1970. His current symptoms began almost immediately after his repatriation. His nightmares, whose content and theme is of being chased by a band of Viet Cong, running away from them as fast as he could, and then becoming trapped and cornered with no where to go, is a distressing and painfully disorganizing experience for him. Flashbacks to dead bodies, to gruesome vocalizations of men shot or being burned by napalm, to firefights are often triggered off by a variety of sounds and smells as well as the sight of trees and heavy foliage. John also expressed his tremendous guilt that half of his platoon which he led had been "wiped out." He blamed himself. He said, "I lost an arm, I should have lost two arms and a leg, or maybe I should have been wiped out with the others." John also reported during the initial interview a poor job history; irritability; rage reactions; autonomic hyperactivity, depression, and anxiety.

John grew up in New York City in a large family, the third of six brothers and sisters. He is from an intact family backround with no evidence of prior psychiatric difficulties. He was a good student, and felt he was well cared for by his parents. He recollects, however, that he was very close to his mother and was referred to by family members as "Mommy's boy." He felt his father never had time for him, and that his success as a businessman was more important than he. Additionally, John had always felt misunderstood by his father, and had craved his father's attention and respect, especially during his adolescent years, but only to be rebuffed and pushed aside as he had most of his life.

John's diagnosis: DSM III—I. Posttraumatic Stress Disorder; II. Passive-Aggressive Personality Disorder, with borderline features.

6. Junior T., who is a 35-year-old Black war veteran, spent the first 15 years of his life in a reform school. He was placed there, not

because he was a behavior problem (for, in fact, he was a very passive child), but because his parents' marriage had broken up, and they neither could nor wanted to care for him. It was "all for their convenience," he said. Visits by his mother were rather sporadic and few, and there was a markedly "incredible coldness" that characterized these visits. Junior could not understand why he was singled out for such maltreatment. He wanted to leave, but could not. His mother said she would consider doing so when he was a "good boy, not before." He noted that other children's parents returned "to bail their kids out of that place" when they were asked to do so. "But not in my case."

Junior joined the Marines at age 17 "to prove myself as the best;" and was sent to Vietnam within 18 months. He saw considerable combat in Vietnam and recollects with tearfulness the grizzly existence he lived for 13 months. He reported symptoms of flashbacks, sleep disturbance, the "startle" response, anxiety, depression, and an explosive, impulsive style of interpersonal relating. Junior is remarried and has two children, a boy with his first wife, and a girl with his second wife. "Neither of them understand me."

Junior's diagnosis: DSM III—I. Posttraumatic Stress Disorder; II. Borderline Personality Disorder, with passive-dependent, impulsive, depressive, and psychopathic features.

Description of the Second-Phase Group Member Additions

7. Jay T. is a 37-year-old white veteran of Armenian background; he was born in upstate New York. He grew up in an intact family with three brothers and two sisters, with no problems either at home or in school. Jay is a Vietnam era veteran: he served in the Army on the east coast and in Germany. Many of Jay's friends he grew up with were sent to serve in Vietnam. They would write letters about their various exploits with danger. He wished to go to Vietnam as well, but he could not get his superiors to comply with his request. Six months, after his friends, Jerry and Harvey, were in Vietnam, Jerry was killed, and two months later Harvey lost an arm and sustained a number of shrapnel in his skull.

Jay's presenting problems centered around the issues of general malaise, guilt, depression, and the seeming inability to "get my life on the right track." Despite the prolonged nature of these problems, he had earned a Masters degree in business administration and had held a number of jobs, each one bringing him higher up the ladder of success. Though talented, however, he engaged in self-defeating characterological behaviors which often resulted in his losing good jobs, and precipitating the breaking up of relationships with women. Jay has never been married, but believes he would like to "give it a try." His expressions were marked by an affectless, detached, controlled, and intellectual character.

Jay's diagnosis: DSM III—I. Depression, Recurrent; II. Compulsive Personality Disorder, with dependency and narcissistic features.

8. Karen K. is a 28-year-old woman who sought help with her recurring memories of her brother, Ken, who was killed in Vietnam. She was very close to him, and when he died "in that terrible place" a part of her "died with him as well." The degree of psychic identification with Ken was profound; however, she denies suicidal ideation or gestures. Karen's guilt and depression over the years have significantly interfered with her personal growth.

Karen grew up in an upper-class white protestant family background. She had enjoyed a close relationship with her father until he died of heart disease when she was 18 years old. "He gave me everything I ever desired," she reported. Ken was her "big brother" with whom she became close after their father's death. He, like father. protected Karen from a psychotically disturbed mother toward whom she felt great pity and ambivalence. She seldom dated, and found it inordinately difficult to establish meaningful and satisfying relationships with men.

Karen is an accomplished tennis player, holds a graduate degree in public health administration, and has a good job with great opportunities for advancement. During the interview she presented herself in a smug, detached, self-centered manner, appearing to need "center stage" adoration from the interviewer.

Karen's diagnosis: DSM III—I. Generalized Anxiety Disorder; II. Narcissistic Personality Disorder, with compulsive, depressive, and dependent features.

Description of the Third-Phase Group Member Additions

9. Toby J., a 29-year-old former wife of a Vietnam veteran, had sought psychological counseling in the past for her inner conflicts instigated by her ex-husband's stress pathology. She now sought assistance with working through and coming to terms with her personality dynamics and masochism. Toby felt that she had suffered immensely as the wife of a Vietnam veteran, but believed that her ex-husband reminded her of her own alcoholic father whom she unsuccessfully attempted to "cure."

Toby recollected her intense fear of her father's violence and moodiness. Her mother was very protective of the father "who could do no wrong." Her feelings of resentment and anger were repressed, so that all conscious sentiments were of pity, and the ardent desire to help him with his problem. After her divorce and initial counseling, Toby was able to resume college and has earned a Masters degree in social work, so "I can help all the people who need me."
Toby's diagnosis: DSM—I. Generalized Anxiety Disorder; II. Passive-Aggressive Personality Disorder, with compulsive and masochistic features.

As outlined above, the multiple-group concept features the progressive diversification of personality and individual psychodynamics by the calculated addition of new group members (as second- and third-phase groups) to the original core "rap" group membership comprised of all combat Vietnam veterans. It is the view here that systematic and careful addition of persons who would provide the group with a full range of character defenses and diagnoses is critical to the enhancement and acceleration of psychic growth and the activation of arrested psychic development. When this occurs, the veteran attains a level of self and structural cohesiveness that protects him from the regressive inclinations characterized by posttraumatic stress pathology. This system of group treatment obviously is equally useful and beneficial to the non-combat veteran as well as to the nonveteran group member. For example, during the third-phase group, though not herself a veteran, Karen was able to address, for the first time, her feelings of longing, loss, and grief over her brother who was killed in Vietnam and over the death of her father. In addition to this accomplishment, Karen, by the group's support and confrontational focus on her narcissistically insensitive, self-absorbed defensive style, gained insight into her unconscious terror of males, while enhancing her sense of womanhood and genuine gender identity.

The Therapeutic Group Interactions

This section of the chapter provides a brief sample of the types of interactions among and between group members at the three developmental group phases. Moreover, at each group phase, specific individual and group issues are illuminated briefly.

The "Rap" Group Interaction: Dealing with PTSD Symptoms. In this affinity group of men with the common experience of having served and suffered in and after Vietnam, Joe, Art, Danny, Tom, John, and Junior met in an effort to reconstruct their lives by engaging in an exploration and sharing of mutual anxieties, fears, grief, and agonies.

The leader's conduct of the group was in a manner characterized by minimal intrusiveness ("ghost presence"), avoiding the use of interpretation, and rather focusing on the vector for the array of symptoms; namely, the experience of the war and its aftermath in each group member's life.

1. *Reactive Numbing of the Self.* For most of the group members this phenomenon began in Basic Training, and culminating in the guerrilla actions of South Vietnam. In Vietnam group members, especially, Art, Joe, and Junior (who lost buddies), and Danny (after his unit's killing the Vietnamese civilians) developed "trained inability to feel" (Egendorf, 1978) in order to cope in an environment immersed in terror and counter-terror of a guerrilla war. Each group member began their group experience with constricted affect and feelings of detachment from self and others, which accompany any survivor's reactive numbing defense to psychic trauma. This writer maintains that psychic numbing is akin to *splitting* (Parson, 1983), a primitive defensive maneuver to allay trauma-related anxieties. Like most primitive defenses, splitting is incapable of generating the psychic protection from anxiety needed by the traumatized ego. The relative failure of this defense results in what this writer refers to as the "somatic accommodation to anxiety." Thus, headaches, nausea, soreness of muscles, general physical fatigue, numbness and tingling sensations, heavy feelings in arms and legs, and pains in lower back are symptoms often reported by persons with posttraumatic stress disorder (Horowitz, 1980). Many of these symptoms were reported by most group members. Somatic involvement of this nature represents a regression to more primitive forms of coping and adaptation, and can become a most intractible form of psychological resistance to the treatment process. As in most instances where splitting is used, aggression is present and functions to protect the vulnerable self from annihilation anxiety.

During the formative period of the group (ie, "rap" group), Joe, Art, and Danny were most expressive of their commonly shared numbing experiences. Later Tom, John, and Junior shared their concerns about their humanity as "unfeeling gargoyles." Knowing that each member had similar problems and concerns regarding their inability to feel, provided a therapeutically rewarding experience for these veterans. The group leader's capacity and willingness to share his own feelings and offering reassurance was also useful. The writer has found it useful to state the following when concerns and sentiments have become a group preoccupation in the beginning of the "rap" group. "I think I know what you are going through. To feel so numb and shut off, is also to feel strange within. You must know this, though, that your numbing serves a very important purpose. Numbing protects you from feeling certain things that you might not be able to bear at this time. This will go away as soon as you have learned to handle your stress symptoms in another way. Numbing is a natural response or reaction to what you have been through in Vietnam." In addition to verbal encouragement and reassurance, the group leader is to be prepared to intervene, on an as needed basis, with cognitive restructuring and behavioral techniques geared toward helping reduce the numbing. Biofeedback, meditation, progressive relaxation, and supervised exercise regime, were of immeasurable value to group members. Other interventions may include referral to a physician with demonstrated knowledge and sensitivity to persons suffering from posttraumatic stress disorder, for pharmacotherapy. In this writer's experience, guided imagery combined with relaxation procedures within the group can often precipitate important abreactive experiences of rage, sadness, guilt, and fear.

2. *Automatic Incursive Phenomena.* All group members had reported episodes of unexpected encroachment of an intrusive idea, memory, affect, or sensation upon their ongoing stream of consciousness. Nightmares and their gruesome details and contents, and the terror-evoking nature of flashbacks, were shared within the group environment of trust, cohesive mutuality, and safety. For the majority of veterans with these symptoms, experience has shown that great symptomatic relief is achieved in a short time in such group environs. The educational component of the treatment group experience is quite helpful in that it offers veterans an intellectual "anchor" by which these symptoms can be made comprehensible to group members. This writer has found that the "mini course" in PTSD and the discussions of related problems through "conceptual labeling" (Horowitz and Solomon, 1978) is a vital aspect of the "rap" group phase of treatment. Imparting intellectual knowledge to group members concerning their stress reactions and disorder is a move in the right direction toward gaining control over impulse-ridden, dissociated affective expressions. In another treatment

context, Brende (in press) found his "educational-therapeutic" approach to work well in a time-limited treatment regime with alcohol and drug-abusing Vietnam veterans. Cognitive and behavioral procedures are also quite useful in regulating incursive phenomena. These procedures brought accelerated symptomatic relief to group members, especially to Joe, Art, and Danny.

    3. *Alienation.* This symptom is akin to numbing and to splitting. It refers to a profound sense of aloneness and cold detachment from self and others. Alienation was especially evident in Art, Danny, and John. The feelings expressed among group members revolved around "feeling different" and "apart from other people." After several months of work, the group came to understand the defensive and protective dimensions of this symptom; that is, being alienated from others meant being relatively unresponsive to others, thus reducing the chances of losing control in the presence of others. Alienation also meant detachment from one's self, which served to dull one's awareness to anxiety, sadness, guilt, and other painful emotions. The alienated veteran has great difficulty in coming to terms with the possibility that someone in the external environment may be able to understand him and his problems. "Only if you were in Vietnam could you possibly understand what we are going through," group members would state for several months during the formative period of the "rap" group. However, during the second- and third-phase group experiences these sentiments had changed to reflect the newly acquired sense of shared human relatedness. Group members had come to learn that their sense of being at odds with culture (Lipkin et al, 1982) was related to their anger over having been narcissistically injured by a culture that had "sold them down the river of disrepute." Anger often prevents a "de-alienation" process. As group members became able and willing to address their anger and resentment over feeling abandoned and rejected by their own country, a longing for closer contact with others was observed.

    4. *The Nontrusting Attitude.* The suspension of trust in other people began in the jungles of South Vietnam for many veterans, where they discovered that children, women, and the elderly of Vietnam were unsuspecting terrorists. Inability to trust is also related to the negative repatriation experience, in which "a rupture in the covenant" between them and their country had occurred. As Danny once stated in this regard, "If an entire country can reject you, blame you, and fail to give you well-deserved respect, how can you trust anyone. When your own World War II hero father and one's mother question the legitimacy of what you did in Vietnam, who in

the hell can you trust?" In the "rap" group, members were able to relax their ordinarily rigid, pathological, fear-determined defenses and allow themselves to be touched by the others' experience.

5. *Rage Reactions.* This symptom can be classified into six types of aggressive drive expressions, with overlap in most instances:

a. *Paranoid Rage* is a form of aggression that eventuates in violent outbursts. It is perhaps the most dangerous kind—for both subject and object—of affective expression. The inherent mechanism is rather complex, and involves an active dynamic interplay between the subject (the veteran) and an object (another person). In what appears to be a vicious cycle, paranoid expressions of rage begin with the subjective experience of *terror* in the subject, who anticipates assault from without. Rather than the expression of rage bringing relief (as in sadistic forms of aggression), it locks the subject into the "terror cycle" of rage expressions, followed by anticipated attack from an object (real or imagined), which engenders more terror, to more paranoid/defensive assault (in verbal-attitudinal or physical modes) by the subject. Paranoid rage is an expression of the endangered self, and its triggering mechanisms are mostly unconscious. From this writer's experience, the veterans most likely to express paranoid rage are those who both saw heavy combat and whose personal developmental history was marked by familial-generated trauma, for example, in the case of Junior who grew up in a home for boys, totally abandoned by his parents.

b. *Narcissistic Rage* is a response, not to inner terror, as in paranoid rage, but rather to the deeply felt sense of injury to the self that comes in the form of *insult.* This insult is not experienced by the individual "as some mild indignity that offends a circumscribed 'part' of the psyche, but a severe, profound assault and a concomitant deep wounding of the self-as-a-whole" (Parson, 1982, p. 6). Narcissistic rage is often expressed toward the United States Government, the Veterans Administration, and other such agencies by the veteran, who has felt cheated, "illegitimate," and insulted by the American people by the harshness of the repatriation experience. There are both conscious and unconscious components to narcissistic rage.

c. *Symptomatic Aggression* refers to "split-off," dissociated, and "de-regulated" anger often observed in persons suffering from posttraumatic stress disorder, whether combat veterans or other survivors of traumatic experiences. As *automatic incursive phenomena,* symptomatic aggression is not regulated by the ego; it is primitive, and internally disruptive and frightening to the subject. All group members reported the sudden, unexpected "going off the handle." The veteran is usually unable to make sense of these angry outbursts; and, for many represents a narcissistic injury.

d. *Self-Maintenance Aggression* is a type of anger used by the self to bring about integration when significant stress and other psychopathology threatens severe fragmentation. "When I expressed anger I felt things coming together; it was strange. I felt in touch with myself and my anger made me touch someone else, as well," Junior once said during a "rap" group session. For some veterans self-maintenance aggression assists them in breaking through the inner affective coldness, and ghastly gargoyle-like "plate-glass" feeling. This anger is for the most part unconscious, and plays a vital role in the maintenance of the self-concept.

e. *"Laundered" Aggression* is a defensive type of anger against the eruption of narcissistic rage, or the dreaded awareness of having committed atrocities, killed, or otherwise harmed someone in Vietnam. This form of aggression is manifested by behavioral denial of unconscious conflict, in which the subject engages in "doing good things for everyone."

f. *Self-against-Self Aggression* is the anger directed toward oneself. It is related to depression and intense guilt, especially survivor guilt and guilt over omission (inaction). Additionally, such self-directed anger has been noted in veterans who committed atrocities, as well as those caught up in impacted grief states over comrades killed in action. Provoking rejection and assault (verbal or physical) from others, dangerous thrill-seeking behavior, one-car accidents, etc. are instances of self-against-self aggression.

6. *Impacted Grief States.* Many Vietnam veterans have experienced much suffering and loss at a relatively young age in Vietnam. They have, for the most part, been unable to mourn fully, partly because of anger and guilt, as well as because they have not been able to forgive themselves for having survived. Most "rap" group members, especially Joe, John, and Art, reported their painful memories of loss, and inability to "come to terms" with lost buddies in Vietnam. For several months, group members grieved with painful tears and heavy hearts over their unusual and extraordinary losses, to include their adolescence, young adulthood years and innocence.

7. *The Authority Factor.* Many Vietnam veterans lost trust in their leaders in Vietnam, and blamed them for much of the mishaps, losses, and the uncelebrated and inglorious reception they received upon returning home. More than other veterans, Vietnam veterans feel that authority persons, agencies of the Government, such as the

Veterans Administration, and others have been unresponsive to their needs. As Joe put it, "It was these authority figures that sent us into the 'Nam, and for what? No, man, not to win. To play a game—a deadly game in which we got hurt, lots of us got hurt. If you can't even trust your leaders in a war, who can you trust, tell me."

The issue about authority came up early in the "rap" group. Each member felt this was central to their lack of trust in persons "over them." The group leader, especially if he is a combat veteran (as in the case of this writer), is spared any direct blame or expressed hostility toward him as authority person. During the second phase of the treatment, however, the leader brought this issue to the fore, while expressing interest in the possible reasons for his being spared of what had been given so freely to other authority persons.

8. *Guilt Feelings.* Intense guilt feelings were expressed by every group member. These feelings were in reaction to "the senseless killings," maimings, and atrocities on both sides. The variety of sources of guilt in Vietnam veteran group members may be classified as follows:

a. *Guilt of Commision* is guilt over having committed violent acts resulting in someone's death or maiming. Men who engaged in atrocities expressed this form of guilt in the group. *Atrocity-related guilt* is extremely painful and damaging to the self.

b. *Guilt of Omission* is observed in men who blame themselves for cowardly, passive, or indecisive action resulting in someone else's death or injury in Vietnam. Group members mentioned regret over not having actively prevented or stopped an atrocity committed by others; or for not making the "right" decision that would have prevented half of his squad from being annihilated by the Viet Cong.

c. *"Gook"-Identification Guilt* is guilt expressed by, but not limited to, minority Vietnam veterans, who report their guilt feelings related to having killed "people of color" with whom they identified in a profoundly personal manner while in Vietnam.

d. *Guilt-About-Guilt* is observed in instances in which group members reported certain acts that made them guilty, but expressed guilt was a cover for a deeper and more anxiety-inducing guilt. Shapiro (1978) gives an excellent example of this king of guilt in his account of Dave, an Army lieutenant, a group member of the early "rap" groups in New York City. Dave had expressed guilt feelings about having killed a dog. Group members asked him why he was so guilty for killing a dog. With passion and tears Dave related earlier experiences with his pet dog and of the innocence of animals.

"Only months later was Dave able to share the more troubling aspects of his guilt; he had killed the dog in a mad frenzy on the day that three men whom he had sent on patrol were killed in an ambush. His guilt for sending them on this mission, whose usefulness he questioned, while he remained at camp, was very intense" (p. 170).

e. *Survivor Guilt* is guilt experienced by the survivor (of combat or other catastrophe) whose life was spared, but someone else's was lost. Art, Joe, John, and Junior explored at length their guilt feelings over having "made it" and their buddies, whose lives they often felt were more valuable than their own, being killed. In survivor guilt, there is a profound identification of the subject with person or persons who lost their lives. This makes the guilt much more difficult to resolve; however, in the "rap" group setting with a skillful group leader, survivor guilt can be understood and integrated.

9. *Intimacy and Relationships with Women.* Group members spoke of their difficulties in relating to women. They believed that the suffering they had both witnessed and brought to the lives of the Vietnamese people disqualified them from being capable to tenderness and human concern for a woman. Joe, Danny, and Junior had expressed their concern that there was probably no woman that would accept them if she were to become aware of what they had seen or done in Vietnam. During the first month Art spoke of his difficulties in getting along with women. He felt that they did not like or respect him, and that he felt they were critical of him. Asking him for specific instances and examples of events with women, it was clear that much of his perceptions of women were distorted by his own relationship with his mother during his earlier experiences. This area was explored more fully during the second- and third-phase groups. Some group members' difficulties with women could not be accounted for by the Vietnam experience alone, but a byproduct of the dehumanized view of women in Vietnam and early problematic relationships with significant women, especially the mother.

Group members expressed their difficulties in getting close to anyone since Vietnam. Those who had lost buddies were especially affected in this area, as well as those members whose past personal dynamics had interfered with the internalization and structuralization of healthy object relations. Much of the "split-off," dissociated rage reactions reported by group members have the effect of keeping people at a distance. "It is really hard to get close to a woman when you are always angry and rageful," one member once said. Group members later learned, especially in the second-phase group that often their anger protects them from getting close to others, especially to a woman. Anger, therefore, keeps the veteran's "counter-tender" defenses intact, and so protecting the veteran from feelings of anxiety and vulnerability. Group members expressed their fears of having someone so close to them as to be able to "decipher" their "guilty souls," and to "take me over completely." Danny, Junior, and Joe wonderedwhether they could ever give, accept or recognize love and affection. As Danny put it, "After having the view of women, as I learned in Vietnam, that they are prostitutes, could be Viet Cong and kill you, that all they wanted was your money and your goods to place on the black market, it's been real hard for me to get that out of my mind." As the leader did throughout the "rap" group phase, he offered emphatic statements intended to engender hopefulness in group members. He told the group that their feelings of detachment, anxiety, fear, and hopelessness regarding women was understandable and expectable given their unique war experience. He went on to indicate to them that he was personally hopeful that their problems in this and other areas of their lives would become more manageable and less painful just as their flashbacks, anxiety, fear, numbing, intrusive ideas, feelings, and memories are now in much better control than when they first began the group.

10. *Anxiety.* This system is the cardinal symptom of PTSD, and it permeates the veteran's entire existence. It forces him into inaction ("petrifies") as well as into maladaptive actions. Anxiety causes the veteran to feel as if his world is coming to an end, which fills him with more apprehension, tensions, while reducing his problem-solving abilities. As Kurt Goldstein (1951) states, "In anxiety, disorganization is clearly apparent. It is . . . experience of the 'catastrophic situation' of danger, of going to pieces, of losing one's existence. . . . [It involves] the inner experience of catastrophe!" (p. 38).

A number of cognitive and behavioral techniques were found helpful in allaying anxiety in group members, during the formative period of the "rap" group. In rare instances anti-anxiety medications were needed. Biofeedback is also quite helpful to veterans with PTSD-anxiety; it brings calm and assists the veteran in achieving the inner experience of being in control.

11. *"Agent Orange" Anxiety.* This symptom has become an important complaint in Vietnam veterans over the past three years. It refers to the apprehension that a number of physical and psychological symptoms are due to dioxin poisoning. Parson (1982) describes this form of anxiety in the Vietnam war veteran. "To have to wonder whether the pains in one's side, the numbness in one's

hand, liver disease, the small cyst in one's back, severe skin rash, ulcers, neuromuscular difficulties, and gastrointestinal pathology, are symptoms of a powerful carcinogen to which one was exposed to while serving one's country a decade ago, is a source of great anxiety indeed" (p. 9).

12. *Depression.* The causes of depression are many for the Vietnam veteran. For group members depression stemmed from a variety of guilt (discussed earlier). The loss of buddies; the hopelessness of self-control; the loss of innocence and one's adolescence; the inability to have found one's niche at 35; difficulties in getting close to others and consummating a love relationship are chief sources of depressive affect. Suicidal feelings and gestures emerged in the group from time to time.

13. *The Pan-Suspicious Attitude.* This symptom is a byproduct of feelings of alienation, lack of trust in others and in the Government, and the general expectation of being humiliated, criticized, rejected, and abandoned by others. The pan-suspicious attitude partakes of both conscious and unconscious mental processes. Unlike stark paranoia, the pan-suspicious attitude is a natural and expectable reaction to psychic trauma where the environment had failed to provide nurturance, hopefulness, and protection. "Pan-suspicious" is used to denote the ubiquitous nature of the veteran's distrust and need to defend himself against "harm" to his inner sense of well-being and self-esteem.

14. *Alteration in Life Course and Its Processes.* Veteran group members demonstrated this symptom by their chronic unsophistication about vocational, educational, and social processes. "Wandering lifestyles and chronic underachieving and instability in education and work . . . settling for less, settling for dullness" (Lipkin et al, 1982, p. 910).

The Second-Phase Group Interaction: Becoming Comfortable and Aware of Feelings

The first-phase "rap" group dealt with stabilizing the veteran's ego functions, building some psychic structure that would be able to tolerate the work of the second- and third-phase group experiences. Whereas the first-phase group focussed on the *then-and-there* of the Vietnam experience, with little emphasis on the *here-and-now* of immediate experience within the group, the second-phase group places a high premium on the here-and-now interaction. Helping the veteran group members (both combat and "era" veterans) to become familiar with their inner life of emotions, and to acquaint themselves with the affective impact they have on others and the effect others' feelings have on them, is central to this group phase. Group members, for the most part, were most inclined to "fleeing from feelings," even though they would talk *about* their inner pain, they were unable to experience this in tolerable dosages. The second-phase group taught the group members how to get in touch with their true feelings, how to suffer controllably, and how to experience themselves in a different way.

During this phase, a notable shift was noticed in the balance between the aggressive and libidinal drive derivatives. Thus, group members' habitual self-experience of fear, panic, disillusionment, doubt, rage, destructiveness, resentment, illness, hostility, hate, distress, anxieties, and anguish were mitigated by re-learning to be comfortable and "at home" with a broad spectrum of positive, essential emotions, such as contentment, passion, concern, care, compassion, protectiveness, excitement, fickleness, happiness, hope, modesty, pleasure, pity, love, and innocence.

Toward the end of the first-phase group, the leader prepared the members for the work of the next phase by giving a "mini" course of emotions and defenses against feelings. For the first time during the treatment experience, the importance of personal dynamics based on early conditionings were explored and given preeminence in the group's work. With the introduction of the new members to the group (in the second-phase group), as discussed earlier, and the subsequent "revolt against the leader," the focus on feelings, individual and group defenses and resistances appeared to be a natural sequel toward the end of the second-phase group experience. Uninsightful defensiveness was pointed out by the leader and/or group members and confrontation was a useful tool of change and growth.

The Third-Phase Group Interaction: Enhancing Growth by Character Change

The third-phase group's focus differs in important ways from the two previous phase-groups. The emphasis is on the systematic analysis of defenses, transference (multiple, hierarchical, and cross transferences with the group matrix among and between group members and group leader), and resistances to accomplish meaningful and lasting character change, as well as the activation of arrested personality development.

The first- and second-phase groups allowed the working through of "freeze dried" images of Vietnam (Blank, 1979), guilt, "instrumental" use of drugs and alcohol, and other symptoms and problems in posttraumatic stress disorder. Especially, during the second-phase group, group themes emerged similar to those reported by Brende (in press). Brende mentions the following group themes during a time-limited group encounter with drug and alcohol abusing Vietnam veterans: encountering death, dehumanization, and the "killer-victim" identification; the "killer identity;" rage about injustice, humiliation, and infantilization by military officers; the "identity split" (Jeckyl-Hyde); encountering the loss of self; and grieving.

In working through these issues in the first two group experiences, only minimal attention was given to individual dynamics within the group, though there were a number of sessions in which the group focussed on a specific individual's pain and Vietnam-related anguish. During the second-phase group, especially during the "revolt against the leader" subphase, the leader directed his interventions toward the *group-as-a-whole* (rather than toward individuals in the group) in an exclusive *here-and-now* structure. However, in the third-phase analytic group treatment the leader's interventions are directed toward both the "horizontal" (ie, the here-and-now group member interactions) and "vertical" (ie, the there-and-then of personal-historical dynamics) axes of the group interactive matrix.

In the psychoanalytic group experience, group members are expected to share in great detail the stories of their lives (Ormont, 1964). This procedure has been found important for two basic reasons: (1) Group members would later be able to grasp genetic-dynamic links between their current group characterological behaviors, and the leader's interventions (especially interpretations); and (2) to promote a sense of individual identity replete with genetic, contemporary, and futuristic dimensions. It is interesting to note how quickly and well group members learn from each other and the leader how to recognize behavior manifestations of character traits in fellow group members.

The group arena proved an excellent forum for the exposure and analysis of *illness-maintaining*, ego-syntonic character defenses in group members; and with the "instrumentalized" diversity of dynamics and diagnoses that comprised the group's formation, acceleration of growth was facilitated for the group. This heterogeneous composition of the group was helpful to members in resolving conflicts with parental, sibling, and contemporary relationships. The third-phase group attempted to break through characterological defenses and armoring to allow growth-arresting anxieties to become released. Many group members pathology was steeped in character resistances (to getting well), making extraordinary demands on this group leader and on the group's observing ego. Group members with impulse control problems (ie, Danny, Art, Tom, and John), within the group structure, had the opportunity to internalize aspects of higher-level ego controls conceivably made available through interaction with obsessive-compulsively organized group members (ie, Jay, Toby, and Karen). Basic terror-stricken character defensive style of Joe and Art were "matched" by the basic calm of John, Junior, and Toby, as well as the terror-"containing" qualities of the group-as-a-whole and the competent, facilitating leader.

Characterological resistances based on repressed intrapsychic conflicts were explored during this phase. Joe's problems with women reached intense proportions in the group. He perceived Karen as powerful and castrating, as well as calculatingly cold, aloof, intellectual and snobby, while the leader was viewed as rejecting of him, but preferring other members and what they had to say. Dynamically, Karen had for several weeks demonstrated an intense attraction for Joe, but viewed him as unstable, that he "might not even be there next week," in spite of the knowledge that Joe had been a group member for over two years. The leader and group addressed these emotional entanglements between Joe and Karen by pointing out that Joe's perception of Karen may be related to his perception of his own mother who disappointed him and used him; and that his feelings toward the leader were motivated by archaic feelings and perceptions of his father as he grew up. Pointed out to Karen was that her ambivalent attraction to Joe was based on her need to find a brother in someone, and so could continue to deny that he and her father were really dead. Her tears were the first ones ever shed for her lost brother and father. She never had allowed herself to cry. Other members of the group who had great difficulty in grieving for dead buddies were empathically touched and deeply affected to observe and experience Karen's pain. In the past, Karen had habitually "offended the group" by her aloof, intellectualized, narcissistic-avoidant position, in which she would tell jokes and flippantly "make light" of serious group issues.

Danny and Tom's explosive character traits, now much more regulated and ego-controlled by this group phase, continued to use intimidation in order to regulate their self-esteem. Their behavior often threatened havoc to the group process. Their covert aggression and potential explosiveness was particularly troublesome to the passive-aggressive personality group members (John and Junior), and group members with paranoid traits (Joe and Art). Group members and leader-directed confrontation was helpful here. Jay asked Danny why was it that he wanted to intimidate him, that he'd always felt intimidated in the group, especially by him. Jay wondered whether it was because he was a noncombat veteran. Other group members (Karen and Toby) shared Jay's sentiment, and said that Danny had a need to be a "super 'Nam vet" because he didn't have anything else to hold onto in his life. Danny seemed visibly "shaken" by this comment. The leader asked Danny for his feelings, noting to him that something was going on inside him. He chose to remain quiet. The leader's subsequent intervention led to Jay's expression of having always been guilty for not having "made it" to the 'Nam. He also revealed an irrational fantasy of omnipotence he had never shared with anyone before. The fantasy was that had he been in Vietnam with his friends none of them would have been killed or made disabled. The group allowed his feelings to be expressed more fully, and members were empathic toward Jay's inner disquietude. Jay felt, also, that combat group members were "very, very fortunate people." Later group sessions helped Jay to work through his rigid, guilt-induced self-defeating characterological behavioral pattern. His obsessive-compulsive defensive rigidity had been experienced by group members as a "turn off," because group members had viewed him as "uninvolved" in the group, and "not wanting to be with us." The leader pointed out to the group that given who Jay is as a person that feelings and getting close to others are very difficult for him as these have been for many others in the group.

This group episode also revealed Danny's intense narcissistic prejudice and anger against "all those who didn't serve in the 'Nam," and helped him connect his feelings to a deeper and more significant source of disapointment and "injustice," namely, to his abandoning and rejecting parents who "didn't serve" him during the years he needed them most. Tom was the group's peacemaker. During this phase it was stated to him directly that he must be "hiding out" (defensively maneuvering) in his avid seeking to make reparation and peace among group members. Toby once said to him, "The war isn't here; why the peacemaker bag?" Other group members from time to time felt and expressed similar sentiments to Tom. Tom had become angry, stating he felt attacked. The leader intervened and reminded the group that in this group phase "all is grist for the analytic group mill," and that group members were only expressing what they felt. Other members were called upon to comment on Tom's angry expression of being attacked. A spirited interaction ensued. Tom said that no one understood what Vietnam veterans have been through. He was cut off by Karen and Toby, who vociferously said that they weren't in Vietnam, but that they understood, felt, and experienced enough to have a good idea what it is all about. Toby mentioned what she'd been through with her ex-husband, while Karen spoke about the loss of her brother in Vietnam and the pain she has endured. The leader pointed out Tom's defensive posturing in feeling misunderstood, and asked for group members' reactions to what they felt was going on. Combat group members said they no longer felt misunderstood and unappreciated, though they stated that they had felt this way for years prior to the "rap" group experience. The leader brought the group's focus back to the original issue; that is, to the possible defensive underpinnings to Tom's habitual peacemaking group behavior, and seeming desire to take care of everyone. The leader later wondered whether Tom's desire to help and care for others was linked to earlier patterns in his life. Danny then asked, "Didn't you say not too long ago that you had to take care of all your family—your mother and brother because you felt if you didn't nobody else would do it?" Tom nodded in the affirmative. The entire group fell silent for a few minutes. Art broke the silence and stated that he has always had a need to care for people also, but that, because of the treatment, he had received some insight suggesting that this pattern for him was due to early pain and humiliation with his father, and his need to care for his siblings though he despised caring for them. A somber and painful countenance appeared in his face; and he yelled, "I needed to be cared for, too, but no one was there for me. My father didn't care, and my mother couldn't have cared less." Group members then proceeded to share their personal feelings of having been humiliated by parents, friends, and other people in the past, and the things they learned about themselves. Tom now spoke up and identified with Art's feelings. He went on to state that he should not express his anger directly toward his father and mother as he would have liked to have done, so he repressed it, but had felt "driven" to be "good." Art again spoke, stating that he hated his passivity and his inclination "to do the good things." Doing the right thing, he noted, made him dull, boring, and empty, and with no sense of being a person.

In a subsequent session, Danny's significant oral character traits of magical omnipotence were mirrored by Jay's omnipotent fantasies of saving his dead and injured friends had he been in Vietnam with them. Group members took note that both these members had a similar issue, though their military experiences were quite different (ie, Danny is a combat vet; Jay an "era" vet). The leader added that much of Danny's oral emphasis was based, not as much on Vietnam, as it is on early childhood deprivations and trauma suffered by parental neglect. This led to a rich interactive exploration of early parental disapointment as well as significant residual transference reactions (within combat veterans) to the Veterans Administration, this writer has referred to elsewhere as the "Big Daddy" transference (Parson, 1981).

In a later session Toby expressed her concern about Vietnam veterans in general; she felt they "were really screwed over." In her first-phase group, this utterance would have been accepted at face value. However, in the second-phase, but especially in the third-phase group such comments take on great importance. The leader asked Toby if she was aware of the possible meaning the statement uttered had for her and for the group. Toby had opened the group session with her comment. She said, "I just feel pity for some vets." "Any vets in the group, in particular?" asked the leader. "Well, I do feel that Danny had been through a lot in life." "What about other group members, have they suffered as much as Danny?" again asked the leader. She replied that "He's suffered the most." Subsequent exploration in the group revealed Toby's transference feelings toward Danny whom she viewed as potentially violent, and being "an alcoholic personality." Toby's distorted and projected elaborations were pointed out to be related to her repressed hostility toward her own alcoholic father for whom she harbored great contempt, but showed, and was aware of, pity for him. Toby then spoke at great length about her ex-husband and their life together. Months later she was able to "make some sense" of her attraction to her ex-husband, and of the masochistic adaptation she had chosen for herself.

Toby's repetitive ego-syntonic masochistic character patterns were further highlighted by her sharing experiences with the group regarding her new boyfriend, George. "Why do you put up with that; he's an animal," Joe stated in a loud voice that betrayed deep feelings. "Get rid of the jerk!" he continued. Various group members addressed Toby's plight with her boyfriend. Later they focussed on Joe's emotion-laden concerns about George. Joe stated that perhaps his anger toward George might have stemmed from something within him; and was helped to see this possibility by the group in a much clearer and meaningful way. Joe had transferentially perceived George as a "bad" father (as he had viewed a number of military officers), while the leader was perceived and experienced as the "good" father. This borderline-type of transference splitting was noted in a number of the combat veterans, and though difficult to resolve, the writer has found that a co-leader (preferrable female or noncombat veteran) is extremely essential in working with borderline patients (Greenblum and Pinney, 1982).

Other Third-Phase Group Issues. When nightmares persisted into the third-phase group, they were approached in the group like any other unconscious product (such as slips of the tongue, dreams, associations, etc.). Thus, John's persistent nightmare of being chased and captured by the Viet Cong was later understood as representing his persecutory and punitive superego related to guilt over repressed hostility and murderous rage toward his father, whose love and affection he had craved, but never experienced with him. John's dissociated anger was also related to his fear of engulfment by his mother, and he blamed her "for infantilizing me and not helping me to grow up and mature." Aspects of John's passive-aggressive personality style was pointed out to him and explored within the group. He subsequently learned to be more assertive and less fearful of his own aggression.

During this group phase, moreover, a number of conceptual, dynamic, experiential, and technical issues peculiar to borderline pathology and narcissistic character problems, were employed in the third-phase group experience (Kernberg, 1975; Teitelbaum, 1980; Drob et al, 1982; Alpert, 1980). Combat group members in this phase group, have achieved a more cohesive self, with less disruptions in their inner world by flashbacks and other *automatic incursive phenomena.* Notable improvement was noted in identity integration and in self-esteem regulation. Group members, both males and females, combat and noncombat veterans, and those without military experience were all able to explore with each other a variety of critical personal issues such as sexuality and sexual functioning, love and hate, authority problems, guilt, separation, death, mourning, loss, etc. as these are linked variously to their individual psychodynamics. The group treatment as outlined in this chapter succeeded in accelerating the integration of trauma, the strengthening of ego defenses, and the maturation and cohesion of the self.

RECAPITULATION AND CONCLUSIONS

This chapter presents a novel group treatment approach to the symptomatic Vietnam veteran. Called the "multiple-group developmental treatment model," this approach features a three-phase group development through instrumental planning and careful selection of group candidates from phase to phase. The phases are conceived as progressive, and intend to meet the changing spectrum of the veteran's needs over time. The ultimate goal of the model is the achievement of integration of defenses, reconnection with the social world, and the building of a cohesive self that would be able to stave off the disabling effects of automatic incursive phenonema (such as flashbacks, nightmares, etc.).

The aims of the first group ("rap" group), composed homogeneously of all combat veterans, is to provide the veteran group members with the opportunity to share mutual experiences with fellow combatants; restore inner calm by increasing the ego's regulatory capability over intrusive ideas, affects, and memories, as well as finding personal meaning for their Vietnam involvement and actions. Behavioral and cognitive techniques and procedures have been found useful; however, the emphasis is on the experiential elements of Vietnam as these emerge in the here-and-now and in the then-and-there of Vietnam. Technically, during the "rap" group phase, the leader discourages the evolution of transference feelings and other regressive group phenomena until at least toward the end of the second-phase group experience, and accelerated in the third-phase group.

The second-phase group is formed by the addition of highly selected group members whose diagnoses and personality configurations are congruent with the immediate goals of the group and its process. The new members are to be noncombat veterans ("era" veterans). The aim of the second-phase group is to provide the group with more diversified dynamic and personality types, with the belief that noncombat veterans are in some important ways different than combat veterans in terms of their relative freedom from incursive phenomena and other stress symptomatologies. The relatively integrated ego of these new members is useful in promoting the growth of other combat veterans, while the noncombat veteran has an opportunity to work through issues that could probably not have been addressed as well in any other forum. The veterans are taught to focus on their emotions and motivational life.

The third-phase group is composed by still adding one or two other persons, with the intention to further expand the diversity and reduce the homogeneity of the group. The belief here is that the more heterogeneous the group, the more it represents a true microcosm of the real world. This is extremely critical for the combat veteran, who, for the most part, is naive about the world of people. The aim of the third-phase group is to effect characterological change by analyzing defenses, resistances, and transference phenomena.

Interpretation, clarification, and confrontation are used in order to bring about the critical dynamic shift in the veteran's psychological relation to his anxieties.

This chapter is written with the belief that the acute, chronic, or delayed sub-types of posttraumatic stress disorder (APA, 1980), as presented clinically by the Vietnam veteran is a conglomerated complexity that defies any easy or superficial approach or intervention. This is because stress pathology involves the entire self—the ego, bodily (somatic) ego, id, superego, ego ideal, and the sociocultural, experiential, dynamic, genetic, and adaptive capabilities. Thus, the "rap" group would not suffice, unless only the most superficial intervention were desired. At the other extreme, the analytic approach would be inappropriate with the combatant since the analysis of defenses and resistances would be premature given the intrapsychic and interpersonal needs of the veteran. This is because the fragmentation of the ego and attendant lack of self-cohesion, lack of trust in any authority person (including therapists), despair, and the impaired narcissistic sense of well-being upon return to the United States after combat, precludes the application of the analytic method.

Approached from the perspective as outlined in this chapter, which utilizes a sequential or phasic pattern to intervention, it is possible to meet the needs of the veteran in a more comprehensive manner, while effecting useful growth and restoration of morale, trust, hopefulness, happiness, and the self.

REFERENCES

Archibald, H. C., Tuddenham, R. D. (1965). Persistent stress reaction following combat: a twenty year follow-up. *Archives of General Psychiatry* 12: 475–481.

Bennis, W. G., Shepard, H. A. (1956). A theory of group development. *Human Relations* 9: 415–437.

Bion, W. R. (1959). *Experiences in Groups.* New York: Basic Books.

Blank, A. S. (1979). First training papers—Operation Outreach. Read before the First Training Conference on Viet Nam Veterans, St. Louis, September 24, 1979.

Bloch, G. R., Bloch, N. H. (1976). Analytic group psychotherapy of post-traumatic psychoses. *International Journal of Group Psychotherapy* 26(1): 47–57.

Brende, J. O. (in press). An educational-therapeutic group for drug and alcohol-abusing combat veterans.

Brende, J. O. (1982b). A psychodynamic view of character pathology in combat veterans. *Bulletin of the Menninger Clinic* 47(3): 193–216.

Beukenkamp, C. (1966). Group process within the group configuration. In: J. L. Moreno (Ed.). *The International Handbook of Group Psychotherapy*, New York: Philosophical Library, pp. 504-510.

Cavenar, J. O., Nash, J. L. (1976). The effects of combat on the normal personality: war neurosis in Vietnam Returnees. *Comprehensive Psychiatry* 17: 647-653.

Cohen, J. (1980). Structural consequences of psychic trauma: a new look at "Beyond the Pleasure Principle. *International Journal of Psychoanalysis* 61: 421-432.

Collins, B. E., Guetzkow, H. A. (1964). *A Social Psychology of Group Process for Decision-Making*. New York: John Wiley and Sons.

Day, M. (1976). The natural history of training groups. In: M. Kissen (Ed.). *From Group Dynamics to Group Psychoanalysis*. New York: Hemisphere Publishing Company, pp. 135-144.

DeFazio, V. J. (1978). Dynamic perspectives on the nature and effects of combat stress. In: C. R. Figley (Ed.). *Stress Disorders Among Vietnam Veterans*. New York: Brunner/Mazel, pp. 23-42.

Egendorf, A. (1978). Psychotherapy with Vietnam veterans. In: C. R. Figley (Ed.). *Stress Disorder Among Viet Nam Veterans*. New York: Brunner/Mazel.

Eisenhart, R. W. (1975). You can't hack it, little girl: a discussion of overt psychological agenda of modern combat training. *Journal of Social Issues* 31: (4).

Fenichel, O. (1945). *The Psychoanalytic Theory of Neurosis*. New York: W. W. Norton.

Festinger, L., Schacter, S., Back, K. (1950). *Social Pressures in Informal Groups*. Stanford, California: Stanford University Press.

Figley, C. R. (Ed.). (1978). *Stress Disorder Among Vietnam Veterans*. New York: Brunner/Mazel.

Fogelman, E., Savran, B. (1980). Brief group therapy with offspring of holocaust survivors: leaders' reactions. *American Journal of Orthopsychiatry* 50(1): 96-108.

Friedman, M. (1981). Post-Vietnam syndrome: recognition and management. *The Academy of Psychosomatic Medicine* 22(11): 1-8.

Friedman, R. M., Cohen, K. (1980). The peer support group: a model for dealing with the emotional aspects of miscarriage. *Group* 4(4): 42-48.

Grinker, R., Spiegel, J. P. (1945). *Men Under Stress*. Philadelphia: Blakiston.

Gibbard, G. S., Hartman, J. J., Mann, R. D. (1974). *Analysis of Groups*. San Francisco: Josey-Bass.

Goldstein, K. (1951). On emotions: considerations from the organismic point of view. *Journal of Psychology* 31: 37-49.

Greenacre, P. (1957). The childhood of the artist: libidinal phase development and giftedness. *The Psychoanalytic Study of the Child*, Vol. 12. New York: International Universities Press.

Grotjahn, M. (1972). Learning from dropout patients. *International Journal of Group Psychotherapy* 22: 287-305.

Haley, S. A. (1974). When the patient reports atrocities. *Archives of General Psychiatry* 30: 191-196.

Hartmann, H. (1950). Comments on the psychoanalytic theory of the ego. *The Psychoanalytic Study of the Child*. Vol. 5. New York: International Universities Press.

Horner, A. (1979). *Object Relations and the Developing Ego in Therapy.* New York: Aronson.

Horowitz, M., Wilner, N., Kaltreider, N., Alvarez, W. (1980). Signs and symptoms of post-traumatic stress disorder. *Archives of General Psychiatry* 35: 85-92.

Kellerman, H. (1979). *Group Psychotherapy and Personality: Intersecting Structures.* New York: Grune and Stratton.

Kernberg, O. F. (1975). *Borderline Conditions and Pathological Narcissism.* New York: Aronson.

Kirshner, B. J., Dies, R. R., Brown, R. A. (1978). Effects of experimental manipulation on self-disclosure on group cohesiveness. *Journal of Consulting and Clinical Psychology* 46: 1171-1177.

Kissen, M. (Ed.) (1976). *From Group Dynamics to Group Psychoanalysis.* New York: Hemisphere Publishing Company.

Klein, J. (1956). *The Study of Groups.* London: Routledge and Kegan Paul.

Kohut, H. (1977). *The Restoration of the Self.* New York: International Universities Press.

Krystal, H. (Ed.) (1968). *Massive Psychic Trauma.* New York: International Universities Press.

Laughlin, H. P. (1979). *The Ego and Its Defenses.* New York: Aronson.

Lifton, R. J. (1973). *Home from the War.* New York: Simon and Schuster.

Lipkin, J. O., Blank, A. S., Parson, E. R., Smith, J. R. (1982). Vietnam veterans and posttraumatic stress disorder. *Journal of Hospital and Community Psychiatry* 33(11): 908-912.

Lowenstein, S., Morrison, A. (1979). The "Newsletter": a catalyst for learning in group psychotherapy. *American Journal of Psychotherapy* 33(1): 128-138.

Mahler, M., Pine, F., Bergman, A. (1975). *The Psychological Birth of the Human Infant.* New York: Basic Books.

Marafiote, R. (1980). Behavioral group treatment of Vietnam veterans. In: T. Williams (Ed.). *Post-Traumatic Stress Disorders of the Viet Nam Veteran.* Cincinnati: Disabled American Veterans.

Mednick, R. A. (1981). Reactivation of arrested development: a theoretical view of the patient-staff "community meeting." *The Hillside Journal of Clinical Psychiatry* 3(2): 163-176.

Money-Kyrle, R. (1950). Varieties of group formation. In: G. Roheim (Ed.). *Psychoanalysis and Social Sciences.* New York: International Universities Press.

Moses, R., Bargal, D., Calev, J., Falk, A., HaLevi, H., Lerner, Y., Mass, M., Noy, S., Perla, B., Winokur, M. (1976). A rear unit for the treatment of combat reactions in the wake of the Yom Kippur War. *Psychiatry* 39(2):153-168.

Neff, L. (1976). Traumatic Neuroses: a syndrome seen in Vietnam War veterans. Read at the American Orthopsychiatric Association Meeting, Atlanta, Georgia.

Parson, E. R. (1980). The CMHC-based treatment of the Vietnam combat veteran: an alternative psychotherapy model. Read at the 32nd Institute on Hospital and Community Psychiatry, Boston, Massachusetts, September.

Parson, E. R. (1981). The Veterans Administration medical center as transference object: implications for the treatment of Vietnam veterans. Invited address to the Continuing Education Symposium. Northport, N.Y. VAMC, April 1981.

Parson, E. R. (1982a). Narcissistic injury in Vietnam vets: the role of post-traumatic stress disorder, "Agent Orange" anxiety, and the repatriation experience. *Stars and Stripes—The National Tribune*, November 18, 1982, pp. 1-15.

Parson, E. R. (1982b). The "gook"-identification: its role in stress pathology in minority Vietnam veterans. Presented at the National Conference on the treatment of post-Vietnam stress syndrome, Cincinnati, Ohio, October 19.

Parson, E. R. (1983). The reparation of the self: clinical and theoretical dimensions in the treatment of the Vietnam combat veteran. *Journal of Contemporary Psychotherapy* 14(1).

Piper, W. E., Debbane, E. G., Garant, J., Bienvenu, J. (1979). Pretraining for group psychotherapy: a cognitive-experiential approach. *Archives of General Psychiatry* 36: 1250-1256.

Rabin, H. M. (1970). Preparing patients for group psychotherapy. *International Journal of Group Psychotherapy* 20: 135-145.

Rapaport, D. (1958). The theory of ego autonomy: a generalization. *Bulletin of the Menninger Clinic* 22: 13-35.

Rome, H. P. (1944). The role of sedation in military medicine. *U.S. Navy Medical Bulletin* 62: 525.

Senft, P. (1966). Clinical data to the phenomenology of the concepts "reality" and "society." In: J. Moreno (Ed.). *The International Handbook of Group Psychotherapy*. New York: Philosophical Library, pp. 284-286.

Scaturo, D. J. (1981). Cognitive factors in group psychotherapy with Vietnam veterans. Read at the 52nd Annual Convention of the Eastern Psychological Association, New York City, April 22, 1981.

Shapiro, R. (1978). Working through the war with Vietnam vets. *Group* 2(3): 156-181.

Shatan, C. F. (1972). Soldiers in mourning (Vietnam veterans self-help groups: the "post-Vietnam syndrome"). *American Journal of Orthopsychiatry* 42: 300-301.

Shatan, C. F. (1973). The grief of soldiers: Vietnam combat veterans' self-help movement. *American Journal of Orthopsychiatry* 43(4): 640-653.

Shatan, C. F. (1974). Through the membrane of reality: impacted grief and perceptual dissonance in Vietnam combat veterans. *Psychiatric Opinion* 11: 6-15.

Shatan, C. F. (1977). Bogus manhood, bogus honor: surrender and transfiguration in the U.S. Marine Corps. *Psychoanalytic Review* 25: 335-349.

Slavson, S. R. (1964). *A Textbook in Analytic Group Psychotherapy*. New York: International Universities Press.

Smith, J. R. (1980). Vietnam Veterans: rap groups and the stress recovery process. Unpublished Paper.

Smith, J. R. (1981). A review of one hundred and twenty years of the psychological literature on reactions to combat from the Civil War through the Vietnam War: 1960-1980. Unpublished Manuscript.

Tropp, E. (1976). A developmental theory. In: R. W. Roberts and H. Northen (Eds.). *Theories of Social Work with Groups*. New York: Columbia University Press.

Van Dalfsen, G. L. (1966). Pedagogic aspects of group psychotherapy with delinquents. In: J. Morena (Ed.). *The International Handbook of Group Psychotherapy*. New York: Philosophical Library.

Walker, J. I., Nash, J. L. (1981). Group therapy in the treatment of Vietnam combat veterans. *International Journal of Group Psychotherapy* 31: 379-389.

Walker, J. I. (1981). Psychological problems in Vietnam veterans. *Journal of the American Medical Association* 346: 781-782.

Wilson, J. P. (1977). Identity, Ideology, and Crisis: The Vietnam Veteran in Transition, Part I. (Unpublished Monograph). Cleveland State University.

Winnicott, D. W. (1958). *Through Pediatrics to Psychoanalysis.* New York: Basic Books.

Winnicott, D. W. (1960). Ego distortion in terms of true and false self. In: *The Maturational Process and the Facilitating Environment.* New York: International Universities Press, pp. 140-152.

Wolk, R. L. (1981). Group psychotherapy process in the treatment of hostages taken in prison. *Group* 5(2): 31-36.

Wong, N. (1981). An application of object-relations theory to an understanding of group cohesion. In: Kellerman, H. (Ed). *Group Cohesion: Theoretical and Clinical Perspectives.* New York: Grune and Stratton.

Yalom, I. (1970). *Theory and Practice of Group Psychotherapy.* New York: Basic Books.

Yalom, I., Brown, S., Block, S. (1975). The written summary as a group psychotherapy technique. *Archives of General Psychiatry* 32: 605-613.

8
Traumatic War Neuroses: Some Pharmacologic and Psychophysiologic Observations

RICHARD B. CORNFIELD, M.D.

The traumatic neuroses of war are clinical states arising from a sudden or prolonged threat to personal survival. An overwhelming external event or series of stresses can flood the individual beyond his tolerance for integrating the experience, especially if he is unprepared for the trauma. Excessive mobilization of psychological and physiological mechanisms for fight-or-flight takes place, and symptoms related to the person's particular emotional vulnerabilities develop. Where neither fight nor flight is clearly available, due either to unpreparedness for a sudden event or to helplessness in a chronic, inescapable situation, psychological regression ensues. A variety of psychoneurotic and psychosomatic reactions with prominent autonomic manifestations may develop. Such reactions are usually acute and self-limiting, but may also progress to long-term invalidism if inadequately treated (Saul and Lyons, 1952; Kardiner, 1947).

Although barbiturates and benzodiazepines have been used to reduce symptoms of anxiety during the acute phases, the pharmacotherapy of traumatic war neurosis in its chronic stages has been minimally investigated or discussed in the literature. This is surprising inasmuch as chronic traumatic neuroses are very difficult to treat psychologically because of the consolidation and hardening of emotional withdrawal and avoidance patterns. However, the patients frequently present with dramatic psychophysiological and psychoneurotic symptoms which seem prime targets for modern psychotropics. Indeed, the biological cast of the disorders prompted Kardiner (1947) to coin the term "somato or physioneuroses" to distinguish them from other neuroses. Finding an effective drug to alleviate chronic symptomatology that has not been amenable to other forms of treatment, including drug and expressive therapies, would be a significant advance, especially because this syndrome is incapacitating to a number of Vietnam veterans and is thus of particular concern today.

In keeping with the general objectives of this chapter, I comment on our recent pilot observations with the medication phenelzine sulfate which we have felt suggestive and promising enough to warrant future carefully controlled trials (Hogben and Cornfield, 1981). I allude to significant contributions to our knowledge of traumatic war neuroses, including more recent work centering on psychological experiences after stress in general. This discussion is followed by a summary of pertinent studies of the effects of phenelzine and other medications on symptoms that are frequently prominent in the traumatic stress reactions. Other biological approaches to the understanding and treatment of posttraumatic disorders will be mentioned.

THE TRAUMATIC SYNDROME

General (Prior Contributions)

Reactions to wartime stresses have been discussed for over a century in the American and European literature. Benjamin Rush warned against fever, in militia officers and soldiers returning from the Revolutionary War, "produced by the sudden change in the manner of sleeping, living, etc. It was prevented, in many cases, by the person lying, for a few nights after his return to his family, on a blanket before the fire" (Fox, 1972). DaCosta discussed the "Irritable Heart" syndrome of many Civil War soldiers, and Oppenheim in Germany used the term "traumatic neurosis" in 1889 to describe the outcome of what was regarded as probable injury to the brain. This concept of neuronal damage in acute traumatic reactions still existed as late as World War I, as indicated by the term "shell-shock." However, Freud in 1922, in "Beyond the Pleasure Principle," proposed his theory of a stimulus barrier (Reitzschutz). He felt that the breakthrough of this hypothetical protective barrier by overwhelming traumata liberated excessive anxiety. The individual rendered helpless would attempt to regain control by the gradual discharge of unmastered excitation through repeated reliving of the trauma through dreams. He thus postulated a repetition compulsion for traumatic experiences and their residues that went beyond the pleasure principle. Kardiner's monumental work with hospitalized veterans after World War I further explored the diversity of psychological and somato-psychic reactions to trauma (1941, 1947).

Recent research by Horowitz and co-workers (1972, 1976) has confirmed the universal tendency for the continual reexperiencing of emotionally traumatizing events in images and memories. In a recent document (1980), he reports on 66 patients referred to a special stress-response clinic. The majority of patients had the well-defined symptoms of intrusive repetition of feelings and thoughts as well as sleep disturbances related to the traumatic event. Other symptoms included emotional avoidance, denial, and sometimes "numbing" regarding the event. An Impact of Events Scale has been devised by Horowitz and co-workers, and his concept of alternating periods of intrusive repetition as well as symptoms of avoidance of emotional pain has had a major influence on the diagnostic criteria for this disorder presented in the current DSM-III.

Description of the Disorder

There are both acute and chronic phases of the posttraumatic syndrome, the former often blending or deteriorating into the latter if allowed to continue without resolution. The acute phase is characterized by such symptoms as disturbed sleep with nightmares, restlessness, poor appetite, perceptual distortions, jumpiness and inability to relax, fear of stimuli with a heightened startle reflex, signs of autonomic over-activity, fatigability, impotence, and difficulty in concentrating. According to Saul in 1945, the syndrome of anxiety, irritability, startle, insomnia, and nightmares represented a common nucleus. Strecker (1945) claimed that the most common traumatic neurosis of World War I was "a relatively simple naive conversion hysteria," while during and after World War II the preponderant psychoneuroses were anxiety reactions, often combined with elements of depression. In addition, somatic symptoms often occurred in parts of the body previously the focus of injury or illness.

Treatment of acute traumatic conditions has relied on the prevention of chronic states through early recognition. Military psychiatry, including the extensive work by Grinker et al with World War II flying personnel (1945 a,b) has contributed significantly through early vigorous rehabilitation of "combat exhaustion" to prevent chronic stress reactions. The immediacy of treatment, the proximity of treatment to the area of battle, combined with expectation of return to the fighting unit, are three well-known concepts of acute care emphasized by Grinker but first developed by Salmon in 1919. Modalities of treatment have included use of minor tranquilizers, sleep, ECT, group therapy, sodium amytal interviews for retrieval of memories and psychotherapeutic abreaction, insulin shock, and various types of supportive therapy combined with rest and relaxation.

In certain persons probably predisposed emotionally (Strange, 1969), the acute stage of a traumatic reaction progresses into a chronic debilitating phase. The chronic posttraumatic stress reaction may occur in previously asymptomatic veterans who lead apparently normal lives, but who showed their first overt symptoms after combat. In many patients symptoms are suppressed by avoidance mechanisms, drugs, or alcohol. The severe forms of the chronic syndrome may be characterized by the following symptom pattern:

1. Recurrent nightmares, often catastrophic, indicating failure of psychological adaptation to the events (Greenberg et al, 1972).

2. Vivid waking visualizations, sometimes in an altered state of consciousness, described as "flashbacks" (day imaging), and frequent intrusive memories and pangs of emotion about the prior disturbing events that have not been emotionally integrated.

3. Generalized anxiety or mixtures of anxiety-depressive symptoms, with certain patients having severe and recurrent acute anxiety or "panic" attacks; the acute and chronic anxiety states often show multiple manifestations of autonomic instability.

4. Chronic irritability and startle reactions to sudden, surprising stimuli such as fireworks or overhead aircraft.

5. A proclivity toward explosive or violent aggressive reactions.

It should be emphasized that many other psychoneurotic elaborations involving autonomic, psychosomatic, sensorimotor, or epileptic-type disturbances may occur.

Outcome Studies

Almost uniformly, such traumatized patients exhibit a marked decline in their general level of adaptive functioning. Kardiner described traumatic neuroses as reflecting the establishment of a new style of adaptation revolving around curtailment of individual resources, and Rado (1942) used the term "traumatophobia" to postulate emergency control (avoidance) mechanisms used by the individual to protect against repetition of the trauma.

Several investigators have studied systematically the long-term course of symptoms. Leopold and Dillon (1963) evaluated the residual symptoms, affect disturbances, sleep changes, and sexual changes, of survivors of a sudden ship disaster. They found 71 percent of the patients somewhat worse after about 3.5 to 4.5 years. Dobbs and Wilson (1960) studied psychological responses to a tape recording of noises of battle in patients with combat neuroses, combat veterans without symptoms of psychiatric disability, and noncombat control veterans. The control patients showed transitory orienting responses to the combat sounds, while combat veterans who were well-adjusted showed moderate or mild physiological behavioral responses. However, patients with combat neuroses showed behavioral responses often almost psychotic in extreme, frequently so exaggerated as to prevent the experimenter from recording and evaluating the physiological responses. Some symptoms were intensified after the experiment in these patients.

In a series of studies at a VA Outpatient Clinic, Archibald and Tuddenham (1962, 1965) found that most patients with a diagnosis of chronic post-combat traumatic neurosis did worse in 15- and 20-year follow-ups in terms of overall psychopathology. They studied the nature of persistent symptoms after an average of 15 years in 67 outpatient veterans. A control group of 48 noncombat, present or prior VA psychiatric outpatients was also studied. While their studies cannot generalize to all patients suffering stress reaction syndromes, but only to those who show persistent symptoms over a number of years, it is significant that symptoms highly specific to the combat situation were checked in self-rating questionnaires and MMPI far more often by the postcombat group (eg, combat dreams and startle reactions, as well as symptoms such as dizziness, blackouts, jumpiness and sweaty hands). Tension, irritability, depression, diffuse anxiety symptoms, headaches, insomnia and nightmares were also prominent in this group.

Chronic traumatic disorders are usually refractory to treatment despite sporadic reports of success (Little and James, 1964; Leehy and Martin, 1967). Once the chronic stabilized states are established, diagnosis may be difficult (van Putten and Emory, 1973). Prominent symptoms mimic such other disorders as drug and alcohol abuse syndromes, hallucinogenic disorders including LSD, schizophrenia, phobic and anxiety conditions, and depressive states. Diagnosis is particularly hampered by the patients' reluctance to discuss traumatic war experiences even if they suffer recurrent visual or auditory flashbacks, intrusive pangs of emotion and remembrance, and nightmares about traumatic events. Frequently, only the most painstaking, carefully focused history-taking uncovers the habitual reexperiencing of traumatic scenes.

In the last several years, Dr. George Hogben and the present author have treated a number of patients showing symptoms of severe, long-lasting, intractable chronic posttraumatic disorders. The patients had not responded to previous multiple therapeutic trials with antipsychotics, tricyclic antidepressants, and psychotherapy with or without medication.

We used a pharmacologic approach that seems to show significant promise based on our open-ended clinical observations. In the hospital and posthospital treatment of patients showing all the symptoms of the chronic stress syndrome described above, including frequent acute hysterical episodes, the MAO inhibitor phenelzine sulfate proved extremely valuable in ameliorating the most disturbing aspects of the disorder (Hogben and Cornfield, 1981). Our sample of patients with these conditions exhibited not only the psychological scars manifested by avoidance patterns or intermittent and recurrent troublesome reminders, but also polysymptomatic complaints. Anxiety-depressive affects, recurrent nightmares, panic attacks often focused on cardiorespiratory organs, and vivid waking visualizations were prominent in the symptom picture. Seeking a medication that might be of benefit, where others had not been, we decided to try phenelzine because of its history of value in individuals who were emotionally overreactive and exhibited anxiety, agitation, somatic complaints, hypochondriasis, general dysphoria, and frequently panic.

We noted the repeated tendency in the patients treated with phenelzine to show a diminution of anxiety and agitation while on this medication; depressive affect fluctuated, sometimes with hypomanic spells, but ultimately the patients' affect stabilized. The most dramatic results were in the termination of nightmares in all patients and in the termination of "flashbacks" in five out of six subjects, with the sixth showing reduced occurrence of flashbacks after 18 days.

We are careful to adjust the dosage of each patient's medication to approximately 1 mg/kg, and most patients showed marked response within 21 days. Panic attacks ceased within two weeks of use of this medication, and by discharge from the hospital the patients felt calmer and had ceased having nightmares and flashbacks of overwhelming traumatic war memories as well as startle reactions and sudden aggressive outbursts. Several patients continued their improvement outside the hospital, and several relapsed shortly after discontinuing the phenelzine. The following are two illustrative case vignettes.

Patient 1   A 29-year-old man was admitted for his fourth psychiatric hospitalization with sweating, tremulousness, and agitation after drinking a quart of vodka daily for almost a year. He was the son of a blind Jewish father and Catholic mother. His mother had frequently punished him for aggressive, impulsive outbursts toward his siblings as a child, while his father showered him with unconditional affection. His father died when he was seven, and he developed a prolonged grief reaction during the next year, waiting frequently at the bus stop for his father to return. Aggressive behavior problems in school led to expulsion before the end of high school, but all through adolescence he maintained an excellent work record. He entered the Army in 1967 and during a year of combat in Vietnam handled dangerous job assignments such as "walking point" and infiltrating behind enemy lines. His first enemy killing involved shooting a booby-trapped Vietnamese child under orders. He was very guilt-ridden over this behavior but claimed, "It seemed to unlock something in me and I went on a killing rampage afterwards." Shortly after his marriage to an Army nurse, his wife was killed by enemy mortar while walking next to him. He stated: "It was my fault; I took cover but I didn't take her down with me."

Shortly after discharge from the service, this man began experiencing chronic anxiety, punctuated two or three times daily by massive panic attacks during which he thought he would die. He had chest pains, palpitations, dyspnea, sweats, and abdominal cramps. He also developed severe nightmares centering on traumatic war experiences. He frequently had intense day images of traumatic experiences in which he heard guns and mortar; he also experienced visualizations occurring before him, blocking out objects in his line of sight. On Independence Day he would become extremely frightened by fireworks. He also showed intense startle reactions and violent behavior if approached unaware. Before hospitalization he developed polydrug abuse and required three hospitalizations for detoxification; gradually, he used only alcohol.

After detoxification in the recent hospitalization, he was logical and coherent but demonstrated the symptoms described above. During the first 15 days of phenelzine treatment with 75 mg/day, he showed an intense abreaction of rage at authority figures and at his father for dying. Day images and panic attacks disappeared in two weeks, while anxiety, aggressiveness, and nightmares took up to four weeks to diminish. Mild nightmare activity was controlled more effectively after discharge from the hospital on phenelzine 90 mg/day with continued supportive therapy.

Patient 2 A 26-year-old Portugese male was hospitalized for severe panic, including fears of dying. He had had similar panic attacks since discharge from the service.

Past history revealed that during his youth he always felt displaced from his mother by his two younger sisters. His alcoholic father worked long hours and did not give the patient much attention except for punishment. The patient was overenergetic and impulsive; he quit school during the 12th grade to join the Marine Corps, where he had nine months of combat in Vietnam.

During combat he killed several enemy soldiers and was frequenty exposed to enemy fire. On one mission his helicopter, mistakenly ordered into an enemy zone, was blown up and two close buddies were killed. The patient stated: "I still hear them screaming." He felt guilty about surviving and noticed a fear of enclosed spaces afterwards for the first time. He became agitated and depressed and was evacuated to a state-side hospital where he received 12 ECT treatments.

The patient's panic attacks started after discharge. He became paralyzed with severe apprehension, palpitations and nausea. Nightmares of traumatic war experiences occurred five or six nights per week, and he slept for only four hours. He also had intense day images of traumatic war scenes which lasted as long as 20 minutes. During these experiences he sat mutely in a chair, unaware of his surroundings. He frequently heard his dying buddies screaming and sometimes a voice commanding him to hurt himself. He could not stay in his house at night with his two children, claiming he was afraid something would happen. He frequently felt like hurting someone and had numerous violent episodes.

During multiple prior VA hospitalizations for panic attacks and auditory hallucinations, this patient was given a variety of psychotropics, including haloperidol 40 mg/day, chlorpromazine 1600 mg/day, diazepam 40 mg/day, amitriptyline 150 mg/day, and doxepin 200 mg/day. Each of these medications was taken for at least a month without therapeutic response. The patient also had several periods of psychotherapy without significant symptom relief. He ultimately turned to narcotics for relief, but he had been rehabilitated and drug-free for two years before this admission.

On admission, the patient appeared terrified, pacing the halls and pleading for medication. He had two to four panic attacks daily, with profuse sweating and nausea. He also spent several periods each day sitting mutely in a chair and staring. He described intense visual images of traumatic war experiences after these episodes. His sleep was sporadic and restless, often punctuated by terrifying war-related nightmares. On awakening he felt paralyzed, but after an interval of pacing he was able to settle back into bed. He had an intense startle reaction and was irritable and abusive. The patient did not respond to a one-month trial of imipramine 200 mg/day. He could not discuss war events without panic.

The patient responded well to phenelzine: "This is the first time I have felt so calm since before the war." During the next two weeks the patient ventilated angry feelings at staff, the government, the war, and his parents. His affect stabilized considerably after the third week. Day images, the screams of his buddies, and voices commanding him to hurt himself stopped completely after the third week. Nightmares decreased markedly after then. These were eliminated completely by raising the phenelzine to 75 mg/day after one month. The patient reported that he did not engage in violence after phenelzine was begun. The patient stopped the phenelzine once, and his symptoms rapidly recurred; they were controlled by restarting the medication. After stabilization as an outpatient, medication was discontinued without incident. Follow-up improvements was demonstrated for six months.

RELEVANCE OF THE MONOAMINE OXIDASE INHIBITORS TO CHRONIC POSTTRAUMATIC REACTIONS

General Information

Our interest in the use of MAOIs, classified as antidepressants, in treating severe posttraumatic disorders stems from emerging concepts regarding the optimal use of these drugs (Tyrer, 1976; Quitkin et al, 1979; Paykel et al, 1979).

Conditions with symptoms somewhat distinct from those of the typical "endogenous" depressions, but approximating the characteristics of our treatment group of posttraumatic stress disorders (PTSDs), seem to have responded most positively. We briefly review data from early reports and from systematic, controlled studies suggesting the effectiveness of phenelzine in certain patients with psychopathology not exclusively or typically depressive, and we discuss more recent lines of evidence with compelling reasons for our trying it with patients with posttraumatic stress disorders.

Monoamine oxidase is an enzyme widely distributed in the brain as well as many other organs in the body (Youdim and Paykel, 1981). There is direct as well as indirect evidence suggesting that more than one form of the enzyme exists; at least two forms, MAO-A and MAO-B, are of interest to the field of psychiatry. In humans, MAO-A catalyzes the breakdown or deamination of chemicals such as serotonin and norepinephrine. These chemicals are frequently implicated in biological theories of major psychiatric disorder, particularly in affective illness. MAO-B type enzyme catalyzes the metabolism of monoamines such as phenylethylamine and benzylamine. Chemicals such as dopamine, tyramine, and tryptamine are deaminated in the human brain apparently by both types of enzymes. Most of the marketed MAO inhibitor drugs apparently work on both enzyme systems, although specific experimental MAO inhibitors (eg, clorgyline with MAO-A only and deprenyl, MAO-B only) are actively under investigation for specific differential clinical effects (Lipper et al, 1979; Thornton et al, 1980).

Thirty years ago Zeller et al (1952) noted that MAO was inhibited by the drug iproniazid. A most interesting chance finding occurred that same year, when other researchers (Selikoff et al, 1952; Bloch et al, 1954) noted feelings of euphoria and well-being in tuberculosis patients treated with the same medication. Thus, early speculation began to mount over the role of MAO inhibitors both in enhancing monoamine availability in central nervous system neurotransmission and in the alleviation of depressive symptomatology.

The initial enthusiasm over this medication's psychic energizing and euphoriant properties (Crane, 1957; Kline, 1958) was soon replaced by over-concern regarding the risk of hypertensive and hepatotoxic reactions. Although the mechanisms for these reactions were soon readily explained (Blackwell et al, 1967), concern about toxicity, coupled with the development of tricyclic antidepressants, lead to a substantial reduction in MAOI use in psychiatric populations. Impressive detrimental evidence on the utility of the MAOIs in endogenous depression came from the British Medical Research Council study (1965) comparing phenelzine, imipramine, ECT, and placebo in 250 inpatients. This authoritative study clearly pointed to inadequate response to MAOIs in patients suffering from the more severe endogenous form of depression.

Atypical Depressive Disorder

Continued interest in the use of the MAOIs, however, was largely due to early reports by Dally, Sargant, West and colleagues in Great Britain. In 1959, West and Dally in a retrospective study reported that certain patients suffering from "atypical depressions" associated with phobic anxiety and hysterical symptoms responded well to treatment with MAO inhibitors (alone or in conjunction with the minor tranquilizer chlordiazepoxide). In a series of 60 cases under their supervision, 72 percent responded favorably to this treatment. Their patients, in general, lacked the endogenous-type symptoms of guilty self-reproach, early morning awakening, or morning worsening; instead, they showed hysterical symptoms, tremor, poor prior responses to ECT, and deterioration toward evening. In 1962, Sargant and Dally discussed a group of anxious depressives who showed both hysterical and phobic anxiety symptoms, often more closely resembling patients with anxiety neurosis or reactive depression. This group had been well-adjusted but decompensated after severe or prolonged stress; in addition, certain patients showed pronounced autonomic responses and prominent phobic, hysterial or obsessive coloring of their clinical picture. These syndromes had frequently been labeled anxiety states or "anxiety hysteria."

Sargant and Dally also mentioned a group of patients who, in their clinical opinion, had done surprisingly well on phenelzine after suffering years of incapacity with "cardiac neurosis" symptoms, including palpitations, hyperventilation, flushing, sweating, and chest pains. Finally, they listed characteristics of those patients (later noted by Pollitt and Young) whose symptoms they felt were responsive to MAOIs: difficulty in falling asleep rather than early morning awakening; reversed diurnal variation of symptoms, with patients feeling worse as the day progressed rather than better; severe lethargy and fatigue; sometimes phobic fears of traveling alone; variation in emotionality from day to day; and premenstrual tension and irritability in women. The authors questioned whether MAO inhibitors were really antidepressant, or whether they were more effective in the treatment of anxiety-related states and acted as delayed psychostimulants. Up to the present time, this question has never been sufficiently answered.

The reports from Britain in the early 1960s were often inadequately designed, retrospective, lacking control groups or sufficient medication dosage or duration of treatment, and to some degree anecdotal (Klein, 1978). Research evidence for the utility of MAOIs was not forthcoming in careful, well-controlled, double-blind studies until more than a decade later in the United States, when a series of studies by Ravaris et al (1976) and Robinson et al (1973, 1978) began to show support for the usefulness of phenelzine in the heterogeneous population of outpatient depressives. These patients, often labeled depressive-anxiety patients, reactive depressives, neurotic depressives, or atypical depressives, showed response not only to depressive mood alterations but also to other troubling combinations of neurotic symptomatology including hypochondriacal, hysterical, and phobic symptoms. We are particularly interested in this heterogeneous group because of its resemblance to the posttraumatic population which we have discussed (Cornfield and Hogben, 1980; Hogben and Cornfield, 1981). The group that Ravaris and colleagues studied consisted of outpatient depressives referred by family physicians. These patients had not responded to the more traditional tricyclic antidepressants or to benzodiazepines in combination. The patients were described as having a mixture of depression and such other neurotic symptomatology as obsessions, depersonalization, and fatigue.

The patients were withdrawn from prior medication, then randomized into two treatment groups receiving either phenelzine or placebo with phenelzine dosage adjusted from 45 to 75 mg/day, depending upon clinical requirements. Phenelzine-treated patients showed especially significant improvement in rating scale determinations of psychomotor change, irritability, and hypochondriasis-agitation. A diagnostic index (DI) was constructed by the investigators from the standardized 23 item Hamilton Depression Scale along with other variables they felt useful in distinguishing between endogenous and nonendogenous depression. Patients were rated in a weighted fashion positively for items of endogenous depression (most positive: suicidal ideation, depressed mood, agitation, retardation, weight loss) and received negatively weighted scores for symptoms the investigators felt least related to endogenous depression (such as psychic and somatic anxiety, early insomnia, generalized somatic symptoms). The two groups were equally matched according to a range of DI scores. The investigators found the highest response rate to phenelzine in those patients who scored toward the lowest end of the diagnostic index, thus suggesting that the best response occurred in the group with fewest endogenous features. This controlled trial was consistent with prior clinical lore suggesting MAOIs effectiveness in atypical or nonendogenous depression.

Further similarly designed studies by the same group have replicated the original findings (Robinson et al, 1978). Of particular interest to us in their recent work is the finding of a positive association between dose, percentage of platelet inhibition, and improvement. They have reasoned that although the ratio of platelet MAO inhibition to brain MAO inhibition is unknown, inhibition in the two sites is roughly parallel. Animal studies have demonstrated that brain monoamines do not increase measurably until 80 to 90 percent brain MAO inhibition. Thus, 80 percent or higher peripheral human MAO inhibition may be desirable if the response to phenelzine in disturbed mood states is due to alteration of CNS MAO levels.

These findings, although intriguing, are unable to specify what particular symptoms are MAOI-responsive or what specific clinical features characterize MAOI improvers. In a recent article on atypical depression, Davidson et al (1982) summarized many of the recent studies, including significant ones by Paykel (1979), Robinson (1978), Shehan (1980), and others who have tried to identify a subgroup of patients most likely to respond to MAO inhibitors as compared with imipramine or ECT treatment. They conclude:

the optimal effects of MAO inhibitors are likely to be seen in the following population subgroups:
1. Patients who exhibit a clear weight gain or increase in appetite or sleep, reactivity of mood, and anergia;
2. Patients with agoraphobia of long duration, and secondary depression;
3. Patients with primary depression in whom pain or somatic discomfort is the leading complaint, and patients with psychogenic pain or hypochondriasis and secondary depression.

Our decision to try the MAOI phenelzine in our group of severe posttraumatic neurotics was also influenced by several other significant clinical and research findings.

Klein (1977) has long advocated the use of phenelzine in the treatment of patients with a condition he describes as a variant of an affective disorder outside the usual range of typical endogenous depression, called "hysteroid dysphoria." He describes such patients as fickle, emotionally volatile, histrionic, prone to excessive emotionality, and who "crash" severely when rejected. In such circumstances they become anxious and morose, and they both overeat and oversleep. These patients are regarded as showing marked and sometimes specific improvement with MAOI treatment (Leibowitz and Klein, 1979).

Interestingly, although our experience has suggested a variety of character types as demonstrating posttraumatic stress disorder, van der Kolk and colleagues in Boston (1982) have recently suggested that the Rohrschachs of patients with nightmares exhibiting a chronic traumatic stress syndrome showed an exceptionally high sensitivity to suggestibility. They mention the patients' strong external response to affective stimuli and a lack of developmentally mature responses, thus highlighting the impulsivity and dependence on external cues in their group of nightmare patients. Overall, the trauma group in their study comparing chronic nightmare sufferers and PTSD nightmare sufferers show a significantly extratensive response, a pattern very suggestive of young adolescents and of people with hysterical character structure.

The MAOI-responsive hysteroid dysphorics discussed by Klein and colleagues, as well as both van der Kolk's population and the phenelzine-responsive patients described many years ago by Sargant (1961) as "hysterical types of depressive reaction," clearly have features in common with most of our patients who showed notable response to phenelzine sulfate. Sargant detailed his group's overall hyper-reactivity, increased emotionality, irritability, and sometimes phobias of traveling alone or going into the street. Roth (1959), in an earlier paper describing a phobic anxiety-depersonalization syndrome ("calamity syndrome"), had similarly described a type of hysterical, overreactive, emotionally immature individual who exhibited close parallels to the type of individual described by Sargant later, also quite responsive to phenelzine treatment.

The following two cases of probable traumatic neurosis exemplify the above-described constellation of personality characteristics and symptoms that was responsive to our trial with phenelzine sulfate.

Patient 3 A 41-year-old patient entered the hospital with sweats and temulousness after drinking one quart of whiskey per day for three months to "calm my nerves." He had entered the Army after graduation from high school in 1955 and had one year of combat in Korea. During combat he was terrified by fighting. He saw buddies killed and was frequently exposed to enemy overruns of his camp.

He developed severe panic states with frightening nightmares and was evacuated to a hospital, where he received eight ECT treatments.

Ever since his discharge, he experienced severe panic states with overwhelming fear, chest discomfort, pain, palpitations and air hunger. He went to hospital emergency rooms on five different occasions with fearfulness, severe chest pain, and choking sensations. He was convinced he had "heart attacks," but no cardiac pathology was found. He avoided elevators and subways. Frightening nightmares of traumatic war scenes occurred two to three times a week. Day imaging of traumatic war experiences happened daily. The patient made intermittent attempts at outpatient therapy. Chemotherapies included chlordiazepoxide 40 mg/day, amitriptyline 150 mg/day, and imipramine 150 mg/day. He had minimal symptomatic response to these treatments: "I drank moderately; that was better—the medications were no good." He attempted several trials of outpatient psychotherapy, but without relief.

Four years before admission, he accidentally killed a pedestrian with his car. After this incident his symptoms markedly increased, and he turned to heavy drinking. He had three hospitalizations for alcohol detoxification and rehabilitation.

On this admission, the patient was agitated and depressed, with impaired concentration. Speech was logical and coherent. Alcohol withdrawal was treated with chlordiazepoxide beginning with 60 mg/day and continuing in diminishing doses. During a drug-free observation period, the patient was panicky and complained of chest pain and shortness of breath. He looked fearful and avoided others on the ward. He had nightmares every night which woke him from a sound sleep. He was able to return to sleep but slept only five hours a night. The patient was encouraged to relate feelings about war-related events, but said "that's all over." Amitriptyline 200 mg/day did not alleviate the symptoms.

Phenelzine was begun, and within one day the patient felt calm: "I don't have chest pains for the first time in 20 years." On the fourth therapy day the patient began to express rage over events in his life. This lasted for nine days, after which he became quite depressed. He then had a brief period of elation, which began on the 18th therapy day. He stopped having nightmares and day imaging on the 14th therapy day. The patient also discussed military events with appropriate fearfulness and anger. Symptomatic improvement continued into outpatient treatment one month after phenelzine was begun; however, the patient dropped out of follow-up shortly thereafter.

Patient 4   A 30-year-old Puerto Rican male was admitted to the hospital for intense panic and increasingly impulsive behavior. His history revealed that he had been sexually abused by his father from four to six years of age. The father, an unpredictable and violent man, deserted the family when the patient was 14. The patient also revealed a history of impulsive hyperactive behavior as a child; he did not finish high school. He handled intense inner tensions by engaging in strenuous physical activity.

After entering the Marine Corps, he had eight months of combat in Vietnam. There he participated in much violence and frequently saw buddies killed by mortar. Enemy mortar burst next to him on one occasion, and he "snapped." He returned to the states, and during a one-month hospitalization was violent and agitated, requiring high doses of chlorpromazine. He refused medical discharge and finished his tour of duty handling body bags.

After discharge from the service, the patient noticed severe, frightening, war-related nightmares for the first time. He was paralyzed on waking from the nightmares but was able to return to sleep. He also had intense, unprovoked day images of traumatic war experiences and heard bullets and mortar whizzing by him. Loud fireworks provoked the visual reexperiencing of war scenes.

The patient developed episodes of intense panic during which he was drenched with sweat and had abdominal cramps. The panic attacks occurred two times a month at first, but gradually increased in frequency to two or three times a day. He was hyperactive and felt boundless energy. He was involved in many violent episodes, both provoked and unprovoked, claiming "I always feel like a time bomb." During the year before admission, he became depressed, disinterested in his usual activities, and impotent. The patient had adequate outpatient trials of amitriptyline 200 mg/day and thioridazine 300 mg/day without symptom remission. Heavy drinking and drug abuse provided symptom relief. The patient worked steadily as a prison guard or cab driver despite his symptoms and substance abuse. During the month before admission he became increasingly impulsive on his job, driving wildly and losing himself on city streets. Two weeks before admission he accidentally shot himself in the hand.

On admission he appeared tense and frightened. His speech was pressured but goal-oriented. Each day he had several panic episodes during which he crouched in his room with sweat running from his forehead. He also had shallow respirations and abdominal pain. He was frequently observed staring out the window looking for the source of bullets and mortar he heard. At times, he cried profusely and looked depressed. He also spent much time restlessly pacing the ward and engaged in physical activities. He had an intense startle reaction and was threatening toward patients and staff when approached unawares. Sleep was restless and characterized by shouting or falling out of bed. He awoke from nightmares several times a night. When he discussed war related events, he was anxious but rarely expressed anger or guilt. The symptoms did not respond to thioridazine 600 mg/day.

The patient looked and felt calmer after phenelzine was begun. He was able to sit for long periods and concentrate on reading. On the fifth therapy day he became angry and spent the next ten days pouring out angry feelings at the war, authorities, his father, and the government. From the 16th to the 20th days, he was depressed and felt lethargic. On the 21st day he became elated and talked optimistically about his future. This state lasted for several days until his mood stabilized. Nightmares, day imaging, and the sounds of bullets and mortar ceased after the 15th day.

As an outpatient his mood remained stable, but he had enormous energy which he controlled by intense physical activity. He had no violent episodes. The nightmares, day imaging, and bullet and mortar sounds did not recur. However, loud fireworks provoked intense visual reexperiencing of war scenes. When he stopped phenelzine for five days, many of his symptoms returned. During this period he became verbally abusive toward the therapist and threatened bodily harm. He ran from this encounter and hit the first person he saw. He started phenelzine again, and within three days the agitated, aggressive symptoms subsided. Lithium carbonate, 1,200 mg/day, helped the patient control the psychomotor pressure.

This combination was maintained for four months and then slowly discontinued. Phenelzine was stopped first, without incident, and then lithium was stopped. The patient became symptom-free, without medication, for five months. He has been stable, except for the brief period described above, for over 18 months.

It is possible that our group of traumatic neurotics with panic attacks are a special subset of posttraumatic conditions; this is an area that should be more extensively investigated. Klein (1978) has noted that acute anxiety or panic attack sufferers usually derive substantial benefit from tricyclic antidepressants for that specific symptomatology. Our group did not seem to show that response but did improve with phenelzine.

Recent research findings by Sheehan et al (1980) strongly support the prior clinical impressions that phenelzine is effective in treating spontaneous acute anxiety attacks with accompanying polyphobic, hysterical, hypochondriacal symptoms.

Earlier studies, in England, had suggested the value of phenelzine in phobic conditions. Specifically, Kelly's retrospective review (1970) of clinical experience suggested its effectiveness with phobic states including panic attacks, while several controlled studies such as Tyrer et al (1973) noted reduction in anxiety related to phobias and modest overall improvement in phobic responses. These reports frequently had had heterogeneous samples including agoraphobics, simple phobics and social phobics who may have derived benefit from the effects of phenelzine on spontaneous panics, with secondary extinction of phobic anxiety. However, in Sheehan's controlled study, phenelzine was clearly superior to placebo on most outcome measures and even superior to imipramine, commonly used in the treatment of panic attacks, on the ratings of symptom severity and phobic avoidance. Of major interest is the finding that elevated scores of depression, including vegetative signs of depression, were not predictable guides to MAOI drug response. Thus, this case of compounds was found effective in the absence of any signs or symptoms of depression.

In essence, these results give strong support to a notion of MAOI (phenelzine) effectiveness in "endogenous anxiety" disorders with accompanying symptoms unrelated to depression. It is likely that the phenelzine-responsive panic attacks and subsequent phobic elaborations after the original panic attacks may be the most specific targets of the drug treatment, with demoralization or depression reactive to the restrictions and chronic fears punctuating the lives of these patients.

SLEEP AND DREAMING

General

Since the mid 1950s, the architecture of sleeping has been studied extensively, and major contributions to our knowledge of dreaming and sleep disorders such as somnambulism, enuresis, and night terrors/ nightmares have been forthcoming. The reader is referred to excellent reviews by Dement (1965), Jouvet (1967), Snyder (1963), Roffwarg (1966), Broughton (1968), Kramer (1979), Hauri (1977), and others. Their research into the nature of sleep has yielded the following basic information: that dreaming is statistically related to a distinct, cyclically recurring type of sleep characterized by bursts of conjugate rapid eye movement (REM). Dream recall following arousal from this stage of sleep has been found to occur between 70 and 90 percent. The other and very different kind of sleep, non-rapid eye movement (NREM) sleep, is usually described as consisting of four stages: stage 1, stage 2, and delta sleep (stages 3 and 4). These stages are progressive, with diminishing vigilance, from stages 1 through 4; stage 1 is a transition between full wakefulness and sleep, and stages 3 and 4 are indicative of deep sleep with slow-delta wave activity. Stages 3 and 4 are subdivided depending upon the number of delta waves; traditionally stage 4 is considered to have more than 50 percent of delta waves with amplitudes greater than 75 mV peak to peak.

REM sleep alternates with NREM sleep at intervals of approximately ninety minutes; physiological parameters are quite different between REM and NREM sleep in normal situations. In the typical sleep pattern of a young adult, there is progressive movement from stage 1 through delta sleep until the first REM, about 70 to 90 minutes after sleep onset; this REM period usually lasts about five minutes. The second sleep cycle begins when stage 2 sleep recurs after the first REM period and is usually characterized by much less delta sleep than took place in the first deep cycle. The second REM period lasts about ten minutes and is more intense than the first. From this second REM period until morning awakening, stage 2 sleep and REM alternate in approximately 90 minute cycles. Delta sleep is rarely seen during these later sleep cycles, having made its major contribution during the first 90 minutes of sleep in the night. As sleep progresses toward morning, REM periods last longer and become more intense physiologically as well as psychologically.

The major sleep disorders have been shown to correlate with stages of sleep. For example, the classic sleep disorders of nocturnal enuresis, somnambulism and night terrors occur preferentially during arousal from slow wave sleep (stages 3 and 4) and are virtually never associated with REM dreaming state (Broughton, 1968). Accordingly, Kramer and others have shown that, for example, the stage 4 night terror (described by Fisher as a combination of extreme panic, flight reactions in the form of motility and somnambulism, and sleep utterances in the form of gasps, moans, groans, cursing, and blood curdling, piercing screams) occur in more than two thirds of instances during the first NREM period, often as early as 15 minutes after the onset of sleep. This finding correlates well with the great predominance of stages 3 and 4 during the first sleep cycle early in the night;

night terrors are not seen during the second part of the night. In comparison to these night terrors, which are fragmentary and poorly remembered with only the briefest glimpses into their content, the more frequent ordinary nightmare, or the REM anxiety dream, occurs later in the night, with a clear mental state on awakening and with usually good and often excellent recall of contents.

Posttraumatic Nightmares

According to virtually all authors, an integral aspect of the classic posttraumatic syndrome is the occurrence of recurrent nightmares, often accompanied by insomnia. Although the nightmares of people with lifelong nightmare conditions seem to occur clearly during REM sleep (Van der Kolk, 1982), it seems that the exact sleep stage location of catastrophic, posttraumatic dreams has not been definitively determined. Schlosberg and Benjamin (1978) made sleep recordings of soldiers who seemed to have their postcombat nightmares during stage 2. Overall, however, traumatic war nightmares have been very hard to study in the laboratory. Harvesting the dreams of these nightmare sufferers during EEG sleep monitoring has produced rather limited results. For example, in the few published studies so far, Greenberg et al (1972) found only two clear-cut nightmares after many nights of sleep recording. Lavie et al (1979) found in their sleep studies that 2 out of 11 patients had nightmares, but that these occurred during REM sleep. The patients in both of these studies had complained of recurrent nightmares of traumatic war experiences.

Dr. George Hogben and the author have regarded the nightmares and sleep disturbances as major target symptoms for medication. The following two case histories are illustrative of the type of disturbed sleep that certain patients with this disorder have shown, prompting us to consider the MAOI phenelzine sulfate for relief of the distressing (nightmare) symptomatology.

Patient 5   The patient, a World War II veteran, entered the hospital for severe panic attacks, nightmares, and deteriorating social functioning. He had been symptomatic since the war.

The patient's mother died when he was five years old. He was raised by an aunt along with nine other children. After several years, he moved back with his father and stepmother. He entered the Army after graduation from high school. The patient's father died shortly after he entered the service.

He had extensive World War II combat experience in the European theater, infiltrating behind enemy lines. On these missions, he killed many enemy soldiers in hand-to-hand combat. He also saw many buddies killed by enemy fire. He was captured, and both his arms were broken by German soldiers. He was hospitalized in a prisoner of war hospital in Italy where he was subjected to many atrocities. German soldiers forced the patient and other sick prisoners into deep, rat-infested pits; healthier prisoners would hide behind dying buddies to protect themselves from the rats. They could hear their dying buddies scream as they were eaten by the rats. As the patient's arms recovered, he served as an orderly in the hospital. He spent hours working with burned and maimed allied soldiers. At this hospital he was forced to witness the German machine gun executions of many patients.

Traumatic war nightmares began shortly after honorable discharge from the service. These nightmares occurred nightly and woke him from sleep. On waking he felt paralyzed, but after several minutes he could return to sleep. He rarely slept more than four hours a night, however. When not sleeping, he heard the voices of his wartime buddies calling out for help. He developed vivid day images of rats scampering around the floor. Other day image contents centered on traumatic war scenes. He also had panic states with paralyzing fear, sweating, chest pain, and dyspnea. The patient was fearful of enclosed spaces and gatherings of people. Whenever he felt his symptoms increase, he drove his motorized home, named "Wandering Jew," around the country.

Five years before admission, the patient stopped traveling and noticed a marked increase in panic and physiological symptoms. The panic became so intense that he was forced to leave his job as a school aide. He was hospitalized three times for severe panic, chest pain with radiation to the left arm, suffocation, and feelings of impending death. Although admitting diagnosis had been "myocardial infarct" on several occasions, no enzyme or electrocardiographic evidence of an infarct were found. Nevertheless, the patient was so symptomatic he had had two cardiac catheterizations, both negative for coronary artery disease. Panic attacks were not suspected and a diagnosis of "angina" was made. He was medicated with propranalol 40 mg/day, isorbide 40 mg/day, nitroglycerine 1/150 g, average dose four/day.

The patient had several unsuccessful periods of psychiatric treatment. Chemotherapy included amitriptyline 150 mg/day and diazepam up to 40 mg/day. These medications did not prevent his nightmares, day images or panic. Diazepam provided some relief of chronic anxiety. Extensive outpatient psychotherapy also did not alter his symptoms.

The patient was an obese man who related in a guarded, frightened manner. He had severe panic attacks three to four times per day. During these he was terrified, diaphoretic, dyspneic, and fearful of dying. Nitroglycerine 1/150 g relieved intense tightness in his chest but not the panic feelings. He had vivid visual images of traumatic war scenes and was often observed swinging a broom under beds at the "rats." Nightmares occurred nightly and interrupted his sleep. Several times a week during the night he was observed listening at the door to his "buddies screaming in another building." On two occasions he broke off conversations with staff, drew back in his chair tense and frightened, and spoke to German officers he saw in front of him, in a clipped, rapid Germanic dialect. Observers conversant in German did not recognize many of the words he used. One of these episodes occurred during an electroencephalogram. Although much of the record was obscured by muscle activity, a few short runs without interference revealed normal waking brain activity.

The patient's speech was logical and goal-oriented except during the two episodes described above. Most of the time he was sad and withdrawn from patients and staff. Doxepin 200 mg/day was given for one month without effect. The patient was encouraged to discuss his feelings about war episodes and his dead buddies. He denied having feelings and related to the therapist on superficial matters only.

Within one day after starting phenelzine, the patient felt and acted calmer. Thereafter, he did not request nitroglycerine. Over the next week, he began interacting with other patients and staff. During the second therapy week, the patient's mood improved and he smiled spontaneously. He openly expressed anger at ward frustrations. Nightmares and day imaging lessened throughout this week. Nightmares stopped completely on the 18th night. Day images of traumatic war experiences also stopped, but the patient continued to see rats infrequently. He also infrequently heard nighttime screams of his buddies. During psychotherapy the patient described with intense anger events in the prisoner of war hospital.

Blood pressure averaged 110/70 mm Hg. All cardiac medications were discontinued during the fifth therapy week, without incident. Blood pressure increased to 120/80 mm Hg after stopping cardiac medication. The patient maintained symptomatic improvement on phenelzine during a three-month follow-up period. He was then lost to follow-up because he returned to his home, which was far from the hospital. Phone follow-up one year later indicated the patient was functioning moderately well without phenelzine.

Patient 6 A 25-year-old Hispanic single male complained of anxiety, panic and aggressive outbursts. The patient had four older sisters, one younger sister, and two older brothers who died when the patient was a young child. When the patient was 16, his parents moved to Puerto Rico, while he lived with friends for two years and finished 11th grade before entering the Marine Corps. There is no history of preservice behavioral problems.

This patient did not see active combat. However, he described being involved in several traumatic combat-like incidents. Two times he witnessed helicopters explode close by him. He stood by helpless while watching the occupants burn and hearing them scream for help, and he assisted in removing their charred remains.

He was a camp guard at one overseas base when a riot by local villagers erupted. He was required to use force to help control the rioters and was exposed to scattered sniper fire. He was also involved in a practice bombing raid during which bombs were dropped near him. This "friendly fire" occurred without warning and was terrifying to him. The patient had two minor physical traumas. He receives 100 percent service-connected disability for his nervous condition.

After witnessing the first helicopter crash, the patient developed nightmares of the incident. These woke him from sleep, and on waking he felt paralyzed. He also became anxious and noticed episodic panic with sweats, breathlessness, and abdominal cramps. He became depressed and took an overdose of diazepam. As more traumatic incidents occurred, his nightmares became more frequent. He also developed intense visualizations of the traumatic incidents when awake.

After discharge from the service in 1974, his symptoms increased in intensity, and he developed thoughts of assaulting others as well as multiple somatic complaints. He began hearing a voice urging him to kill himself. He startled easily and lost his temper with little provocation. He felt helpless and flew into blind rages in VA facilities over "not being helped." Chemotherapeutic agents taken by the patient before phenelzine included chlorpromazine 400 mg/day, loxapine 40 mg/day, and amitriptyline 100 mg/day. These agents did not alter the symptoms. Psychotherapy centered on his feelings about traumatic service events, but discussing these did not alleviate his symptoms.

The patient was a thin, anxious man who related in a suspicious and frightened manner. He appeared depressed and cried readily. He was treated as an outpatient with phenelzine 60 mg/day. Within two days he felt and looked calmer. He stopped having catastrophic dreams on the fifth therapy day. Daytime flashbacks stopped at one week. On the seventh day he began expressing rage at former Marine Corps officers and VA officials. He ventilated angry feelings for several weeks and then became depressed. The depression lifted after one week. Thereafter, the patient responded with appropriate affect. The patient tested his response to the medication two times by stopping it. All the symptoms came back within two days and were rapidly controlled by restarting the medication. A ten-month follow-up report indicated that he continued to do well with phenelzine.

Inasmuch as the patients we treated complained of frequent, often severe, well-remembered and recurrent nightmares, we considered the pharmacologic effect of phenelzine on sleep architecture. A number of studies have suggested that phenelzine can totally inhibit REM sleep in normal as well as depressed patients; therefore, we regarded phenelzine in sufficient doses to be of potential value in either diminishing or abolishing dream activity. In earlier significant studies, Akindele et al (1970) had demonstrated delayed suppression of the signs of REM-sleep with phenelzine and noted that the delay of the beginning of mood elevation in three depressed patients was chronologically related to REM sleep suppression. It was felt that REM suppression and mood elevation may have been associated manifestations of more basic changes in brain chemistry. Wyatt et al (1971) repeated similar observations in treating six anxious-depressed patients. However, there was only one patient who showed a clear temporal relationship between mood improvement and REM sleep suppression. Dunleavy and Oswald (1973) demonstrated a mean delay of 16 days for total REM suppression on a 60 mg/day phenelzine dose, and an eight-day delay on a 75 mg/day dose. In 9 of the 22 depressed patients, restoration of normal mood coincided with the delayed abolition of the signs of REM sleep. Thus, these three studies strongly suggested that phenelzine could not only abolish REM (dream related) sleep in one to four weeks, but might also have delayed mood elevating properties in certain depressed patients. Although very recent studies (Vogel, 1980) have pointed to improvement of depression by REM sleep deprivation, clearly phenelzine's low effectiveness in the majority of endogenous depressions, despite its capacity to eradicate REM sleep, leaves certain questions largely unanswered.

The time course of cessation of nightmares parallels the time course established by EEG studies of the suppression of REM sleep by phenelzine. This cessation of recurrent nightmares of horrifying combat experience may be an important factor in patients' favorable therapeutic responses. Kramer (1982) has suggested that perhaps the physiologic basis for chronic traumatic neurosis is the disturbance of sleep itself; he feels that insomnia, irritability, nightmares, and depression may be the major characteristics of a more basic circadian rhythm disturbance. There have been suggestions in the literature (Kleitman, 1963; Friedman and Fisher, 1967) that the sleep-dream cycle may be part of a continuous ultradian biorhythm that cycles over a 24 hour period. Thus, the REM stage of sleep may possibly have a counterpart in the awake state. To date, documentation of an awake REM state has relied on demonstrating cycles of physiologic instability and drive activity similar to those observed during REM sleep.

The flashback activity observed in a number of the patients whom we have been describing may have been a manifestation of an awake REM state. Each patient described three to five periods of intense visualization while awake. Although these periods seemed to follow a regular order in some of the patients, precise measurement of the time sequences was not possible. Most of the patients stopped having flashbacks completely during phenelzine therapy, the rest had fewer visualizations. The suppression of flashback activity during phenelzine therapy may thus have resulted from the inhibition of an awake REM state or analogue.

OTHER SIGNIFICANT AREAS OF RESEARCH

Tricyclics

The effects of tricyclic medications deserve carefully controlled trials in this condition. The tricyclic antidepressants have a capacity to suppress or diminish REM sleep as well as tending to increase the percentage of time spent in stage 2 sleep. However, it seems generally agreed, especially with imipramine, that REM suppressive effects lessen over the course of several weeks, although complete tolerance has not developed. Usually, a pronounced REM rebound occurs with the tricyclics as well as MAO inhibitors. However, most studies with tricyclics have been done in normal individuals. Studies in depressed patients do not necessarily point to clear-cut suppression of REM sleep with most of the tricyclics. The only tricyclic producing a profound REM suppression in normals as well as depressives is chlorimipramine (Passouant et al, 1975), which clearly deserves a pilot study with the traumatic neuroses.

In a series of five patients in clinical practice, Burstein (1982) has suggested that the tricyclic drug imipramine has produced favorable results in patients after automobile accidents and exhibiting symptoms of impotence, fatigue, increased startle, heightened nervousness, poor sleep with recurrent nightmares, as well as a tendency towards flashbacks of the accident when approaching the geographic location. He claims that imipramine has an overall calming effect as well as a pronounced effect on the sexual dysfunction. It also helps reduce the intensity and frequency of recurrent nightmares of the accident. Friedman (1981) has discussed administering tricyclic antidepressants "as a treatment of choice in questionable situations . . . with considerable success, especially with amitriptyline." He quotes Hauri as suggesting that in patients with nightmares that may arise out of stage 1 or stage 2 sleep, REM suppression is incidental and that the success of treatment is derived from the use of this medication that deepens sleep; nightmares may occur but do not awaken the patient.

Lithium Carbonate

The role of lithium carbonate in the treatment of posttraumatic stress disorders or chronic traumatic neurosis also merits exploration. There is a substantial literature, primarily represented by the works of Sheard and Marini (1978), suggesting its value in modulating intense aggressive feelings and behavior, particularly in aggressive prisoners. Most sleep reports are in agreement that, in therapeutic doses, lithium reduces REM percentage sleep but increases deep or delta sleep, without a REM rebound on termination of the drug. The diminished REM sleep time is due to shorter REM sleep periods. However, it seems to lack the massive REM suppressant effects that the powerful MAO inhibitors exhibit. Van der Kolk (1982), in recent pilot work with lithium carbonate with chronic traumatic neurotics, in both group and individual settings, suggests that lithium-stabilized patients are able to respond appropriately to a stimulus that had earlier provoked the dramatic startle or over-reactivity so often seen in these syndromes. Most of his patients who had complained of a "short fuse" showed, over time, the capacity to differentiate present unexpected sounds, such as a car back-firing, from wartime-type sounds. Their responses on lithium lacked the dramatic dissociative and hysterical features so often seen with over-intense startle reactions. Thus, if his preliminary findings are born out in controlled studies, the role of lithium in poorly modulated aggressive outbursts frequently leading to dissociative panic states could be a significant one.

Arousal, Startle Response

Other recent studies at the pilot stage show promise in enhancing the understanding of these disorders at the biological and physiological levels. For example, Kramer and co-workers in Jackson, Mississippi are finding in sleep laboratory studies that posttraumatic neurotics seem to have NREM sleep disturbances as well as REM disturbances that are noise-sensitive. These patients have shown a hyper-responsiveness to a modest 70 dB of noise during NREM sleep, showing an intense arousal similar to that of a night-terror (see Kramer, 1979). He claims that this intense arousal by ordinary sounds during NREM sleep is very similar to the heightened startle reaction of these patients while awake. Keane (1982), from the Jackson, Mississippi VA Medical Center, has recently used "flooding" techniques for desensitization of traumatized patients, with diminished arousal responses, progressively and over time, to images and traumatic, emotionally intense memories. Kolb (1982), in the Albany VA Medical Center, has suggested, in pilot work recently, the existence of a Conditioned Emotional Response to combat sounds, induced frequently by a meaningful auditory stimulus relating to combat sounds. He and co-workers are attempting desensitization by repeated but gradually increasing exposure to these sounds in over-reactive, heightened-startle patients, with a progressive reduction in symptoms in these patients with accompanying psychotherapy and pharmacotherapy. He feels that the primary disturbing factor in a group of combat-experienced posttraumatic neurotic patients is this conditioned emotional response, against which patients attempt various mechanisms of defense and avoidance.

CONCLUSION

At the present time there is an obvious scarcity of well-controlled studies into psychophysiologic aspects of the traumatic neuroses or posttraumatic disorders. Even psychopharmacologic clinical studies in carefully chosen populations are absent from the psychiatric literature, with the exception of pilot and anecdotal reports. That a syndrome of multifaceted psychiatric dysfunction could avoid careful investigation at basic and clinical research levels is curious, particularly in an era of sophisticated research methodology. Hopefully, the future will see reports in the professional scientific literature that may begin to enhance our understanding, in depth, of biological and physiological parameters of these conditions. Carefully targeted clinical pharmacologic approaches, if initiated, may hopefully provide an effective means of treating the chronic traumatic syndromes.

BIBLIOGRAPHY

Akindele, M. O. et al. (1970). Monoamine oxidase inhibitors, sleep, and mood. *Electroencephalography and Clinical Neurophysiology* 29: 47-56.

Archibald, H. C. et al. (1962). Gross stress reaction in combat: a 15 year follow-up. *American Journal of Psychiatry* 111: 317-322.

Archibald, H. C., Tuddenham, R. D. (1965). Persistent stress reaction after combat: a 20 year follow-up. *Archives of General Psychiatry* 12: 475-481.

Blackwell, B., et al. (1967). Hypertensive interactions between monoamine oxidase inhibitors and food stuffs. *British Journal of Psychiatry* 113: 349-365.

Bloch, R., et al. (1954). The clinical effect of isoniazid and iproniazid in the treatment of pulmonary tuberculosis. *Annals of Intern Medicine* 40: 881-900.

Broughton, R. (1968). Sleep disorders: disorders of arousal? *Science* 159: 1070-1078.

Burstein, A. (1982). Personal communication.

Cornfield, R., Hogben, G. (1980). Traumatic Neuroses of War. *Weekly Psychiatry Update Series* 30(3): 1-7.

Crane, G. (1957). Iproniazid (Marsilid) phosphate, a therapeutic agent for mental disorders and debilitating disease. *Psychiatric Research Reports* 8: 142-152.

Davidson, J. et al. (1982). Atypical depression. *Archives of General Psychiatry* 39: 527-534.

Dement, W. (1965). In Vol. 2, New Directions in Psychology. Newcomb, T. (Ed.) New York: Holt, Rinehart and Winston, p. 165.

Dobbs, D., Wilson, P. (1960). Observations on persistence of war neurosis. *Diseases of the Nervous System* 21: 686-691.

Dunleavy, D. L. F., Oswald, I. (1973). Phenelzine, mood response, and sleep. *Archives of General Psychiatry* 28: 353-356.

Fisher, C., et al. (1973). A psychophysiological study of nightmares and night terrors. *Archives of General Psychiatry* 28: 252-259.

Fox, R. (1972). Post-combat adaptational problems. *Comprehensive Psychiatry* 13(5): 435-443.

Freud, S. (1922). *Beyond the Pleasure Principle*. London: Hogarth Press.

Friedman, M. J. (1981). Post-Vietnam syndrome: recognition and management. *Psychosomatics* 22(11): 931-943.

Friedman, S., Fisher, C. (1967). On the presence of a rhythmic, diurnal, oral instinctual drive cycle in man. *Journal of the American Psychoanalytic Association* 15: 317-343.

Greenberg, R. et al. (1972). War neurosis and the adaptive function of REM sleep. *British Journal of Medical Psychology* 45: 27-33.

Grinker, R. R. (1945). Psychiatric disorders in combat crews overseas and in returnees. *Medical Clinics of North America* 29: 729-739.

Grinker, R. R., Spiegel, J. P. (1945). *Men Under Stress.* Philadelphia: Blakiston Co.

Hauri, P. (1977). The sleep disorders. Kalamazoo, Michigan: Scope Publishers—Upjohn Co.

Hogben, G., Cornfield, R. (1981). Treatment of traumatic war neurosis with phenelzine. *Archives of General Psychiatry* 38: 440-445.

Horowitz, M. J., Becker, S. S. (1972). Cognitive response to stress: experimental studies of a "compulsion to repeat trauma." *Psychoanalysis and Contemporary Science* 1: 258-305.

Horowitz, M. J., Wilner, N. (1976). Stress films, emotions, and cognitive response. *Archives of General Psychiatry* 30: 1339-1344.

Horowitz, M. J. et al. (1980). Signs and symptoms of posttraumatic stress disorder. *Archives of General Psychiatry* 37: 85-92.

Jouvet, M. (1967). Neurophysiology of the states of sleep. *Physiology Review* 47: 117-177.

Kardiner, A. (1941). *The Traumatic Neuroses of War.* New York: Hoeber.

Kardiner, A. (1947). *War Stress and Neurotic Illness.* New York: Hoeber.

Keane, T. (1982). Personal communication.

Kelly, D. et al. (1970). Treatment of phobic states with antidepressants: a retrospective study of 246 patients. *British Journal of Psychiatry* 116: 387-398.

Klein, D. (1964). Delineation of two drug-responsive anxiety syndromes. *Psychopharmacology* 5: 397-408.

Klein, D. F. (1977). Psychopharmacologic treatment and delineation of borderline disorders. In Hartocollis, P. (Ed.) *Borderline Personality Disorders: The Concept, The Syndrome, The Patient.* New York: International University Press, pp. 365-383.

Klein, D. et al. (1978). Antidepressants, anxiety, panic, and phobia. In Lipton, M., DiMascio, A., Killam, K. (Eds.) *Psychopharmacology: A Generation of Progress.* New York: Raven Press, pp. 1401-1410.

Kleitman, N. (1963). *Sleep and Wakefulness.* Chicago: University of Chicago Press.

Kline, N. (1958). Clinical experience with iproniazid (Marsilid). *Journal of Clinical Experiential Psychopathology* 19(Suppl 1): 72-78.

Kolb, L. (1982). Personal communication.

Kramer, M. (1979). Dream disturbances. *Psychiatric Annals* 9: 7.

Kramer, M. (1981). Personal communication. In Friedman, M. J. (Ed.). Post-Vietnam Syndrome: Recognition and Management. *Psychosomatics* 22(11): 931-943.

Lavie, P. et al. (1979). Long-term effects of traumatic war-related events on sleep. *American Journal of Psychiatry* 136: 175-178.

Leahy, M. R., Martin, I. C. A. (1967). Successful hypnotic abreaction after 20 years. *British Journal of Psychiatry* 113: 383-385.

Leopold, R. L., Dillon, H. (1963). Psychoanatomy of disaster: long-term study of post-traumatic neuroses in survivors of a marine explosion. *American Journal of Psychiatry* 119: 913-921.

Liebowitz, M., Klein, D. (1979). Hysteroid dysphoria. *Psychiatric Clinics of North America* 2(3): 555-575.

Lipper, S. et al. (1979). Comparative behavioral effects of clorgyline and pargyline in man: a preliminary evaluation. *Psychopharmacology* 62: 123-128.

Little, J. C., James, B. (1964). Abreaction of conditioned fear reaction after 18 years. *Behavior Research Therapy* 2: 59-63.

Marini, J. L., Sheard, M. H. (1977). Antiaggressive effect of lithium ion in man. *Acta Psychiatric Scandinavica* 55(4): 269-286.

Medical Research Council. (1965). Clinical trial of the treatment of depressive illness: report by the MRC Clinical Psychiatry Committee. *British Medical Journal* 1: 881-886.

Oppenheim, H. (1889). Die traumatischen neurosen. Berlin: Hitschwald.

Passouant, et al. (1975). *International Journal of Neurology* 10(1-4): 186-197.

Paykel, E. et al. (1979). Depressive classification and prediction of response to phenelzine. *British Journal of Psychiatry* 134: 572-581.

Pollitt, J., Young, J. (1971). Anxiety state or masked depression: a study based on the action of monoamine oxidase inhibitors. *British Journal of Psychiatry* 119: 143-150.

Quitkin, F. et al. (1979). Monoamine oxidase inhibitors. *Archives of General Psychiatry* 35: 749-760.

Rado, S. (1942). Pathodynamics and treatment of traumatic war neurosis (Traumatophobia). *Psychosomatic Medicine* 4: 362-368.

Ravaris, C. L. et al. (1976). A multiple dose controlled study of phenelzine in depression-anxiety states. *Archives of General Psychiatry* 33: 347-350.

Robinson, D. S. et al. (1973). The monoamine oxidase inhibitor, phenelzine, in the treatment of depressive-anxiety states. *Archives of General Psychiatry* 29: 407-413.

Robinson, D. S. et al. (1978). Clinical pharmacology of phenelzine. *Archives of General Psychiatry* 35: 629-635.

Robinson, D. S. et al. (1978). Clinical psychopharmacology of phenelzine: MAO activity and clinical response. In Lipton, M., DiMascio, A., Killam, K. (Eds.). *Psychopharmacology: A Generation of Progress.* New York: Raven Press.

Roffwarg, H. et al. (1966). Ontogenetic development of the human sleep-dream cycle. *Science* 152: 604-619.

Roth, M. (1959). The phobic anxiety-depersonalization syndrome. *Proceedings of the Royal Society of Medicine* 52: 587.

Salmon, T. W. (1919). The war neuroses and their lessons. *New York State Journal of Medicine* 109: 933-944.

Sargant, W. (1961). Drugs in the treatment of depression. *British Medical Journal* 1: 225-227.

Sargant, W., Dally, P. J. (1962). Treatment of anxiety states by antidepressant drugs. *British Medical Journal* 1: 6-9.

Saul, L. (1945). Psychological factors in combat fatigue. *Psychosomatic Medicine* 7: 257-272.

Saul, L. J., Lyons, J. W. (1952). Acute Neurotic Reactions. In Alexander, F., Ross, H. (Eds.). *Dynamic Psychiatry.* Chicago: University of Chicago Press.

Schlosberg, A., Benjamin, M. (1978). Sleep patterns in three acute combat fatigue cases. *Journal of Clinical Psychiatry* 39: 546-549.

Selikoff, I. et al. (1952). Toxicity of hydrazine derivatives of isonicotinic acid in the chemotherapy of human tuberculosis. *Quarterly Bulletin of Sea View Hospital* 13: 17.

Sheard, M., Marini, J. (1978). Treatment of human aggressive behavior: four case studies of the effect of lithium. *Comprehensive Psychiatry* 19: 37-45.

Sheehan, D. V. et al. (1980). Treatment of endogenous anxiety with phobic, hysterical, and hypochondriacal symptoms. *Archives of General Psychiatry* 37: 51-59.

Snyder, F. (1963). The new biology of dreaming. *Archives of General Psychiatry* 8: 381-391.

Strange, R. E. (1969). Effects of combat stress on hospital ship psychiatric evacuees. In Bourne, P. G. (Ed.). *Psychology and Physiology of Stress*. New York: Academic Press.

Strecker, E. A. (1945). Psychiatry and War. In: *Fundamentals of Psychiatry*. Philadelphia: J. B. Lippincott.

Thornton, C. et al. (1980). The effect of deprenyl, a selective monoamine oxidase B/inhibitor, on sleep and mood in man. *Psychopharmacology* 70: 163-166.

Tyrer, P. et al. (1973). A study of the clinical effects of phenelzine and placebo in the treatment of phobic anxiety. *Psychopharmacologia* 32: 237-254.

Tyrer, P. (1976). Towards rational therapy with monoamine inhibitors. *British Journal of Psychiatry* 128: 354-360.

van der Kolk, B. (1982). Personal communication.

van Putten, T., Emory, W. H. (1973). Traumatic neuroses in Vietnam returnees: a forgotten diagnosis? *Archives of General Psychiatry* 29: 695-698.

Vogel, G. W. et al. (1980). Improvement of depression by REM sleep deprivation. *Archives of General Psychiatry* 37: 247-253.

West, E. D., Dally, P. J. (1959). Effects of iproniazid in depressive syndromes. *British Medical Journal* 1: 1491-1494.

Wyatt, R. J. et al. (1971). Total prolonged drug-induced REM sleep suppression in anxious-depressed patients. *Archives of General Psychiatry* 24: 145-155.

Youdim, M., Paykel, E. (1981). Monoamine oxidase inhibitors: The State of the Art. New York: John Wiley and Sons.

Zeller, E. et al. (1952). Influence of isonicotinic acid hydrazide (INH) and 1-isonicotinyl 2-isopropyl hydrazide (IIH) on bacterial and mammalian enzymes. *Experientia* 8: 349-350.

9
Fear of the Dead:
The Role of Social Ritual
in Neutralizing Fantasies from Combat

HARVEY J. SCHWARTZ, M.D.

Blood hath been shed ere now, i' th' olden time,
Ere human statute purged the gentle weal;
Ay, and since too, murders have been performed
Too terrible for the ear. The times has been
That, when the brains were out, the man would
Die, and there an end; but now they rise again,
With twenty mortal murders on their crowns, and
Push us from our stools. This is more strange
Than such a murder is.

Shakespeare *Macbeth* III, iv

Traumatic neuroses have been part of the human condition since the beginning of time. The horrors of war have always left their mark on its combatants. Civilizations in the past have respected the psychic crisis that combat inflicts on its soldiers. The fears, fantasies and guilts of battle have been integrated into cultural mythology that acts as a collective secondary process for the overwhelmed soldier. Through this mechanism of community ritual, the veteran is helped to progress from his regressive acting out of aggression to his more mature precombat ego functioning.

The major wars of this century have been characterized by a deep social commitment to the moral righteousness of the cause. The perception was of evil being challenged in a necessary struggle for survival. The country was mobilized and its preexisting moral self-image was consistent with the activities of its soldiers. At the conclusion of hostilities treaties were signed, families rejoiced and heroes were welcomed home. The collectively shared and dependable concept of the war led to a religious embrace of the courageous warriors.

I suggest that an important factor in the soldier's reintegration into civilized life is the compatibility of his precombat moral self-image, his wartime activities as perceived and defined by his supporting culture, and his continued acceptance upon his homecoming. These dependable social forces act as a trustworthy "holding environment" during the regression of battle. The primitive and stimulating fantasies that are unleashed by combat are thereby tamed by the soothing of an accepting culture. The absolution that society can grant from its valued position of respect is an essential feature in the soldiers' rehabilitation.

The recent war in Vietnam differed fundamentally from the earlier wars of this century. On the homefront, the political and moral precepts that led to the conflict were seen as bankrupt and self-serving. The social and military leadership were perceived as untrustworthy and dishonest. This breakdown in the supporting social matrix was reflected in the disorganized concept and conduct of the war. For the soldier, the enemy was unclear, the purpose vague, the aggression unguided, and righteousness irrelevant. Thus, failure of the society to provide a respected and coherent schema for the war on a macro level led to micro failures of leadership, guidance and direction for the everyday activities of the infantryman.

I believe that this failure of structure has contributed to the large number of Vietnam veterans whose lives remain overwhelmed by their traumas. The unconscious fantasies and conflicts stimulated by battle have not been tamed by the coherent and loving forces of the community. The failure to provide the veteran with a welcoming home ceremony symbolizes the broader failure at sustaining him with a dependable and moral concept for his activities.[1]

---

[1] The therapeutic power of external life events has not been well studied. From an epidemiologic perspective, Tennant (1981) researched the role that these "neutralizing" events have in countering the effects of trauma. He found that these events "substantially negated or counteracted the impact of an earlier threatening event or chronic difficulty," and were associated with a more favorable outcome. Tennant considers the postcombat welcoming home ceremony to be a "major and profound neutralizing event" (personal communication; see also Davidson, 1979). I address the possible unconscious meaning of these events in the discussion, pp. 262-267.

While the fantasies stimulated by combat are as primitive and varied as the act itself, I focus our attention in this report on a specific fantasy system and illustrate its role in the chronic disability of a Vietnam veteran. My purpose is to underscore the importance of repressed fantasies in the war neuroses and thereby reemphasize the role of unconscious forces in this condition. As mentioned, I believe that these stimulated conflicts need attending in order for the veteran to reenter civilized life.

A word about the patient is in order before the clinical material. Mr. C. represents an extreme example of postwar disability. His fantasy of attack by the vengeful dead is an all-consuming nightmare. I believe he is an "exception that highlights the everyday." I do not present him as an example of a patient who necessarily would be helped by a cultural ceremony. He is, unfortunately, a patient who reveals to us in relatively undisguised fashion the power and primitiveness of the unconscious fantasies stimulated by war. I believe it is his failure of repression rather than the fantasy itself that makes him unusual. He serves as a reminder to us of man's most ancient fears.

CLINICAL MATERIAL

Mr. C., a 31-year-old white man, presented himself lying stretched out on a couch, disheveled, unshaven, and sleeping. I awakened him to come to my office and he rose mechanically as if in a daze. He lumbered his large frame slowly and with difficulty. His eyes were glazed and he seemed to be in another world. He sat, began smoking, and with some hesitation mumbled a few words about Vietnam. There were long pauses between his phrases and it seemed as if speaking was a new experience. While his voice was soft and distant, his thoughts were coherent and without signs of a thought disorder. Slowly his muttered fragments began to form sentences and I carefully listened and inquired. He spoke of being afraid to sleep, for the moment he closed his eyes he heard screams and saw dead bodies. He said he kept his mind blank because that way the bodies can't get him. He lived alone in his car and stole his food. He reported no human contact for one and a half years since he left his wife and three-year-old son, whom he had begun to beat. He did not know his age though the records showed his birthday to be three days earlier. He reported long periods of forgetfulness—he could not remember where he was or what he had done. In addition to his multiple somatic complaints, he painfully spoke of feeling unappreciated for the job he had done for the Marine Corps.

Throughout this introduction, I was both interested and confused. This was clearly a man in a severely regressed state with primitive ego functioning. However, despite his apparent schizoid adaptation, I was impressed that he was returning for treatment after a previous failed therapy. I also noted that although his affect was mostly blunted, he slowly began to relate warmly to me and seemed to appreciate my quiet interest in him.

His previous records answered many questions. The patient had been discharged from Vietnam against his will ten years prior, after working in Grave's Registration for over two years. His job there was to examine and process all the dead bodies of American soldiers. His records show that since his discharge, he has been chronically depressed and unable to hold a job or relate comfortably to friends. He had been hospitalized twice and had not responded to various psychotropic medications.

I agreed to work with this man as he had nowhere else to turn. I also was fascinated by his presenting condition and hoped to learn about the forces that brought him to this state. I was concerned that I knew nothing of his prewar and childhood life, but he was unable to give a history. (I was to later learn that he had not had any major psychiatric disorder before the war. There were signs, however, of severe and lifelong conflicts over primitive aggression.) The patient's relatedness to me was both a potentially hopeful sign and a foreshadowing of the powerful transference images that would emerge. I allowed myself to be emotionally available to him and I wondered what our future together would be.

Over the course of our next sessions, he became more animated and engaged. He spontaneously spoke at great length and in great detail of his job in Vietnam. I was struck by the immediacy of these events for him. They were with him as if he were still doing them today and not ten years ago. Looking back, I see this as another premonition of our difficult future.

His job in Vietnam was to collect, transport, examine, record and piece together the bodies of dead and almost dead soldiers. The bodies were generally burned, decomposed, mutilated or in pieces. Limbs would be unattached, faces blown apart, and gut and genitals ripped open. During busy times, the bodies would be stacked up like logs and he would work around the clock. The morgue became this man's home for two years. He ate there, played there, had sex there and often slept on the body tables. His early reaction to the carnage was to vomit continuously. This receded and he learned to keep his mind blank.

The details of this patient's macabre activities need not be spelled out in this report. Suffice it to say that this man engaged in work that put him in intimate and continuous contact with the most primitive and bizarre aspects of war. I will report only the specific instances that relate to his fear of the dead bodies.

On one occasion the patient was sent a 'body' that was still alive, screaming and begging to be killed. For three hours the patient stood by this man, who had his chest blown apart and his arm detached. Finally, he could take no more and he smothered him. After that "I heard him screaming even when he wasn't. All that night I felt he was coming out of the refrigerator to jump me."

At another time the patient recalled being locked in the darkened morgue refrigerator for 14 hours. He screamed in terror that the bodies would rise up and attack him.

This fear of the dead was an everpresent concern to the grave workers. A standing routine was for one of them to hide in the refrigerator in a body bag. As an unsuspecting coworker would enter the room, the 'dead man' would jump up, terrifying the friend and chasing him from the room. The others would laugh in reassured relief. They repeated this sequence over and over without any diminution of affect.

Gradually, the men learned that they could manipulate others through this fear. They would illegally bring prostitutes into the morgue and hide them in body bags. When the officers would search for the women, the men knew that they were afraid and would never open the bags—and they never did. The women in the bags as well served to further blur the boundary between the dead and the living. In time the distinction would be almost entirely lost.

There were other social consequences to working in the morgue. The ubiquitous fear of the dead generalized to fear of those who touched the dead. The grave registration workers were looked upon as contaminated lepers by the other soldiers. They were isolated from group activities and were subjected to verbal abuse. Most importantly, they were denied access to the mess hall and were forced to eat inferior food by themselves. They were untouchables. This outcast status drew them closer to each other and to their work.[2]

---

[2] This social isolation has been well known since primitive times. Freud (1913, p. 51), quoting Frazer (1911, p. 138) notes: "Among the Maoris anyone who had handled a corpse or taken any part in its burial was in the highest degree unclean and was almost cut off from intercourse with his fellow-men, or, as we might put it, was boycotted. He could not enter any house, or come into contact with any person or thing without infecting them. He might not even touch food with his hands, which, owing to their uncleanness, had become quite useless."

After many months, I began to learn about Mr. C.'s life in Vietnam before his stay at Grave's Registration. He was sent to war as an infantryman and was desperately afraid of hurting others, "I tried not to think of what I was doing, I'd shoot back, but hope that no one got hurt. That's the worse thing to do on earth. I think of someone's mother, father, and husband and what the people have to go through."

Finally, not long after his arrival he witnessed his first death, that of his best friend, "I wish it were me—I wish I never came back." He soon thereafter learned of the Grave's Registration position. This was a volunteered-for job, available to any soldier. One could leave the front lines for the safety of the morgue at will. Many infantrymen tried this work, only to return to the danger of battle in a day or two. Mr. C. never left. He consciously saw this as helpful work and took great pride in the respect with which he treated the bodies.

In time, however, his guilt emerged and mushroomed. "I feel like the lowest thing on earth . . . it was different over there . . . when I was a kid, when the other guys did something wrong, I didn't do it . . . over there you had to do it . . . everyone acted like they were crazy . . . I did it, too . . . I acted crazy . . . I turned into a monster . . . I'll be there for the rest of my life . . . I came back physically, but only one-half of me . . . I still eat, sleep and act the same."

Self-destructive guilt was a common phenomena among Grave Registration workers. I was told that they all came to dramatic ends. One friend drove wildly about the country-side until he smashed into the circulating propeller of an airplane. Others stayed permanently drugged, drunk, or jailed. Others killed themselves. For Mr. C., his punishment was never to leave Vietnam. He hides in his car from the bodies chasing him. "This way I can see when they come after me and I won't be trapped. The gooks will get me sooner or later. The dead bodies are punishing a lot of people." His ability to discriminate past from present was, at best, tenuous and frequently nonexistent.

Throughout the early part of his treatment, Mr. C. continuously described his terrifying dreams. The vengeful, attacking dead bodies would haunt him throughout the night. Often he would awaken only to experience his greatest fear—the nightmare would continue while his eyes were open. Occasionally, he would actually flee his car and run down the street in terror of the pursuing bodies. At times, the dreams would contain other graphic images from his unconscious. More than once he dreamt he was eating flesh from the bodies. Other times, he dreamt that doctors were cutting the legs off still alive bodies.

These transference images grew until one session when he anxiously walked into my office. He, as usual, failed to acknowledge my presence and my greeting. He spoke slowly and in a daze and began describing his dream in which I was allied with the dead bodies and was trying to hurt him. He saw my meetings with him as a means to trick him, "You're not going to outsmart me—I'm on to you!" The infantile basis of these images was suggested by the dream as he described looking through a keyhole and seeing me plotting with the dead bodies. However, the imminent issue became his ego. In reciting the dream, he slowly became transported to another world. His look became distant, his agitation mounted and I felt as if I'd entered someone else's nightmare. My efforts to ground him in the reality of our meeting were meaningless and I saw myself becoming transformed in his eyes. These eyes began searching the office for his attackers and, as they materialized to him, he grew pale. His fears gelled into terror and he began screaming that I was trying to kill him. He leaped from his chair and fled the office in fear for his life. Significantly though, he was then able to speak coherently to two female secretaries and recount these events. The psychosis at this moment was limited to the transference.

One month later he returned and did not recognize me. It was as if I was a new doctor. He was in a daze and described the intervening month as being filled with attacking dead bodies. In fact, he exclaimed, "I tore the liver out of one of those damn bodies when it snuck up on me!" He described living "as if I'm in a dream" and felt he was in Vietnam.

Soon thereafter he came to the office in a dissociative state and was in Vietnam. I was his Lieutenant Colonel and it was 1971. He was pleading with me, as he did in Vietnam, to be allowed to stay here and continue working at Grave's Registration. He was enraged that he was being sent home against his will. His sole purpose for coming to my office was to try to remain here in Vietnam. This dissociative state lasted the entire session. He looked confused when I told him he was in the United States and had been here for ten years. As I persisted, he became anxious and screamed, "You're trying to fuck my mind up!" Indeed, when I told him I was a doctor, he sat quietly, puzzled a moment, and as if in a flash of insight, laughingly declared: "You've been around these bodies so long they have you believing you're a doctor!"

This state came and went. When he was not in it, he had no memory of it ever occurring. At other times, it would last four to five weeks. It was a bewildering period for me. The result of my transient regressive identification with him left me in a state of deep confusion. There was no shared ego with which to safely anchor myself. Either I too was in Vietnam, or I was out of empathic contact with him. Verbal interventions, other than agreeing with his reality, produced agitation. Besides, I began feeling foolish in speaking of mundane present reality; it seemed make-believe and beside the point. Indeed, it felt unreal. I found myself drawn into joining him in Vietnam. The alternative to this wholesale regression would be for me to both hold on to present reality and also to reach out and identify with his psychic reality. This demanding undertaking would expose me to the chasm of time and space that separated us. It would open me to the vast emptiness that his denial and regression had created. I felt frightened of this netherland of consciousness and feared for my ability to contain it. It was as if I was being exposed to the vacuum of awareness that he defensively retreated to in his horrifying work. I sensed that this terrifying absence of time contained a rage and a grief too awesome to bear.

I chose to remain mostly silent throughout this period and did my best to maintain an affective accessibility to him. Later there would be evidence to suggest that one of the precipitants to this regression was his rage at me for not seeing him when he came at the wrong time for his appointment. This rage transcended his integrative capacity.

Mr. C.'s treatment continued to be difficult. However, throughout the turmoil specific themes underlay his difficulties. The guilt over the death of his friend, as well as the chronic stimulation and guilt over his experiences with dead bodies was everpresent. The intractable fear of the vengeful attack by the dead bodies contained many overlapping elements. These include primary guilt, self-punishment, projected and identified-with rage, including cannibalistic and castrating impulses, as well as warded-off separation and mourning.

Fundamentally though, Mr. C.'s central difficulty was the predominance of a regressive ego state that left him passively at the mercy of his drive organized fantasies. This archaic dream-like schema resulted in distortions of reality, a compulsion to reenact, a loss of self-awareness and a blurring of self-nonself boundaries. Verbal interactions lost their value as he was oriented towards a visual and pictorial form characteristic of primary process (Rubinfine, 1967).

Throughout all the patient's regressions, absences, prolonged silences and dissociations, I made an effort to accept and contain his distortions as well as my own sense of reality. While it is difficult to prove that my consistent "holding," or "diatropic attitude" (Spitz,

1956) was specifically therapeutic, and it is not my purpose here to try to do so, it has become apparent in recent months (after 16 months of treatment) that the patient has undergone significant change.

Mr. C.'s nightmares have decreased in frequency and real-life intensity. He has begun to attempt initial encounters with other people. In addition, he now sits waiting for me awake and alert. He looks at me clearly, greets me on occasion and I feel more alive in his presence.[3] He is beginning to be aware of who I am as a separate and real person. He remains suspicious, but less delusional. When upset he declares, "You *act like* a dead body." This recent transference contains neurotic elements and is quite fragile. He is often on the verge of slipping into a transference that is essentially psychotic, "Sometimes I wonder if you ain't one of them."

Most significantly though, I am able now to separate myself from his distortions and work through their resistant elements. Upon doing so, there is a great outpouring of memories, guilt, and affect from the war. He has begun turning away from using me to relive his past, to having me share in his remembering. He speaks and shouts of the meticulous details of his horrifying work. He desperately attempts to communicate the odors he smelled, the mangled bodies he touched, the conversations he had with dying men and his constant fear. He exhorts me to feel his feelings and wishes for us to return to Vietnam together so he can show me the morgue. "I've got to put myself there (in his overwhelmed feeling state) in order to tell you what it feels like . . . I want you to be there . . . I want you to feel like I felt."

Mr. C. also spontaneously brings up his guilt, "I dream these guys are going to kill me . . . I'm always scared . . . It's a payment for fighting, for wanting others to die . . . I'm dying a slow death . . . I'm serving time."

Finally, Mr. C. has raised for himself for the first time the fundamental question that has long been on my mind. "Why did I stay at this job . . . I could have left at any time . . . I kept doing it even though I hated it . . . Why?"

This gradual and delicate change in the patient is essentially a shift towards a secondary process orientation. He is beginning to remember the past using verbal representations with an acceptance of

---

[3] It was only many months after writing this that I realized the full meaning of my feeling "more alive in his presence." Only in retrospect did I become aware of the degree to which I had begun to experience myself as an inanimate "body."

the reality principle. His guilt and self-punishment remain overwhelming. His projections are borderline psychotic. However, there has
been a slowly budding awareness of me, not as an attacker, but as an
interested helper.

DISCUSSION

The tragedy of Mr. C. and his very uncertain future lies in his
inability to tame his fantasies from the war. While more regressed
that most other Vietnam veterans, he has in common with them a
failure to reintegrate into civilized life. Whether it be nightmares,
flashbacks, or more subtle failures of intimacy, the veteran of the
past war remains mired in his unconscious reactions to death.

Freud addressed this issue in *Thoughts on War and Death* (1915,
p. 296). He asked, "What . . . is the attitude of our unconscious
towards the problem of death? The answer must be: almost exactly
the same of primaeval man. In this respect, as in many other, the
man of prehistoric times survives unchanged in our unconscious." He
continued somewhat later (1919, p. 242), ". . . it is no matter for
surprise that the primitive fear of the dead is still so strong within us
and always ready to come to the surface on any provocation. Most
likely, our fear still implies the old belief that the dead man becomes
the enemy of his survivor and seeks to carry him off to share his new
life with him."

In *Totem and Taboo* (1913), Freud turned his attention to primitive civilization in order to study their reactions to wartime killing.
In this same work he acquainted us with the complex social responses
the societies offered to their returned warriors. From his examples
we see that many of the proscribed community ceremonies were
created to drive away "the ghosts of the victims that are pursuing
their murderers" (p. 38).

On the island of Timor, returned soldiers were required to participate in rites of appeasement which involved sacrifices to the souls
of the men whose heads had been taken in battle. ". . . a part of the
ceremony consists of a dance accompanied by a song, in which the
death of the slain man is lamented and his forgiveness is entreated.
'Be not angry,' they say, 'because your head is here with us; had we
been less lucky, our heads might now have been exposed in your

village. We have offered the sacrifice to appease you. Your spirit may now rest and leave us in peace" (p. 37).[4]

This collective ceremony seems created out of a recognition of the individual feelings of guilt elicited by combat. Again, in Timor, when the leader of an expedition returned home he was forbidden to "return at once to his own house. A special hut is prepared for him in which he has to reside for two months, undergoing bodily and spiritual purification. During this time he may not go to his wife nor feed himself, the food must be put into his mouth by another person" (p. 39).

This period of sanctioned regression condensed many elements of mourning, passivity, punishment, and cleansing. This social isolation was carried even further by the Monumbos of New Guinea who declared anyone who killed a foe in battle as "unclean." "He may touch nobody, not even his own wife and children; if he were to touch them, it is believed that they would be covered with sores" (Freud, p. 40, quoting Frazer, 1911, p. 166).

I suggest that these seemingly harsh proscriptions grew from an exquisite intuition into the unconscious fears in veterans of combat. They contain a respect for their ordeal, titrated punishment (castration), a temporary and healing regression, and finally, a reacceptance back into society. Intrinsic to these ceremonies is a controlled time limiting factor which would undermine any tendency toward chronic regression and disability.

At this point, it would be helpful to step back from this anthropoligical digression and address the psychological question head on. Why the need for public ceremony? What is its intrapsychic function? My beginning thoughts in this area took me back to a patient I presented elsewhere (see Chapter 3). Upon his return from many months of jungle warfare, this veteran, like many others, wandered about the countryside aimlessly for one year. He then settled in a hut alone in a remote region of Hawaii. He cut himself off from the local villagers, ate only vegetarian food, and was celibate. After one year's time, he returned to civilization.

---

[4] It is not only the ordeal of war that elicits this fear of the returning dead. As Fenichel noted, civilians as well contain these fears and have also created ceremonies to tame them. Specifically, the "pious rituals of holding vigils at the side of the bier and of throwing sand into the grave or of erecting monuments of stone . . . which are intended to prevent the dead from coming back" (1945, p. 395). Brenner has stressed that in addition to the defensive-aggressive elements, these rites also manifest the libidinal attachment to the dead (1983, p. 134).

One may consider that this patient attempted a self-proscribed, cleansing ritual quite similar to the ancient and time-honored rites of atonement and purification. What is most noteworthy though is not its remarkable resemblance to the past, but how it differed.

For this and many other Vietnam veterans, this self-imposed exile *failed* to grant them relief from their ghosts. It is this failure that leads us to consider that it is the missing *public participation* in the ceremony that is the key ingredient for therapeutic success. We are then led to ask what is it in this public ritual that affects the psyches of returned soldiers?

In *The Ego and the Id*, Freud comments (1923, p. 58):

> . . . to the ego, therefore, living means the same as being loved— being loved by the superego . . . the superego fulfills the same function of the *protecting and saving* that was fulfilled in earlier days by the father and later by Providence or destiny. But when the ego finds itself in *overwhelming danger of real order* which it believes itself unable to overcome by its own strength, it is bound to draw the same conclusion. It sees itself *deserted by all forces of protection* and lets itself die (italics mine).

I believe these thoughts bear directly on the question before us. The community's participation in the welcoming home ceremony serves the same function as the "protecting and saving" father. Without this loving, the soldier perceives himself as again deserted by the caring and protecting parents as he was at the moment of the "overwhelming danger" of battle. There is a reexperiencing by the ego of this frightening state of abandonment and anomie. If this condition persists without a 'therapeutic' intervention by the community (or failing that, via a therapeutic object relationship), the ego becomes fixed in a chronic regressive state of fear and helplessness. In severe cases, the abandonment by the caring 'parents' may lead the ego to give "itself up because it feels itself hated and persecuted by the superego, instead of loved" (p. 58).[5]

In contrast, when the community offers its love and appreciation to the returning soldier through public ritual, his sense of abandonment is undone. He thereby becomes able to assume an identification

---

[5] As Bettleheim simply stated it: "One cannot meet catastrophic events and survive when deprived of the feeling that somebody cares" (1979, p. 102).

with the cultural lineage of revered (phallic) warriors.[6] In addition, the culture's caring becomes internalized as a more accepting superego. The regressive and punishing superego that threatens retaliation for his acts of war takes in the acceptance and forgiveness of the parent culture. This includes the 'fathers'' sanctioning of the displaced oedipal crime. This intercession by the elders repairs the tear in generational continuity and strengthens the sons' affiliation with "the historic traditions and values of the group or community; that is, to the values of the father's generation and those which preceded it" (Arlow, 1951).

To pursue the specifics of this community intervention somewhat more thoroughly, I would like to propose an additional conceptual basis for its role in the 'treatment' of a specific defensive system. For many ex-combatants the overwhelming trauma of their experiences, possibly combined with a developmental predisposition, has led to their use of the regressive defense of pathological splitting. Within this distorted framework, the 'system' becomes the all-bad persecutor that they must defend against by attacking. Beneath this rage lies an all bad guilt-ridden self-image that characteristically lacks any elements of a modulating self-love. A veneer of all-good grandiosity is used defensively to ward off this cataclysmic state. The resultant cycle of narcissistic aloofness and suicidal depression not only wreaks havoc upon their emotional equilibrium, but also results in a painful alienation from life-sustaining object relationships. I suggest that the great power of the community's acceptance can accomplish what we strive for in the early phases of treatment. The validation and containment of these part-objects through the consistent caring and neutralized observing strength of the community's holding, or therapist's ego, can offer an experiential model for the "mending" of the split. In both situations, the patient experiences a new relationship that derives from the ability to *symbolize* what was previously acted out. Thus, the power contained in becoming part of the historical mythology of the culture has the ability to reestablish the primacy of the secondary process in the same fashion as the discovery of the 'illusion' of the transference.

---

[6] This fear of abandonment often becomes a central issue in the therapeutic relationship. Any failure in empathic relatedness and certainly any absences can provoke powerful affective responses. The patient's ability at these times to draw upon past sustaining images, their "evocative memory" (Adler and Buie's use [1979] of Fraiberg's [1969] concept) is fundamental to their continued sense of integration. I cautiously raise the possibility, fully aware of the theoretical obstacles raised by such a proposition, that becoming part of a respected cultural heritage may serve a similar function in providing the veteran with historical sustaining objects.

This psychic space of illusion is a common element in man as a social being as well as a psychological one. In the best of circumstances, these two frames are dialectically joined to help create the capacity for symbolic meaning. This metaphorical level of consciousness can serve as a subliminatory container for overwhelming impulses. However, mental play and ambiguity are only possible when archaic frustration and aggression are no longer imminent. For many patients, particularly those who have experienced actual trauma, the establishment of this real/not real space, becomes *the* therapeutic task.

It is in the discovery of the possibility of fantasy that the veteran of combat can transcend his concrete *action* orientation. He can use this creative arena to explore the meaning, power and grace in *words*. His impulses and wishes can be transformed from dangerous reality to symbolic thought.

The culture at large helps create this illusory space through its historical mythology. Doctors rely on "the relational process through which illusion operates" (Khan, 1973)—the transference.

Khan addresses the continuity between the community and transference frames when he quotes Cassirer:

> It was a long evolutionary course which the human mind has to traverse, to pass from the belief in a physico-magical power. Indeed, it is the Word, it is language, that really reveals to man that world which is closer to him than any world of natural objects and touches his weal and woe more directly than physical nature. *For it is language that makes his existence in a community possible; and only on society, in relation to a "Thee," can his subjectivity assert itself as a "Me"* (Cassirer, 1946).
>
> For this usage of the Word Freud provided a new human laboratory and a new function: namely, that of cure. *The use of the Word is dependent on the capacity of the analytic situation and process to sustain illusion. When the latter breaks down, then the usage of the Word has to yield to other forms and styles of relating and experiencing* (Khan, 1973) (italics mine).

This suggestion of 'therapeutic' cultural forces is not intended as a departure from more traditional analytic conceptualizations. Indeed, it is my very respect for the depth and universality of the unconscious fantasies that are stimulated by battle that leads me to study collective healing forces. We are faced by prohibitively vast numbers of disabled patients whose defensive use of projection and withdrawal have left them beyond the reach of traditional treatment.

On a technical level as well, I believe this population is well suited to social intervention. The therapeutic task with some of these men is not one of de-repressing structural conflict. This would in fact demand the careful individual analysis of layers of drive-defense configurations. Instead the problem often is of *de-regressing* the overburdened soldier who lacks an adequate "container" for his overpowering fantasies. I have suggested that induction into a cultural mythology can act as a "retrospective stimulus barrier."

REFERENCES

Adler, G., Buie, D. H. (1979). Aloneness and borderline psychopathology: the possible relevance of child development issues. *International Journal of Psychoanalysis* 60: 83-95.

Arlow, J. (1951). A psychoanalytic study of a religious initiation rite: Bar Mitzvah. *Psychoanalytic Study of the Child* 6: 353-374.

Bettleheim, B. (1979). The holocaust—one generation later. In: *Surviving and Other Essays*. New York: Knopf.

Brenner, C. (1983). *The Mind in Conflict*. New York: International University Press.

Cassirer, E. (1946). *Language and Myth*. New York: Dover Publications.

Davidson, S. (1979). Massive psychic traumatization and social support. *Journal of Psychosomatic Research* 23: 395-402.

Fenichel, O. (1945). *The Psychoanalytic Theory of Neuroses*. New York: W. W. Norton.

Fraiberg, S. (1964). Libidinal object constancy and mental representation. *Psychoanalytic Study of the Child* 24: 9-47.

Frazer, J. G. (1911). *The Golden Bough*. London: St. Martin.

Freud, S. (1913). Totem and Taboo. *S.E.* 13.

Freud, S. (1915). Thoughts on War and Death. *S.E.* 14.

Freud, S. (1919). The 'Uncanny.' *S.E.* 17.

Freud, S. (1923). The Ego and the Id. *S.E.* 19.

Khan, M. M. (1973). The role of illusion in the analytic space and process. *Annual of Psychoanalysis* I: 231-246.

Rubinfine, D. L. (1967). Notes on a theory of reconstruction. *British Journal of Medicine Psychology* 40: 195-206.

Spitz, R. A. (1956). Countertransference—comments on its varying role in the analytic situation. *Journal of the American Psychoanalytic Association* 4: 256-265.

Tennant, C., Bebbington, P., Hurry, J. (1981). The short-term outcome of neurotic disorders in the community: the relation of remission to clinical factors and to 'neutralizing' life events. *British Journal of Psychiatry* 139: 213-220.

10
Understanding and Treatment of Combat Neurosis:
The Israeli Experience

RAFAEL MOSES, M.D. AND IMMANUEL COHEN, M.D.

In wanting to share with you our experience in Israel of the understanding and treatment of combat reactions, we are basing it on experiences which began in the War of Independence of 1948-1949 and went through the wars of 1956, 1967, the War of Attrition in the early 1970s, up to the Yom Kippur War in 1973 and impressionistic information from the Lebanon War in 1982. Clearly, our view of combat reactions in Israel changed in these 35 years, and what we will present to you is our view as of today, using a retrospective glance which perhaps allows us to perceive more clearly some of the ways of viewing combat reactions as time progressed and both people and behaviors changed. We present our thoughts in three main parts. The first part is a focussing on the Israeli context and some of its social and cultural aspects and the special influence which we think this has had on the soldiers in battle and therefore on the possibility of their breakdown. The second part deals with our understanding of the various factors which impinge upon the soldier at the time of battle.

We attempt to describe the forces on both sides within the soldier, which on the one hand help him to overcome the serious stress to which he is exposed and on the other hand predispose him towards a breakdown, and the interplay between the two kinds of

Copyright © 1984 by Spectrum Publications, Inc. *Psychotherapy of the Combat Veteran,* edited by H. J. Schwartz.

forces. In the third part, we describe methods of treatment which are in part based on our understanding of what goes on within the soldier. We take into account a deeper psychodynamic understanding of the person at the period of crisis as he is exposed to the various social factors which influence his reaction at that particular point. We supplement this point of view by that which represents the needs of the social unit within which the soldier functions, namely, the army. We will stress two aspects of the army—its needs and its capabilities. Any army psychiatrist must—to function effectively—combine as fruitfully as he can, the needs of the soldier's unit at the time of battle with his view of the needs of the individual. The treatment considerations, however, depend not only on these two views—of the individual and of the social system within which he functions, the army. These must necessarily take into account the resources of the social system for providing appropriate treatment.

ISRAEL—THE SOCIOCULTURAL CONTEXT OF THE WARS

All Israeli wars, except the recent Lebanon War, were fought by Israeli soldiers when there was a general consensus that this was a war of survival. Israelis, and therefore the soldiers, faced a threat by Israel's neighbors; the aim of the war was to defend Israel against this threat and to ensure its survival. The need to ensure the survival of Israel at times touched upon recollections of the holocaust and the threat to the survival of the Jewish people which the holocaust had posed (Brecher, 1980). It is true that in retrospect one war, the Suez Campaign of 1956, is not seen by all so much as a survival war as it was conceived of at the time. At the time, however, the perception of Israelis and Israel's soldiers was that the small country was surrounded by enemies who outnumbered Israelis by at least ten to one, and who were in the early days and the early wars, much better equipped than the Israeli army. In other words, Israelis conceived of themselves until after the 1967 war as the underdogs; the need to fight was therefore strictly one of self-defense and survival. This state of affairs, then, can be seen as influencing the *specific* motivation of the soldiers, which they brought with them to the battle. We differentiate from this the *nonspecific* motivation which varies more with socioeconomic background, education and perhaps the cultural background and values of the soldier. By and large, higher socioeconomic background and education correlate with a stronger identification with the national unit, the state, and its needs. The nonspecific motivation of the Israeli soldiers was highest in the War of Independence in 1948 and gradually decreased to some extent as the population changed its composition during these 30 to 35 years. It was, however, counterbalanced by other factors, which we will refer to later. It is perhaps interesting to note that the perceived danger was greatest in the three and a half weeks' waiting period before the Six-Day War in June 1967. At this time there was among most of the population of Israel a strong fear of being overrun and either killed, brutalized, or thrown into the sea. This leads also to the perceived image of the enemy, which during that particular period was fueled by the television pictures of frenzied mobs in Cairo shouting for a holy war and for the destruction of the Jews. However, this was only a special case of the general perception that Egyptians and Syrians were implacable and brutal enemies from whom no quarter could be expected. With regard to Egypt, this image continued until President Sadat's visit to Jerusalem in 1977; then this image changed dramatically. With regard to Jordan, the image was more moderate. But before the Six-Day War, the fears by inhabitants of Jerusalem—adjacent to Jordan's army, the Arab Legion—were as great and intense (probably because of the closeness in this case) as those regarding the Egyptians.

Let us examine briefly the connection between the kind of war and the number of combat reactions. First, in the War of Independence, the number of recognized combat reactions was small. Two small psychiatric units were set up; there was no treatment of psychological casualties in or near forward areas. This fact seemed surprising in view of the fact that the war broke out relatively unexpectedly, Israelis—or, at the time, Jewish Palestinians—were totally unprepared for fighting a war. Many units of the army were not sufficiently trained, and at the same time many new immigrants, including numerous holocaust survivors and refugees from Arab countries, were inducted into the army and sometimes had to be sent into battle without any training. Let us at this point describe as an example in somewhat more detail the Battle of Latrun.

THE BATTLE OF LATRUN

Ten days after the State of Israel was proclaimed, the battle for Latrun began. Latrun lies astride the highway from the coast to the capital, and had to be captured in order to break the siege of Jerusalem. A special brigade was set up for this task. It was composed of

one hastily assembled half-track battalion and two infantry bat-
talions, one drawn from existing formations and one made up of new
immigrants who had just arrived in the country, and who had
received some training with dummy weapons in the displaced persons'
camps in Europe and in the immigrant camps of Cyprus. There were
three attempts to capture Latrun: one on May 25th, one on May
30th, and a final one on June 9th, 1948, before the ceasefire took
effect on June 11th. Latrun was a well-defended police station. The
firing power of the well-trained Jordanian legion that manned the
police station was five to one against Israel. The new immigrant battalion included many holocaust survivors which had spent time in
Cyprus. They did not know Hebrew. Commands were given in a
variety of languages, understood by some but not by everyone. One
group of soldiers spoke only Arabic and no Hebrew. The group
cohesion in the battalion was obviously quite limited. Since at that
time in the Israel Defense Forces most of the officers did not wear
insignia of rank, many of the soldiers could not recognize their commanders, whom they did not know personally, nor could they recognize their voice. Therefore, one could expect very little, if any, automatic behavior to take over in the heat of battle.

The number of casualties was high. In all, there were about 400
killed, and roughly 1,500 wounded in the battle itself. Among the
killed was a high number of commanders, for whom there were very
few replacements. We would assume that all these factors further
undermined the already tenuous self-confidence of the soldiers on
the basis of their training and their relationship with their commanding officers. On the positive side of morale, we can assume that there
was a high motivation with regard to the overall goals of the war.
Against this weighed very serious doubts of some of the senior army
officers as to whether this battle was indeed necessary and worthwhile. It was a desperate battle, and as such we would assume that it
would raise the identification threshold for psychological problems
and casualties. In addition, there was at that time practically no
awareness of psychological reactions to battle. Also, as is known of
Israel generally at that time, there was no social legitimation of
personal feelings. In this context we might quote General Moshe
Dayan who had been known to say, perhaps around that time:
"Don't explain (failures), don't complain (about difficulties)." In
other words, it was felt that failure should not be explained, and suffering not complained about; only results count. Yitshaki (1982)
who described the battle of Latrun in a recent book, called it the
greatest failure in the history of the Israel Defense Force. Under

average circumstances, one would have expected that with the number of casualties at about 2000, there would have been approximately 240 psychological casualties in this battle of three weeks' duration. The circumstances surrounding it—the lack of training of the soldiers and of the units being outequipped five to one in firing power, the lack of adequate communication between commanders and soldiers at least in the immigrant battalion, the lack of previous joint training, the relatively large number of casualties, especially of commanders—would lead us to expect a higher than average number of overt psychological casualties, that is definitely more than the usual 12 percent. Although no definite figures are available for psychological casualties of that particular battle, we do know that the number of overall psychological casualties in the War of Independence who were hospitalized or treated in an ambulatory way was quite small. There were two small units, one for psychoses, one for neuroses, set up several months after the Latrun Battle. Therefore, it would seem safe to assume that during this battle no more than 30 psychological casualties were identified. Such a small number of identified psychological casualties could be due either to a high breakdown threshold (successful coping leading to a low number of breakdowns) or a high identification threshold (many soldiers with psychopathology not being identified as casualties).

We would explain the small number of casualties in the War of Independence by two factors: One, the high motivation to defend oneself in a war of survival fought totally on one's own territory and secondly, a concept which we would like to elaborate on a little more, namely, the identification threshold for combat reactions.

The identification threshold (Cohen) is determined by the level of psychopathology which can be borne by both the individual and the unit without requiring labelling of a soldier as a combat reaction, as a battle casualty, and therefore his extrusion from the unit and his relegation behind the frontline for diagnosis and treatment. This threshold depends on the estimation by both the person and his environment as to what is normal or acceptable pressure under the circumstances and when treatment by the Medical Corps is indicated. It is therefore not identical with the severity of the clinical picture. In that sense it is an indication of the range of tolerance of psychopathology by the individual soldier as transmitted to him by the overall environment, including his buddies and his commanders. To put it another way, it is the ability of the particular unit to serve as a holding environment for the upset soldier which will determine the identification threshold. The level of the identification threshold can, of course, be determined by an order from above, passed on to the various levels of command. For example, the awareness of the existence of combat reactions in 1948 was exceedingly low, whereas in the Lebanon War in 1982 the expectation of having such casualties and the readiness to treat them was higher than it had ever been before—mainly as a result of the experiences of the Yom Kippur War in 1973. In addition, the identification threshold is indirectly also a function of the morale of the unit, because the morale determines at what point a specific individual is more likely to break, namely, a high morale will lead to a higher breaking point and a lower one to a lower point. A soldier may feel much psychic suffering without identifying himself as a casualty; alternatively, a soldier might see himself as a casualty with relatively minor suffering while his environment views him differently. It is thus conceivable that if an army is very much aware of combat reactions and in that sense creates a low identification threshold, and if on top of this the morale in a certain unit is low, this would then lead to a high incidence of combat reactions. There are, of course, other factors which also influence the identification threshold, such as how desperately the battle is being fought: the more desperate—the higher the threshold will be.

Although there is more to be said about the identification threshold and its intricate relationship to a large number of other social variables within the army, our aim here is to discuss the term in its relation to the different Israeli wars, particularly in light of the extreme differences that exist between the War of Independence in 1948 and the Lebanon War in 1982.

The Suez Campaign in 1956, the second Israeli war, was a short war; because it was both so short and so successful, the number of psychological casualties was very small—considering also the fact that the identification threshold was still very high in the Israeli army at that time.

The next big war in the Arab–Israeli conflict was the Six-Day War in 1967. One of the important functions of the three and a half weeks' waiting period before the Six-Day War was to allow a more intensive preparation for dealing with psychological casualties than had existed at any time before in the Israel Army. For the first time, detailed instructions were printed and issued which were designed both to provide know-how for preventive as well as therapeutic action, but also to enable a wide-range of people in the army and in civil defense to recognize psychological casualties and to learn basic steps in how to deal with them. The purpose was to decrease their otherwise very great sense of helplessness vis-à-vis frightening phenomena. This process, we assume, considerably lowered the identification threshold. In fact, it turned out that while there were some psychological casualties in the waiting period before the outbreak of war, as the war broke out, the number of recognized and treated casualties was very small indeed. It was only six years later, during the Yom Kippur War that we met a number of soldiers who had reacted in 1967 in typical psychological ways to the trauma of battle, but had preferred to—or even been able to—live with their recurring nightmares and anxieties without seeking treatment.

It was perhaps the next war, known as the War of Attrition, in the years 1969-1971, that first began to focus attention more seriously on the psychological reactions of soldiers to the vicissitudes of this static war. Indeed, at this time the social orientation had also begun to move away from a strong emphasis on the group, and a discouragement of the individual from introspection, toward a larger openness to the individual, his needs, and his feelings (Moses and Kligler, 1966; Moses, in press). This is thus one reason why more attention was paid around 1969 to the psychological state of the individual soldier within the fortifications of the Bar Lev line, where he was exposed to repeated shelling and occasional commando raids.

The Yom Kippur War in Israel did for psychiatry and for the recognition of psychological problems what World War II did for the same in the United States. For the first time, there was a considerable number of identified combat reactions, which were diagnosed and treated first in forward positions; if necessary, soldiers were sent back to rear units specially formed for the treatment of these soldiers. This was a war that broke out totally unexpectedly for the Israeli population and most of its soldiers. Israel was initially overwhelmed by attacking armies both on the Southern Egyptian front and the Northeastern Syrian front. As a result, then, of a lower identification threshold and a total lack of preparation for the onslaught which occurred, the number of identified casualties was relatively high. Attention was focused on soldiers with combat reactions more than at any other previous time in Israeli history. This was also a time when the population of Israel vented its disappointment and fury on its leaders who were responsible for this failure— for which there was now a new national term (Meh'dal). The soldiers, including those with combat reactions, were of course an integral part of this. After 1967, there had been a large expansion of the territory under Israel's control, and along with it an almost similarly large expansion of the national ego (Moses, 1982). Along with this change in size and in image of Israel, both in the eyes of its citizens and of outsiders, went the loss of the status of an underdog. These then, sketchily, were the circumstances under which the Yom Kippur War began. It gives some indication of how unprepared Israel's soldiers were psychologically for the severe attack and the difficult fighting with all the horrors of warfare at close quarters which took place (for a more comprehensive discussion see Cohen, 1979).

It was at the beginning of this war that we had an opportunity to study a total sample of a population of soldiers evacuated to a hospital where the less severely injured were treated. The unique opportunity to interview all soldiers thus admitted helped us clarify some of our thinking about the incidents of psychological symptoms in soldiers with and without physical injury—a topic which since Freud (1921) had been decided unequivocally, namely, that soldiers who had physical injury did not develop combat reactions. In contrast to this finding, we discerned a psychological reaction ranging from mild to marked severity in almost all the soldiers admitted to this hospital. This made us think more about the social function of the combat reaction in that it serves for the soldier as an alibi, and removes him from the frontline without additional physical injury. Whereas on the other hand, a soldier physically injured, even if only mildly so, has an "alibi" through such an injury itself. By alibi we mean the social and superego legitimization for evacuation, which makes the soldier's peers and the soldier himself accept the evacuation as "all right" (Moses, 1978).

PSYCHOLOGICAL AND PHYSICAL INJURY

A 24-year-old officer ("Zalman") was in a tank that was hit by an enemy shell and began to burn. He and a buddy jumped out and doused the fire in sand. The third tank crew member tried to get out of the tank but could not and died. Zalman was evacuated to the hospital because of burns. In the burn unit he was routinely seen by a psychiatrist. His blatant manic denial was quickly punctured by his talking about the war experience and his intense guilt feelings about not having been able to save his buddy. He became gradually more depressed. After ten days he was released from the hospital and resumed his studies in the university. Several years later he contacted the psychiatrist whom he had then seen in the general hospital and asked for psychotherapy. He was concerned mainly about his self-image and his self-esteem, but also about his relationship with the opposite sex and his quite close attachment to both his parents, particularly a very rivalrous attachment to his father. During a year and a half of psychotherapy, the following facts relating to the army trauma emerged. It was only several months after his war experience that he and some of his buddies from the unit began to spend their nights talking about the horrors of the war. In order to push away the intensely frightening aspects of this, they would drink in order, as he put it, "to drown" their feelings. At the time, most of them had recurring nightmares of the war in general, and he of the traumatic event where he had been wounded in particular. After about four months of getting together fairly regularly once to twice a week in this way, they were able to distance themselves both from their experiences and from each other. Although the psychotherapy did return a number of times to the special and traumatic aspects of the war service, this was clearly a marginal event. Psychotherapy focused on how he related to himself; on how he related to his father, his boss, his psychotherapist; on his need to conquer women and his difficulty in holding onto a woman. As a result of therapy, changes occurred in all of these three areas. Obviously, however, we could not tell, and hopefully will not know, whether he would react any differently to a similar traumatic war experience after the psychotherapy.

It was also at this time that we were able to observe a number of soldiers who had developed combat reactions in the Yom Kippur War and thus came to our attention, and who, it turned out, had had previous psychological reactions, again of various intensity, sometimes beginning during the Six-Day War and repeatedly stirred up again during the War of Attrition. In other words, these were masked reactions which had appeared in 1967 or in 1969–1971 and had not then led to the soldier either being removed from the battle-zone (which probably had not been necessary at all during the short Six-Day War), or even led him to seek treatment after the battle was over or after he was removed from the battle zone. These masked reactions, we feel, are important in that they should be taken into account when assessing the overall incidence of combat reactions.

MASKED PSYCHOLOGICAL REACTION
(BELOW THE IDENTIFICATION THRESHOLD)

A 30-year-old sociologist was a member of a tank crew when the tank was hit by enemy fire and put out of action. While the other two crew members were injured, he was spared physical injury but was brought to the nearest medical post for evaluation. Not having been diagnosed as a psychological casualty, he was told to rejoin his unit, which was no longer involved in battle. He suffered from recurring nightmares and was concerned about his ability to go back into a tank and function again. However, he did not discuss this with anyone, knowing that he was a reserve soldier assumed to be discharged. In addition, he did not want his army record to be marred by such information. Two weeks later he sought psychological help. This sociologist identified himself as a psychological casualty but was not so identified by the environment. Such masking by the person is an indication of strength whatever the motivation for the masking. In discussing his reaction to the traumatic event, he was able to talk about his strong need for control and his fear that he had lost it, or had been on the verge of losing it. In the psychotherapy sessions, too, control was exceedingly important to him. Although much of the material focused on the traumatic battle event and his reaction to it, it soon tied up also with earlier events relating to other experiences with death and injury as well as earlier childhood and family events. This reserve soldier emerged from a time-limited psychotherapy, strengthened in his ability to contain his, to him, untoward reactions to the stress of battle. Perhaps he emerged also with a feeling that he had been able to talk about himself, about his bad and difficult experience now, and about other difficult experiences in the more recent and early past. Therefore, it seems likely that he might return for further therapy at some future date—in spite of his considerable intellectualizing defenses.

DELAYED PSYCHOLOGICAL REACTION

A 22-year-old ex-soldier sought out psychiatric help in response to a recent traumatic event: he had encountered four weeks previously a street gang in his neighborhood who had taunted and threatened him and there had been a mild fistfight. He did not see any connection with his army service during the recent fighting. In reply to questions, he related that indeed he had seen some of the battle results, killed and wounded, although he had not been directly involved in the fighting. In talking further about the youngsters he encountered, he quickly became aware of his intense aggressive feelings toward them, and soon also of his wish that they might die or, more clearly, his wish to kill them. Ongoing psychotherapy related this acute anxiety attack to specific experiences during the war. At the same time, it was gradually possible to make connections between the experiences during the war, experiences in the neighborhood, and early childhood experiences related to growing up in his family.

The last war about which we know least at this point is the Lebanon War, officially known as Operation Peace of Galilee which began June 7, 1982. In terms of the aims of the war and in terms of the identification of the soldiers with the leaders of the country and the cause for which they were sent to fight, there was for the first time an important difference. For the first time there was no national consensus about the war as there had been for all previous ones. It would be reasonable to assume that this difference in the motivation, from this point of view, of the soldiers to fight would have left an imprint on the readiness to develop combat reactions. Information available thus far does not tell us much about this question. The readiness to deal with psychological casualties was greater than ever before, implying a lower identification threshold; the type of warfare was at times quite difficult—house-to-house fighting in urban areas. While the war was going on and while siege was laid to West Beirut, the argument raged in public—particularly on television—whether it was justified and made sense to take Beirut by force. A senior army commander resigned around this question. However, we are not in a position at this time to say anything about any impact this might have had on the incidence of psychological casualties in the Israel Army during this war.

We have given a brief outline of the six wars which took place as part of the Arab–Israeli conflict from 1948 to 1982. We have thus presented our view of how the various social and cultural factors which impinge upon the point where a combat reaction may occur can be expected to interrelate with the various specific circumstances surrounding a specific war, and therefore the motivation of the soldier to serve in the war. To phrase it differently, we believe that the emphasis should be placed on motivation factors in soldiers, as they derive from the specific circumstances of the social and cultural milieu; the aims of a war; the ideological support which a population gives to a war decided on usually by the government; the balance of forces; the intensity of fire; the trust that a soldier puts both in his peer group and in his commanders; and what we have called (following Cohen) the Identification Threshold. We shall now go on to the next topic—how we understand the development of a combat reaction.

OUR THEORETICAL UNDERSTANDING OF
HOW A COMBAT REACTION OCCURS

The first question to be asked, of course, is whether there exists an early predisposition for the development of this syndrome. Freud (1940) has said that "the relations of the traumatic neurosis to determinance in childhood have hitherto eluded investigation" (p. 184). One of us (Moses, 1978) has considered in some detail the question of whether an early predisposition and vulnerability exists in the acute traumatic neurosis in general and in the combat reactions in particular. He has found that while an early predisposition was expected by the time of World War II, selection procedures particularly during that war showed themselves to be generally unreliable for weeding out persons who would be at risk as soldiers. Today, however, armies have found one reliable factor for weeding out potential breakdown soldiers: it is related to a lack of motivation to fight in a very general way. Such a lack of motivation may of course be a result of a variety of different factors which may have to do with the social and cultural background of the individual or with the specific personality factors which are not spelled out. One study has found a clear correlation between certain stressful life events which cause a person to be at risk (Holmes and Rahe, 1967). This finding can, we believe, be similarly applied to soldiers in battle; namely, that recent events such as a marriage recently contracted or a divorce which has taken place recently or a pregnancy all affect the soldier's ability to function. All such acute upsetting events which require an adaptation to change thus would seem to make a person belong to the at-risk population in and out of the army. Most armies still take into serious consideration the fact that there must be some correlation between peace-time adaptation of the potential soldier and his functioning in battle.

In his 1978 paper, one of us (R.M.) describes how a number of preventive methods used with soldiers showed that by preparing soldiers, the threshold of trauma was increased, a narcissistic support was provided both through bolstering the soldier's self-esteem and through legitimizing his psychological reaction, and that, finally, by using group methods, a sense of group belonging and cohesion of the group self was strengthened. These methods of preparing soldiers were by and large efficient and thereby made three relevant points: (1) that the self of the soldier, his narcissistic needs and supplies and his being open to narcissistic hurt were an important factor to be taken into consideration and a factor which also opened up a preventive avenue; (2) that, as expected and as is well known, preparedness for a possible trauma works to raise in an important way the threshold to trauma; and finally (3) that group cohesion, group support, and a cohesive group self are also important factors in raising the threshold against traumatic breakdown. This meant paying particular attention to groups but also to the group self, that is to narcissism in the group (Moses, 1982). In his 1978 paper, Moses also showed that since traumatic reactions show a marked tendency to become chronic, often for years and decades, this must indicate the exertion of a strong pull towards chronicity and decompensation of functioning, as well as strong regressive phenomena, of id, of ego, and of super-ego: of structure and of function. Such regressive modes with intense feelings of helplessness and marked dependency would again indicate the likelihood of early fixations exerting a strong regressive pull. In addition, they also point to the importance of the helplessness-omnipotence axis. The marked stereotype of the symptoms as a result of ego impoverishment and constriction also would indicate that there must have previously existed in the ego a similar readiness, at least. Mainly through experiences in psychotherapy with soldiers who had broken down, it appeared that the trauma of battle easily and quickly connected with other traumata, usually losses, of earlier periods; these it turned out, had usually not been adequately worked through. This, then, was another indication that there had been latent problems that were rekindled, as it were, through the battle trauma. In some cases, as we know, people seemed to be actively seeking out traumata, a behavior which also had a repetitively similar character. The counter-phobic seeking out of heroic situations by quite different personality types of soldiers, or indeed other people is analogous. Finally, the refractoriness to treatment, particularly of the chronic instances of combat reaction, seemed to present another strong indication that here was a basic attribute of these individuals, namely, a strong motivation against introspection, against examining one's own feelings and intrapsychic processes. From this list of six clinical characteristics which must have dated from early on in the development of these individuals, a previous susceptibility and vulnerability dating back to childhood was assumed. This was understood to be based on the general tendency for earlier patterns of coping and problem-solving to persist, yet to be inhibited as they are superceded by newly acquired patterns. Later on they reemerge at a time when the existing psychic organizations cannot cope effectively with new external stresses (Sandler and Joffe, 1967). A comparison of injured soldiers with psychological casualties was used to point out the importance of self-esteem, narcissistic supplies, and narcissistic wounding in soldiers in battle. Though both groups were exposed to the same kinds of external and internal stresses, the injured group was legitimately evacuated from battle and the care of their bodies, their temporary dysfunction and obligatory regressions were sanctioned, while the psyche of the soldiers with combat reactions could not thus be cared for. Their removal from the battle zone was not legitimized, their self-esteem was not maintained, but rather seriously hurt by their "breakdown." To phrase it differently, the injured soldiers were given an "alibi" for nonfunctioning, which was totally adequate to sanction evacuation, while the psychological casualties needed to make up for themselves an "alibi" for the painful narcissistic wound of having "failed." The same paper also reports a number of detailed mechanisms which can be observed in the acute appearance of the combat reaction. The long prevailing view that traumatic neuroses are a result of the unexpected flooding of the ego by excessive overwhelming stimuli seemed to work against the search for such more detailed mechanisms. One such mechanism is related to transitory identifications with either the aggressor or the victim in battle through a temporary loosening of ego boundaries, and in line with other temporary loosenings of ego boundaries and brief identifications and dis-identifications which take place at many moments in our everyday life. Thus, sudden strong identificatory feelings of guilt or helplessness may be generated which overwhelm existing ego functions (Sandler as quoted in Moses, 1978). Such identifications also emphasize two other aspects: First, the ups and downs in our everyday psychic activity which is dominated not only by deep unconscious conflicts, but takes place to quite an extent in response to more preconscious conflicts related to developmentally later structures in the ego which respond to minor narcissistic hurts (for this see also Kohut, 1971), and feelings of shame or conflicts between different feelings which come up from one moment to another (Sandler, personal communication). Secondly, this mechanism again points up the importance of narcissistic supplies and their waxing and waning during everyday life, but also the particular more acute and more intense forms of narcissistic reactions which should be looked for in the breakdown of soldiers, as also in other acute psychic reactions.

Two further mechanisms also serve to stress the importance of the impact of the breakdown on the soldier's self-esteem. For example, it seems suddenly to upset a previous precarious balance about his own worth between a positive and a negative self-esteem;

just as a child feels that he must be bad if he is attacked or abandoned. So must a soldier revive this feeling, albeit in part unconsciously, in battle. To sum up, then, we would adopt the view on the
early predisposition, on a more present-day view, following Sandler,
of conflicts which fluctuate from day to day and from moment to
moment which are often conflicts between one wish and another
wish, rather than a deeper more basic structure of conflicts between
a drive and the superego which opposes its discharge. In the context
of these conflicts which become acutely exacerbated during the
breakdown in battle, we feel that narcissistic esteem and narcissistic
hurts are very important factors for both the individual and the
group. Such a view obviously has clear implications for both prevention and treatment.

We have looked in some depth at what has also been called the
readiness to develop trait anxiety which the soldier brings with
himself to battle. We have mentioned previously the importance of
some of the individual social and cultural characteristics which are
codeterminants in what we have previously called the breakdown
threshold. Here we must specify socioeconomic class and education
which have been shown as relevant factors. We have also mentioned
the importance of the morale of the unit which related to discipline,
group cohesion and the group self, and also to leadership as it is
exercised in the unit. We have connected this with the trust of the
individual in his commander, but also with his ability to recognize
the commander in battle, and similarly with his trust in his peers.
We now know that many of these factors can be augmented through
training and through being examined and emphasized regularly
during recurrent training periods of the soldier. If previously we had
been talking about what has been called trait anxiety, we are now
talking about what has been analogously called state anxiety: this
is the anxiety which is related not to the traits which the soldier
brings with him to the situation, but rather to the situation itself, to
the state in which the soldier finds himself. Here we must focus again
on the identification with the goals of the society generally and with
the goals of the war or of this specific battle, but also such basics as
whether the soldiers had been given reliable trustworthy arms and
ammunition, etc. Experience has shown that, after appropriate
screening, state anxiety seems to be a more powerful determinant of
being at risk, and to be more overwhelming than trait anxiety: this
fact has led to more intensive training to try and counteract state
anxiety in the Israeli Army as well as in other armies. Among the
various external and internal support systems which can help increase

the threshold to trauma of the soldier, information provides an important measure of cognitive control which is decidedly helpful. This includes information about the enemy, and about the decision-making on one's own side, as well as the ability to predict stressful events. The more a soldier knows what to expect and when to expect it, the more prepared he will be and the higher his trauma threshold will be.

An interesting sideline on this issue is the importance of a soldier having enough sleep and enough food—seemingly elementary facts. However, some soldiers did not, because of their intrapsychic state, allow themselves either enough sleep or enough water and food (although, at times, battle conditions did allow this) and sometimes smoked incessantly in addition. Such soldiers, then, were more likely to develop combat reactions. This raises the more general question of how such behavior by the soldier facilitates the development of combat reactions, but also what personality factors lead to such behavior. The first can be answered in a very general way: that such activities—lack of sleep, not enough food or fluid intake, too much smoking—weaken the ego and its ability to resist trauma. The question as to what brings this about, leads us into perhaps more general statements about adaptability and flexibility, again related to coping behavior or to a healthy ego, whatever that may be. These findings, however, would seem to indicate that persons, on the other hand, who are free enough to make the best out of difficult situations and find what they need even under difficult circumstances—for example, sleep under fire, or food in difficult circumstances—are people whose general psychic adaptability and flexibility are greater. This means that their options under stress are increased.

A comprehensive view of the etiology and genesis of combat reactions should, we believe, include both early and later individual factors as well as individual attitudes in the present, which at the same time relate to and result from a variety of social and cultural factors on large and small group levels. Such a view will also provide some indications for prevention and treatment of combat reactions.

We would have been delighted to be able to follow the suggestion of our editor and discuss some of the interrelations of individual genetic predispositions with the situational context. How do these two fields interact and interweave as they meet in battle? Unfortunately, in our opinion, present knowledge is not yet able to deal anywhere near systematically with this complex question. Clearly, beginning answers would not only be of much help in understanding the development of combat reactions, but would at the same time clarify this same largely unanswered question for all psychological disorders and decompensations: How do the propensities of the individual and the way he has managed to move along the developmental track influence his meeting with the situational context as it impinges upon his particular strengths and particular sensitivities? War and the army provide conditions which, difficult and complex as they are, allow for relatively more analyzable and isolable factors than most other life situations.

SYMPTOMATOLOGY AND CONTENT OF SYMPTOMS

There seems to be little difference in the symptomatology of the combat reactions in Israel compared to Vietnam, Korea, or other war experiences in recent years. There are the same main groups of dissociative, depressive, anxiety and predominantly autonomous symptoms and few psychotic reactions. Phenomenologically, then, we would see no difference worth mentioning. When we look at differences in terms of content, it seems worthwhile to ask questions, even if we do not have answers to them yet. For example, it would be interesting to know what kinds of fantasies about battle are more prevalent in Israel as compared to other cultures. Or equally, what is it in a traumatic event that a specific individual or a group of individuals remembers over other aspects of the same traumatic event. In part, self-selective memory will relate to the individual's past and therefore to his conflicts and his predispositions: but they may also relate to sociocultural aspects of the content of symptomatology. There is one further area which we would like to single out in terms of content and/or specific symptoms in Israel, that is, guilt. Guilt feelings have been described as a predominant symptom by some of the Israeli authors (Levau et al, 1979; Moses et al, 1976; Neuman, 1974). If indeed this were a true finding, namely that there were more overt guilt feelings of soldiers in combat reactions in Israel than in other wars, such as Vietnam, then one might conjecture about possible reasons for it. On the one hand the identification with the war being waged throughout most of the Israeli wars would lead to a war superego more demanding and in that sense more adapted to the circumstances of battle than in a war with which the soldier is not fully identified (as was the case in Vietnam?). The other area where we would look for factors increasing guilt in Israelis, would be the cultural one, namely whether guilt is more prominent in Judaism than in other religions or ideologies. One would look for example at the culture of the Shtetl (Zborowski and Herzog, 1962) and in documents transmitting general Jewish values such as *Portnoy's Complaint* (Roth, 1960) and *How to be a Jewish Mother* (Greenburg, 1965). However, one would also want to search more specifically for guilt mechanisms in the Israeli population (Moses, unpublished manuscript).

TREATMENT

It is of interest to compare the emotionally more distant psychotherapeutic and abreactive treatment of Israel battle casualties during the War of Independence in 1948 with the much more emotionally close brief psychotherapeutic treatment carried out in a rear unit established in the wake of the Yom Kippur War (Moses et al, 1976). It seems that here it is not so much the treatment modality as the social climate, which has changed, related to many other factors affecting the psychological and social climate in Israel during that period (Moses, 1982). Such a change in emotional distance paralleled a change in the attitude towards immigrants and holocaust survivors over this period of time (Moses, in press). The new development during the Yom Kippur War was an intensive 24- to 72-hour treatment in a forward psychiatric station placed adjacent to a field hospital near the frontline which used abreaction, either hypnotically or spontaneously induced, accompanied by desensitization procedures to war noises, (tanks and shooting), using for both these methods both individual and group methods (Arieli, 1974). The percentage of soldiers returned to battle was described as very high, but not specified. Only a small number of soldiers had to be sent to the rear for further treatment. However, we do not know what percentage of soldiers broke down once more after having been sent back to their units. This contrasts with reports by the US Surgeon General, in the second half of World War II, where on the one hand there was strong pressure to return everybody to the front line, and on the other hand units were told that they would be given no replacements for evacuated soldiers—a strong incentive not to evacuate them as psychological casualties. After the efforts to send almost everybody back to duty, about one-third of these became psychological casualties a second time.

This is an interesting finding in terms of what happens to battle casualties who are sent back to the front line immediately. We do not, of course, know whether any of them were wounded or killed after having thus been sent back.

During the Yom Kippur War, there were two rear Israeli units for the treatment of combat reactions which were both situated in military installations, where soldiers then lived under a military regime. Both units used a very short period of treatment, namely, from two to three weeks. In one unit, therapy consisted of individual, small group and large group therapy. Individual and group therapy took place every day six days a week and large group meetings were held twice a week. In the other unit less emphasis was placed on group therapy. In neither of these short-term treatment units was there any emphasis on family therapy, which however became more of a focus later on, as the soldier-patients became more chronic. Even during the short-term period, the obligatory visit home became an important crisis, because it was here that the patients had to choose between loyalty to their buddies and a newly to be restored bond with the civilian population, namely their families.

We should like to present here an illustrative case as reported by one of us (I.C.) (see also Cohen and Cividalli). We believe that this soldier's case, even though presented in a very succinct form, is a vivid illustration of almost all aspects of etiology, dynamics and treatment of combat reaction.

This was an "unidentified case," in that it stayed below the identification threshold during the war and was finally brought up by a lower identification threshold in his family, after the war.

Ya'ir, a 27-year-old infantry soldier, married and father of a two-year-old boy, was separated from his company and attached to another company. Thus, he arrived at what he called the "wrong position" on the Bar Lev line in 1973, two days before the Egyptian attack.

His father had immigrated from Yemen in 1932, had no formal education, worked all his life as an unskilled laborer. The family story is that, while in the army during the War of Independence, the father broke down after seeing friends killed by Arabs. He was hospitalized in a mental hospital, and died two years later from Buerger's disease. One brother is two years older. His mother, a housewife, is very close to him.

Ya'ir's unit was heavily shelled as the war began. He happened to be outside his position, ran toward it and just as he entered a shell exploded near him. His mortar was blown away by the explosion. He went into the fortified position, was shaking all over, felt as if paralyzed and refused to go out even though his commanders called him. He heard over the intercom that his buddies' position was overrun, and "everybody killed—where is the army?" Refusing to leave the bunker, he was yelled at "You're not a man." Four days later he was extricated by Israeli tanks to the rear.

Afraid of death, particularly at night, still shaking and feeling paralyzed, he managed to continue as a soldier for two months, when he was released. He now had the following symptoms: an anxiety state with night fears, irritability, inability to concentrate, lack of sexual interest and ability to function, sleeplessness, lack of appetite, passivity, lack of initiative, sad looking. He spoke little and quietly, avoided people. He was totally dependent on his wife.

He also reported starting quite heavy drinking during this period in order "to quiet himself, to forget and to conceal his symptoms."

Three months after discharge he was called again to the reserves, which led to an immediate exacerbation of symptoms. He refused to seek medical help but was finally brought to a psychiatric clinic by his wife.

He was assigned to group therapy (Cohen and Cividalli) with 12 other ex-soldiers, of whom 10 remained. They met once a week for 1.5 hours. After 15 group meetings, the wives joined the group. They had been meeting in a separate group previously. The group was terminated by mutual agreement after 1.5 years, when much improvement occurred in all participants, except in Ya'ir, whose improvement was quite limited and shaky.

Ya'ir grew up with his mother since his father's death at age two, when his brother was given to an aunt to be brought up. He was a bad student at school, and barely completed three classes. He changed jobs frequently, and continued to be "kept by mother." Their relationship was always a very close one. He grew up as "the only man at home." Ya'ir was always quite passive and obedient toward his mother. So was he in the army, "doing what he was told to," although he was highly motivated, but with no initiative.

Ya'ir's description of his older brother, a father of two children, but divorced ("probably because of his mental disturbances," in Ya'ir's words), sounded psychopathic and, as reported by Ya'ir, probably had a police record. Ya'ir expected him to be a father substitute but was always bitterly deceived. Actually his brother treated him with cruelty, many times "beating him to death."

Shortly before his regular army service, Ya'ir started a steady relationship with a girlfriend, which lasted about four years but finally "they had to separate" because of both families objections. Later on (at the age of 23) he married his present wife who "was brought by my mother, but I did not love her." In spite of that, he managed to function quite well after his marriage, holding a steady job as a repairman and even working many additional hours in a second one. He was "very active" and "devoted to his family and work." At intake, both spouses stated that "life was fine" before the war. About one year after their marriage (and three years before the war) they had their first child, a boy.

At intake Ya'ir made the impression of a very retarded depression, with chronic anxiety exacerbated by his recent new call to the reserves. Psychodiagnostic tests were performed, after some of the staff raised the possibility of malingering. The tests revealed "a rigid personality" with a borderline IQ (about 80), a severe constriction of ego functions due to depression, but possibly also to a psychotic process, which still had to be ruled out.

Indeed, during treatment, Ya'ir showed many times psychotic-like regressions, with heightened anxiety and paranoid ideation, but always managed to reorganize from them.

Treatment was instituted with a moderate amount of sedative medication, and (as mentioned) with group therapy which later on emerged as a couples group. This treatment concentrated upon the couple's relationship as an enactment of previous conflicts in childhood and war. During this treatment, a very problematic marital relationship came into light, aggravated by the reaction of both of them to the trauma of war. At the beginning, all this was masked by a repetitive and compulsive need to concentrate upon the battle situation only, while separating it from family life in past and present— as Ya'ir's unique and private experience, not understandable by any significant others, close as they may be. Ya'ir and his wife were quite passive and scarcely verbal in the group, showing much resistance to therapy in general and to "a mixed-couples" group in particular. The communication between them was very limited and Ya'ir felt completely dependent on his wife, feeling "not a man anymore."

Later on, they became more involved in treatment, more verbal, and their communication improved. Gradually, feelings of anger toward his wife came into expression, and a connection was made with feelings toward his mother.

The present situation in the group and at home links the conflictual position of helplessness and "castration" in war with the complicated family relations in his traumatic childhood, as with his mother, brother and wife today.

The world and language of fantasy, nightmares and symptoms, interconnected and integrated gradually with his feelings and behavior at home and in the group. His fantasies of "what could have happened, had he been taken prisoner," his nightmares about his comrades being killed while he was separated and unable to help them, and of himself being overrun by enemy tanks, while his buddies,

commanders and family are of no help, or his fears, when in darkness, that someone will catch him—all these were accompanied by
the constant fear of "going crazy" like his father "because of the
Arabs," in the 1948 war.

Helplessness, and fear of losing control paralyzed him and brought
to a culmination the unverbalized anger, anxiety and depression, as
observed in his passive-aggressive position at home and in treatment.
These processes were at times aggravated by his strong resistance
to change each time that some progress was made in treatment.
There were ups and downs in the treatment, with absenteeism and
sometimes with psychotic-like regressions, both partly due also to his
low capacity for insight and verbalization.

During treatment, the intermingling of facts and fantasy, symptoms and functioning, past (distant and immediate: childhood and
war), and present (as a husband and father) was made clear, but only
partially worked through by Ya'ir.

His childhood and adolescence background, being "left alone by
father" and of being heavily dependent on his mother and cruelly
abused by his older brother, added to his military experience. He
started as a well motivated fighter in the Six-Day War (1967). He
reported being "slapped by the commanding officer" while "trying
to stop [me] from punishing Arabs who still had weapons at home:
I wanted to avenge my father." All this be brought with him to the
Yom Kippur War (1973). Then he was separated from his original old
buddies and best friend, and two days later he heard about their
deaths, while he was "at the wrong position" and his mortar destroyed
by enemy fire, leaving him helpless, afraid of death, and unable to
move.

Not being with "his own buddies" aggravated his situation. So
too did the reaction of his "new comrades": one officer cursed him
for "exaggerating the situation" and others shouted at him: "You're
not a man!" These reactions stirred, in him, old feelings of abandonment, disappointment, helplessness, and impotent anger, which had
to be repressed, and aggravated his isolation.

Guilt and shame were mixed: toward his dead buddies, his father,
and his new comrades from whom he distanced himself for fear of
being laughed at again.

Toward the end of his treatment, his brother became very ill and
weak. Soon a diagnosis of advanced gastric cancer was made. Ya'ir's
longstanding death wishes towards his brother now came very close
to fulfillment, broke into his consciousness and were verbalized in
treatment, accompanied by vividly aroused guilt feelings. During

treatment some change was attained in the couple's communication patterns, mutual understanding and acceptance. The war trauma helped to open up heavily defended childhood and marital conflicts, which existed albeit, without awareness, before the war. One of the results was that feelings of hostility and sometimes hate towards his wife managed to be openly verbalized due to Ya'ir's increased openness, and brought about frequent and more intense quarrels, but also less pathological dependence in the couple's life.

After 1.5 years of a very difficult treatment in the group, heavy resistance—at times very regressive—and of Ya'ir's struggle against "going crazy like my father," Ya'ir's state and function improved somewhat, but he was still symptomatic and in need of treatment. Indeed, he continued individual and drug therapy (including moderate doses of major tranquilizers), for an additional half year, with one of the therapists of the couples group (a female psychiatrist). At this point, due to technical reasons, he had to change therapists, and continued in an abreactive insight-oriented individual therapy, this time with a male psychologist. After three more years of quite drastic ups and downs, and discontinuation of drug treatment, he probably reached a new steady state in feeling and function, equivalent, although very different, to the prewar equilibrium. We believe that this equilibrium was again, a relatively fragile one, prone to eventual breakdown if exposed to new psychic trauma.

Indirect follow-up in these days, indicated a continuation of this steady state, with a reasonable social readjustment.

In this case, the treatment approach was in all stages an analytically oriented one. This seems to be the preferred treatment orientation, but it soon became clear, especially during the war but also afterwards that the number of experienced psychotherapists was not large enough for such an ambitious plan. At the same time, even some of the experienced psychodynamically trained psychotherapists did not sufficiently believe in short-term psychotherapy. Thus, more emphasis began to be placed on behavioristic therapies, which existed side by side with the psychodynamic ones. It was unfortunate that adequate and comprehensive published follow-up results are not available on either the treatments of 1973, or later treatments comparing different treatment modalities. It would have been an unusual opportunity to compare such different therapies. The only available follow-up study by Levav et al (1979) is not sufficiently informative from this point of view.

The treatment of soldiers with combat reactions which have become chronic, ie, after they have been discharged from the army, has been in the hands of the various psychiatric clinics throughout the country. Here again adequate and reliable follow-up information is not available. However, the general experience seems to be that treatment of such ex-soldiers is very frustrating. Halmosh (1982) reports on the difficulties; his findings are in line with an earlier study by Mann et al in 1965. Unfortunately, we do not know how many of these ex-soldiers were given competent regular psychotherapy which tried to deal with their problems in the light of our knowledge, rather than by supportive means or combinations of supportive and medication approaches. However, from our experience we do know that the treatment of such soldiers over the long term is difficult in that it is not easy for them to work well in introspective exploratory psychotherapy. The use of group psychotherapy seems to have been an easier and preferable tool of treatment perhaps for both patients and therapists. Yet we do not know enough about treatment results to be able to make any valid comparison between the treatment modalities. The later developed view that the chronic psychological illness of the ex-soldier is really a "family affair" and as such warrants family therapy has led to some interesting experiences. But again, unfortunately, there is no sufficient information that allows us to compare its effectiveness in any meaningful way.

At this point we would like to present an additional and last clinical vignette, dealing this time with the group therapy of the postcombat reaction veteran.[1]

Twelve freshly discharged veterans were referred to the therapy group while their wives were concommitantly seen in a parallel, separate group. They had no previous history of psychiatric diagnosis or treatment and included no psychotic patients. They were all married. The therapeutic contract included a "preparation" period of six months as a "men only" group, to be merged thereafter with the parallel group of their wives. Our group was started about six months after the ceasefire while most of the army was still at the front.

The patients had had a different medical history in the army: some of them were identified as combat reactions during the actual fighting, and after brief treatment close to the frontlines, were evacuated and treated at a rear military psychiatric treatment unit for up to three additional months. Others were immediately discharged

---

[1] Special mention should be made here of the fact that this couples group was treated conjointly by an experienced female psychiatrist who was also the initiator of this therapy group (N. Cividalli, MD) and one of us (I.C.). The conjoint treatment proved to be an important asset for the process, but is discussed elsewhere (Cohen and Cividalli).

after little treatment; and still others managed to continue with borderline functioning until after their unit was discharged; they "broke down" only when they arrived back home.

The merging of the two groups occurred only after a self-selection: only five couples were able to overcome their resistance and formed the stable couples group which continued for another year. Five other couples were not able to reach an agreement as to their joint participation in the group. Therefore they continued their treatment as a group of men only. Two couples dropped out.

We deal here only with the initial men's group, mentioning very succinctly some of the presenting symptomatology of the patients. It was fairly uniform with some individual variation. It included sleep difficulties and nightmares, overt anxiety, sweating palms and palpitations, depression, irritability and lack of concentration, sexual problems, various degrees of work difficulties up to total inability to work, feelings of guilt and worthlessness, and a permanent, compulsive and exhausting preoccupation with the war experiences and trauma.

Their great difficulties on the interpersonal level, mainly within the family unit, were not presented as main complaints; they were even concealed. The family had ceased to constitute a support system and became instead a painful source of conflict.

Our therapeutic approach was a group analytic one, which we tried to adapt to the specific situation and people treated. We were aware from the beginning, of the limitations imposed upon the length and depth of treatment by two facts: First, the ego strength, the psychological-mindedness and the motivation for in-depth, explorative and interpretative treatment were assessed as very limited. Second, the specific psychopathological entity warned us against a tendency to prolong such a dependent-therapeutic relationship. We considered that a link exists between the chronification of symptoms and the "chronification of treatment." Therefore we preferred a shorter treatment; we conducted our explorative and interpretative activity in close parallel to the vicissitudes of the patients' ego strength and defenses.

The focus of this therapy was in two main areas: the marital and social interactions in the "here and now," and the trauma of war as remembered and reexperienced in the "here and now" of the family and the group. We wanted to show that those two areas are not disconnected, as they protested, but on the contrary, are one the result of the other. However, the marital reality is more available to observation and influence than the war trauma.

The constant compulsion of the ex-soldiers to "stick to the battle" and to keep its experience separate from their other experiences, was evident from the first session: everyone's "carte de visite" was his war story. This meant not only "this is me, that's who I am," but also instituted a competition in the group, based on the intensity of their war experiences. Most of the patients had previously undergone abreactive treatment, or narcoanalysis, and now longed for this kind of catharsis. We dealt with this problem in therapy in two ways. We did not encourage abreaction, yet nor did we prevent ventilation or spontaneous abreaction when it occurred. Instead, we encouraged their connection of this war material with the current interaction at home and in the group, thus helping the group to struggle with the resistances to the transition from war to family and group life. The presence of the wives, later, was of much help in this direction. The termination of this therapy was mutually decided upon by patients and therapists, one and a half years after it began. One of the veterans achieved only limited improvement and needed additional treatment. As regards the others, there was considerable improvement in all areas, and treatment was evaluated as successful. So far, eight years after termination, none of them applied or was referred for treatment again.

As an illustration of the main points made, we would like to present some extracts from the verbatim transcription of the group therapy. We chose representative parts from the initial stages of the men's group, when the two groups (the men's and the wive's) were still separated.

Extracts are from the first, ninth, and 15th sessions, while the 16th was already the first session of the merged couples' group.

Our illustrations are to serve two main purposes: the first is to communicate some of the atmosphere in the group. The second is to emphasize the principal focus which arose in this group therapy: the struggle and the interlacing between the two central themes, namely, the war experiences and those between the spouses, after the return home of the veteran. We must perforce leave aside the more general details of the group dynamics, of the group analytic approach and of our techniques and interventions. In addition to limitation of space, those details are less relevant, since they are by no means specific to this group compared to others elsewhere.

The two *specific* aspects of this psychotherapy are the context and the content. By the context we mean a couples' therapy group where both spouses are suffering from post-combat reaction. The specificity of the content lies in the combination of both combat trauma and family conflict.

Verbatim Transcription*

First Session [Men Only], *Seven Participants, May 1974* In the opening words the therapists make clear that "we will not limit ourselves here to the battle experiences, but we shall try also to understand what happened after the war, here and now, at home, at work, in the group, and how all those connect with prewar family life."

After a short silence and the invitation by the therapist to start, the first speaker takes the initiative:

Uri: Only some days ago I left the military treatment unit. I was there in a similar group. I can say that I'm quite OK now—only a few small problems . . . (talking with a hardly audible voice) . . . I don't know how to explain it: I'm not a hero and all of a sudden it comes out that I was a hero. *This* is my problem: I'm usually afraid and all of a sudden I did things which I cannot understand, that are not usual for me. It all came out after the war—I became indifferent, I didn't care to live, nothing could scare me and nothing was important anymore.

I haven't returned yet to live at home after the war. (Uri explained elsewhere that since the war, he lives with his parents and sometimes at his sister's, while his wife and children are at home). I have no patience for no one. I lost my self confidence at work. I spoil things, I'm afraid to do harm, to forget checking the brakes or some other motor . . . (Uri is a mechanic, but didn't return to work since the war). I don't want to endanger anyone.

At home? . . . that's foolish, but I don't miss anyone . . . (silence). [Meanwhile, Eli talks about his outbreaks at home and asks Uri why can't he do the same at his home. We shall return now to Uri.]

Uri: I couldn't do this at home. There I feel like it's easier to break everything than to talk about anything. Indeed I broke so many things at home . . . and it's at my own expense. And when I think of that I'm sorry, it's not reasonable and not worth going home at all. At home they expect me to be a father—I have obligations, and that's very annoying.

Eli: Maybe home is the right place to get it all out? . . . To let steam off?

Uri: I have already managed to break everything at home . . .

---

*The verbatim quotations do not form a continuous sequence, but they are only separate (although sequentially related) fragments, which we deemed relevant and representative.

Eli: At home I can throw everything at my wife—I mean words—and calm down—not violently . . . I know I'm not right, but I have no other place to do it . . . Oh yes, I was also at this treatment unit in the army—of course they helped me. I felt there like in a good home. [And some 15 minutes later:]

Benny: In the last war (1967) I was wounded . . . I mean physically . . . and now my psyche is injured—there's no difference for me. But if people think that a visible bandage is a proof of heroism and an internal one is not . . . let them think whatever they want!

Ofer: But you can't convince people that you are hurt: they *see* that everything is in place with you on the outside. Why do you think I grew a moustache? It's because I didn't want people to think that I wasn't in the army . . . When I was in the military treatment unit, my head was swollen from talking everyday: psychologists, doctors . . . but I felt OK there, with all this headache it felt good when they gave me this injection to talk and I was groggy for a couple of hours.

Therapist: And what happened when you returned home?

Ofer: It was OK for about two months and then it all came back again: I couldn't sleep at night, I didn't care and my palms were sweating . . . I prefer not to mix my family life with these things.

Therapist: Because it hurts?

Ofer: Maybe not because of that. I just don't want to . . .

Therapist (to Eli):   And you said that you could let it all out at home when you are angry?

Eli: In the military treatment unit, in the treatment group, we talked about telling everything at home, but it didn't work. Out there at the unit, there was always somebody to listen to you, to calm you down. It was good . . . at home I said to myself that I should try to manage and control myself—to be OK—but I felt that it isn't OK. It's even worse . . . I am more tense, and everything Ofer told us just now. My palms also sweat. I can't sleep and I have so many, so many thoughts.

Therapist: And what is your wife's reaction?

Eli: At the beginning she understood . . . but now she says "To hell with it! How much can I take?!" and so she hits back with anger at my anger and tells me "to keep my nose out of her business." If she doesn't prepare my coffee in the morning, it's big trouble! Before? I didn't care! I try not to remember. Now I feel that when I shout at her it's to forget other, more serious things . . .

Therapist: And did you talk about what you experienced in battle?

Eli: No, from the beginning I didn't tell her. I didn't want her to know. She doesn't really listen and isn't really interested. She doesn't care and that's why I keep those things to myself . . . She says that I thrash at night, while asleep. Afterwards I was afraid to fall asleep . . . yes . . . let her see me like that at night! . . . No, I'm telling you, she doesn't understand. She would say that all this happened to everyone in the war, and then why should I take it all to heart . . . but she doesn't understand that a buddy of mine died next to me.

[And later on:]

Uri: . . . the war is for me like a closed book: I finished reading it and put it aside.

Therapist: So you closed the book. Do you want to close something else now?

Uri: Yes, but they never let you close anything. It's either the planes or the army calling you back or coming to give you a promotion. I don't want to listen to the radio. What do they talk about there? This one is dead, the other wounded, and both sides shoot at each other. The war goes on, it isn't over, it's all the same now at home, only without the helmet . . .

Session 9, Ten Participants, July 1974   After Haim described in brief his feelings and symptoms after the war:

Benny: Let us be clear, we are all like Haim, and the feeling is like we're born anew, because we were close to death. And anyone who's born anew needs warmth just like a newborn baby. We're like the Phoenix, born again from ashes—you see the fire and the smoke and the comrades and the ashes. We feel like we were given our lives as a present, but it's hard for us to forget the price, and that's why we are here. It all went too deep.

Therapist: You mean what happened to you in the war?

Michael: You may think of it like that, but . . . it's more of an obsession . . . a nightmare . . .

Session 15 (The Last Session With Men Only) 12 Participants, August 1974

Therapist: So, what do you think about the wives joining our group and talking together?

Uri: The earlier the better. Each one of us has to see the problems of both spouses, deep down to their roots. We should hear each other's side in their own words. If we can both talk here—we might understand things better. There are always two sides to any coin.

Benny: So we can judge who's right!

Uri: It's not a courthouse here.

Therapist: Do you think that family problems which started before the war and are aggravated now, should be discussed together, here?

Uri: I would shoot all those wives. Eli told me that they are right, they demand what is their due, but they should understand that you want to, but you just can't.

Therapist: You mean sex?

Uri: It's very important!

Therapist: So she feels as if you don't want her?!

Uri: Yes! And the trouble is that you can't, it just doesn't happen somehow, it doesn't mean anything to you. In spite of all, after the war the wife doesn't attract you as before, and that brings up lots of other problems.

Benny: Why don't you call a spade a spade! Don't be afraid . . . Now I want to tell you what happened to me after the war. I went with my wife to the funeral of one of my buddies. She felt very badly, as if she were a widow. She seemed to want to punish herself for my returning home: "Did she really deserve to win me back from war?" At home she was very tense, explosive sometimes, and turned her back to me.

Therapist: You mean that what happened to you is the reverse of Uri's story.

Yossi: And now you want to bring all those things here, to the group?! How can you expect a man to hear somebody tell him that he is not a man—and yet when other women are listening? And they will all know?!

Benny: Everyone tells his or her secrets in his own group here (meaning the two separate groups of the men and their wives).

Haim: Maybe there are problems at home, quarrels, but not with me. My wife got some brains from her group and now it's going better. So, now I'm looking for the point I'm interested in—that I'm afraid to death from the army—I am still confused and I can't sleep. My wife can't help me sleep at night. I had a problem and I consulted Benny and Uri here (group members) and that's all I need: to rest from the army!

Therapist: You told us that since you shared your fears with your wife, things are better.

Haim: OK, but my problem is still there. So what if we keep quarrelling? She won't divorce me—she has no parents . . . And besides, I'm telling you, I don't care what she thinks of my masculinity!

Benny (to Haim): You don't appreciate your wife. She seems pretty low in your eyes. One can see that.

Uri: My problem is also with the army, like Haim. I sweat a lot when I see a tank or a cannon. If we go back there we can go crazy, I've seen this before with one guy in our battalion . . .

Therapist: And what do you expect from the group?

Uri: I came to the group because after the war I had become only half a man. I can't work, I'm nervous and people can't talk to me. I'm not afraid of anyone. That isn't normal. I asked the doctor to send me to the madhouse and I tried to hit a policeman. I didn't want to, but I came to this group. When I came back from the war, they sent me to (names military treatment unit)—I had injections there and pills . . . I came back 60 percent . . . Until two weeks ago I didn't work. Now I'm better and I agree to have my wife back home. We never tried to understand what happened to us, how all this mess came about.

[After about 30 minutes, Uri talks again about his battle experiences and his related symptoms, and here we intervene] :

Therapist: But how does this connect with your relationships at home?

Uri: That's exactly what I was trying to tell you. When you come back home finished, broken, and after you've seen so many dead, your buddies died near you, and you took them to the grave by pieces, then you come back without any will to live. There is no value in life or in the world. You see your wife, your children and home and you say to yourself: "What does all this help, what does it matter? Tomorrow we'll go back and die." So, when I returned from the front I asked my wife for some hours to myself, to think, but then she started to demand things from me—even shoes for the children! What the hell! Is this what bothers me just now? This is what makes trouble with your wife—and she thinks you're crazy.

[Later on, a plane is flying by and sudden and intense noise of its jet engines penetrates the room. Uri is the one who immediately reacts verbally and talks about his fears in such cases.]

Therapist: But now you aren't afraid anymore.

Uri: Yeah! Because all are here with me. If you sit with me, I can go on talking all day: I promise you I won't go to sleep.

Benny: Uri, give us a hint about where and when all that really started.

Haim (interrupting): I'll tell you—it all started on the ceasefire day near Ismailia (the most remote post of the Israeli Army at the northern end of the West Bank of the Suez Canal in Egypt).

Therapist: What do you all think? He told us that after being treated in the army he was OK for two months and then . . . what happened?

Haim: That's right! Until I got called up again to the reserves. Then you start sweating and all that again . . .

Ya'ir: Me too—I was better when I came back home, but then I ran away from home, I walked around in town and when I came back an argument was started between us, and then, problems . . .

Uri: Let's forget the family story for a moment! When I came home angry after the war, after I saw so many dead, can I then have sex with my wife just for pleasure? Back from hell! Ha! It just doesn't work that way! The wife didn't understand that at all and that's how war started at home . . . I can't stay home alone. I'm afraid of the darkness.

Therapist: Could you explain all this to your wife?

Michael and Yossi (vehemently and at unison): But she must know all that!

Uri: Do you know what our first quarrel after the war was about? I couldn't get to sleep. I wandered through the house, but it didn't work. I got drunk. I told my wife that she can't return my buddy to me. And then she said that I can go too—me and my buddy. I don't know. I'm fed up. I have to let steam off somewhere. I'm afraid of jet noises even in the movies. Last week I went to check my heart. I can assure you I am not ill, but all this makes you sick. At first I thought I can't see at all. Maybe this happened before the war too, but I thought so much about the war that I connected it with the war. My hearing too . . . today I blame the war for it. I don't want any friends. I'm afraid tomorrow they'll die at war. That's why it's too early for me to go back to the army.

[The group goes on discussing the pros and cons to the merging of the two groups due to take place the next meeting.]

Therapist (to the whole group): How do you think your wives can help if they were here? Do you think you can help them too here?

Michael: You want her here to make her understand, but my wife understands already; then why should she come?

Therapist: Is that what she's telling you, that she understands, or is that what you really feel?

Michael: That's what I think . . . but actually . . . (silence).

Benny: People know me as a man without family problems, and now my wife and I find that we do have problems. I thought before that everything is OK, but now I have discovered important things . . .

Haim (interrupting): I don't like your going on with this. You can come back to it later. Now I want you to deal with *my* problem: the army!

Therapist: You probably have come to a stage at which you don't want to talk about your family.

Haim: Because it doesn't bother me!

Benny (to Haim): I'm still sure it all began before the war.

Yossi: OK! So I want to tell you: I can't sleep without a light, and my wife understands and leaves the light on, so she helps me, and we don't have any problems.

Therapist: And what about her?

Yossi: Maybe she suffers . . .

Ya'ir: If she'll talk about the problems with him, they'll just get worse. Everything will go from bad to worse.

Haim: I don't have any need to talk about my wife.

Therapist: I understand that your wife also came to a point in her group (the wives' group) at which she feels that it's dangerous for her to go on.

Haim: I heard that in the wives' group they talk too much about what happens in the bedroom, and not everyone likes this. But I don't want to talk about this! It's true that a few times I spoke to my wife and I felt better, but just now, talking about home, I came to have a headache. I remember here a session in which Benny recalled that during the war he remained only with his underpants, and then I felt identified with him. But now look, I'm losing weight every month—I can prove it, look at my belt. It's true that with my wife things go better, but this doesn't solve my problems. I don't care about anyone, although some things do matter to me. This indifference is quite peculiar. I'm afraid to go back to the army. Others had a number of wars and in the last one broke down. For me one is enough.

[The session ends with a general discussion about the reluctance to go back to the army. The more silent members, who didn't speak before, now join in. This theme brings "solidarity" to the group and "solves" their problems about the decision to have their wives join the group at the next meeting.]

* * *

In terms of treatment then, we would summarize by saying that the most effective treatment of combat reaction seems to take place as soon as possible, as close as possible, that is in line with the immediacy and proximity concepts which have been formulated in the

U.S. Army. Once an actual breakdown has been established and the soldier had to be moved back to rear hospitals or units, his chances of improving decrease considerably. However, it does seem well worthwhile to institute a short-term army-regimented psychotherapeutically oriented treatment that emphasizes the needs of the self and the importance of self-esteem, the previous traumata which the soldier-patient recalls in the course of such an intensive psychotherapy as well as group approaches. Once discharge from the army becomes necessary, the chances for improvement decrease further, in part because there is now a wide diversity of treatment approaches, but also because none of the known approaches, including the psychodynamic one have proved very efficient with this kind of psychological problem. This is all the more reason, then, to place much emphasis on preventive approaches which will in the first instances utilize all the group approaches. The emphasis is on morale and on preparedness, and the provision of reliable information. In addition, such preventive measures take into account the narcissistic needs of the individual and of the group to the extent that they can be optimally met within the group situation of the army. However, we do feel that the problem of how to treat the psychologically disabled veteran has not yet been solved any way approaching optimal conditions. In our view, more energy and resources should be devoted to comparative studies on the subject which take comparable populations and treat them by different modes, by well-trained psychotherapists or psychiatrists in a milieu which; in any case, is fully identified with the particular mode of treatment.

REFERENCES

Arieli, J. (1974). *Harefuah* (Hebrew). Vol. 85, Dec. 15, 1974.

Balint, M. (1969). Trauma and object relationship. *International Journal of Psychoanalysis* 50: 429–435.

Brecher, M., Geist, B. (1980). *Decisions in Crisis*, Israel 1967 and 1973. Stanford, California: University of California Press.

Cohen, I. (1980). The Identification Threshold of the Combat Reactions (unpublished manuscript).

Cohen, I. (1979). The Symptoms and Treatment of the Combat Reaction Casualties in the Arab-Israeli Wars since 1948. Invited Opening Lecture at the International Symposium on War Psychiatry, Munich.

Cohen, I., Cividalli, N. Group Therapy of the Post-Combat Reaction Couples, 1974–1976 (unpublished manuscript).

Freud, S. (1919). Introduction to Psychoanalysis of War Neuroses. *S.E.* 17: 207.

Freud, S. (1940). *An Outline of Psychoanalysis. S.E.* 23: 141.

Greenburg, D. (1965). *How to be a Jewish Mother.* Price Stern.

Halmosh, A. F. (1942). Some dynamic aspects of treatment resistant emotional war casualties. In Speilberger, Ch.D., *Stress and Anxiety.* University of South Florida, Tampa: I. G. Sarason, University of Washington, and N.A. Milgram, Tel Aviv University. Vol. 8: Hemisphere Pub. 171-175.

Holmes, T. H., Rahe, R. H. (1967). The Social Readjustment Rating Scale. *Journal of Psychosomatic Research* 11: 213-218.

Kohut, H. (1971). *The Analysis of the Self,* Hogarth Press.

Levav, I., Greenfield, H., Baruch, E. (1979). Psychiatric Combat Reactions during the Yom Kippur War. *American Journal of Psychiatry* 136: 637-641.

Mann, K., et al. (1965). The progress of disabled veterans. *Archives of Environmental Health* 10: 754-760.

Moses, R. (1978). Adult psychic trauma: the question of early predisposition in some detailed mechanisms. *International Journal of Psychoanalysis* 59: 353-363.

Moses, R. (1982). The group self and the Arab-Israeli conflict. *International Review of Psychoanalysis* 9: 55-65.

Moses, R. (1983a). Emotional response to stress in Israel: A psychoanalytic perspective. In: S. Breznitz (Ed.) *Stress in Israel.* New York: Van Nostrand and Rinehold.

Moses, R. (in press). An Israeli psychoanalyst looks back in 1983 in *Psychoanalytic Perspectives on the Holocaust.* S. Luel, P. Marcus (Eds.) New York: Columbia University Press.

Moses, R. A psychoanalytic view of unconscious guilt on the Israeli side of the Arab-Israeli conflict. Unpublished manuscript.

Moses, R., Kligler, D. (1966). The institutionalization of mental health values, A comparison between the United States and Israel. *Israel Annals of Psychiatry* 4: 148-161.

Moses, R., Bargal, D., Calev, J., Falk, A., Halevi, H., Lerner, Y., Mass, M., Noy, S., Perla, B., Winokur, M. (1976). A rear unit for the treatment of combat reactions in the wake of the Yom Kippur War. *Psychiatry* 39: 153-162.

Neumann, M. (1974). Combat reaction and its treatment (Hebrew). *Harefuah* Vol. 85, Dec. 15.

Sandler, J., Joffe, W. G. (1967). The tendency to persistence in psychological function and development. *Bulletin of the Menninger Clinic* 31: 257-271.

Sandler, J. (1967). Trauma, strain and development. In: S. Furst (Ed.) *Psychic Trauma.* New York: Basic Books.

Sandler, J. Personal communication.

Zborowski, N., Herzog, E. (1962). *Life is with People, The Culture of the Shtetl.* New York: Schocken Books.

Index

Abandonment, 95, 265
Abreaction, 286
Adolescent development, 110-111
Affective illness, 230
Agent Orange, 55
Agent Orange anxiety, 175, 206-207
Aggression
  combat veterans exhibiting, 48, 57
  combat, types of, 109
  in delayed psychological reaction,
    278
  guilt and, 72
  laundered, 203
  noise hypersensitivity and, 68
  paranoid rage and, 202
  in posttraumatic stress disorder,
    202-203, 224
  self-against-self, 203
  self-maintenance, 203
  splitting and, 199
Agoraphobia, 233
Alienation, 165, 166, 201
Amitryptyline, 246
Amnesia
  in combat psychopathology, 27
  with night terrors, 104
  in stress response, 128
  from traumatic experiences, 1
Animal magnetism, 5, 6
Anti-hero syndrome, 165
Antidepressants, 229, 245-246
Anxiety
  Agent Orange, 175, 206-207

[Anxiety]
  barbiturates and benzodiazepines
    for, 221
  in combat psychopathology, 27, 50
  in delayed psychological reactions,
    279
  group therapy for, 206
  of nightmares, 114, 115
  phenelzine sulfate for, 226
  in posttraumatic stress disorder,
    224
  separation, in war neurosis, 107
  somatic accommodation to, 199
  state, 283
  support groups for allaying, 167
  trait, 283
Authority
  group therapy for problems with,
    203-204
  guilt and, 77
  transference and, 87-89
  as underlying theme of rap session,
    170
Azam, Eugene, 10, 16

Barbiturates, 221
Battle fatigue, 126
Battle of Latrun, 271-276
Benzodiazepines, 221
Benzylamine, 230
Bibliotherapy, 175
Bioenergetics, 153
Bourne, Ansel, 10

Braid, James, 7
Breakdown
    group cohesion against, 271
    stages of, 27
    threshold for, 283
Briquet, Paul, 13

Calamity syndrome, 234
Castration, 57, 69
    helplessness of war linked to, 289
    masochistic regression and, 75
Character disorders
    analysis of, in group therapy, 156
    chronic regressed, 42-44
    delayed regressed, 42
    psychoanalytic psychotherapy for,
        40-41
    rap group members with, 176
    in traumatic neuroses, 164
Charcot, Jean-Marie, 10, 15, 16, 17
Chlordiazepoxide, 231
Chlorimipramine, 246
Clorgyline, 230
Cognitive techniques in group therapy,
    161-162
Combat aggression, 109-110
Combat neuroses
    categorization of, 40
    history of, 26-27
    from Israeli wars, 269-302
        in battle of Latrun, 271-276
        delayed psychological reaction
            in, 278-279
        masked psychological reaction
            in, 277-278
        mechanism of reactions in, 280-
            285
        psychological and physical
            injury and, 276-277
        symptomatology in 285-286
        treatment of, 286-302
    predisposition and vulnerability to,
        280
    psychotherapy of, brief, 125-150
        anxiety barometer in, 139-142
        focus of, 137-139
        outcome of, 148
        patient selection for, 131-133
        technical considerations for,
            137-146
        work-up for, 133-136

[Combat neuroses]
    reciprocal images of masculinity
        with violent action in, 147-
        148
    regression of id, ego, and superego
        in, 281
Concentration camp survivors
    countertransference reactions in
        therapy for, 81
    psychic structure alterations in, 167
    psychopathology of, 33
Conversion reactions
    in survivor syndrome, 19
    from traumatic experiences, 1
    of Vietnam veterans, 25
Countertransference
    definition of, 96
    in therapy for guilt, 52, 81
Cryptamnesia, 10
Cultural factors in Israeli wars, 285-
    286

Death
    fears relating to, 253-267
    Freudian theory on problems in
        dealing with, 262
    guilt and, 258
Death instinct, 29, 100
Delta sleep, 239
Deprenyl, 230
Depression, 48
    atypical disorder, 231-233
    drug therapy for, 229, 245-246
    fear of dead and, 256
    group therapy for, 207
    guilt and, 73
    hysteroid dysphoria, 233
    monoamine oxidase inhibitors for,
        230-234
    in posttraumatic stress disorder,
        224
    rap sessions for treating, 174
    self-against-self aggression with, 203
Desensitization procedures, 286
Despine, Antoine, 10
Diazepam, 242
Dopamine, 230
Dreams
    ego psychology of, 114-116
    Freudian theory on, 113
    function of, 116-118

[Dreams]
 nightmares. *See* Nightmares
 as outlet for unconscious impulses,
  114
 preconscious in, 113
 in REM sleep, 239
 rhythm of cycles, 245
 self-psychology of, 118-119
 self-punishment and, 76
 stress and, 116
 traumatic experiences evoked via
  imagery of, 103
 wish fulfillment theory of, 114
Drug therapy, 226, 229-248
 case studies with, 291
 with lithium carbonate, 246-247
 with monoamine oxidase inhibitors,
  229-238
  for anxiety and nightmares,
   226-227
  clinical studies of, 232-233
  dosages for, 227
  for flashbacks, 245
  sleep effects of, 245
 with phenelzine sulfate, 227-229,
  234-238, 240-245
 with tricyclic antidepressants,
  245-246

Education, patient
 vs breakdown threshold, 283
 on group therapy, 175
 on transference, 95-96
Ego
 autonomy of, in group therapy,
  187
 in dream theory, 114-116
 in fear of dead, 260
 in guilt therapy, 78-79
 libido and, in war neurosis, 108
 in nightmares, 104, 114-116
 in persecutory guilt, 73
 regression of, in war neuroses, 281
 self-punishment and, 73
 traumatic experiences affecting, 19,
  28, 30-31
Ego strength
 definition of, 115
 in dream and nightmare
  psychology, 115
 for psychotherapy, 131

Emotional adjustment, postwar, 49
Encounter therapy, 153
Enuresis, nocturnal, 239
Erikson, Erik, 12
Exorcism, 2, 3-4, 6
Experiential group therapy, 160

Fantasies of combat, 254
 in case study, 290
 neutralization of, social ritual in,
  253-267
 repressed, in war neuroses, 255
Fantasy-imagery, 153
Fear of dead
 analysis and treatment of, 253-267
 Freudian theory on, 262
 guilt and, 258
Flashbacks
 in awakened REM state, 245
 phenelzine sulfate for, 227, 245
 in posttraumatic stress disorder,
  224
Flourney, Theodore, 10
Freud, Sigmund
 on death, 262
 dream theory of, 113
 in historical overview of war
  neurosis, 12-13, 16, 18
 hysteria studies by, 28
 trauma defined by, 28
 on traumatic neurosis, 28, 29
 on unconscious guilt, 71

Gassner, Johann Joseph, 3-6
Genetic predisposition to combat
  neuroses, 284
Grief
 in group therapy, 161
 group therapy for, 203
 rap sessions for treating, 174
 in stress response, 126
Group games, 153
Group therapy. *See* Psychodynamic
  group therapy
Guilt
 case presentations of, 54-70
 of commission, 204
 counter-guilt character and, 71
 depressive, 73
 in Freudian theory, 71
 gook-identification, 204

[Guilt]
  group therapy for, 204-205
  about guilt, 204-205
  in Israeli wars, 285
  literature review of, 48-54
  masochism and, 75, 76
  of omission, 204
  origin, manifestation and treatment
    of, 47-82
  persecutory, 73
  primary vs secondary, 73
  projection of, 71-72
  rap sessions for treating, 174
  self-against-self aggression with, 203
  survivor, 205
  in survivor syndrome, 75
  therapeutic value in exposing, 75-
    76
  in working on dead, 258

Hallucinosis, 19
Hostility
  to authority, 88
  in combat aggression, 109
  combat veterans exhibiting, 48
  guilt and, 72
Hurst, Arthur, 15-16
Hyperaesthesia, 27
Hypervigilance
  in survivor syndrome, 19
  from traumatic experiences, 1
Hypnosis, 2, 7-8, 11
Hypochondriasis, 233
Hysteria
  mental and physical disturbances
    with, 15
  psychic origins of, 13
Hysteroid dysphoria, 233, 234

Id, 281
Identification
  in combat reactions, 273, 282
  father, and superego, 73-74, 76, 77
  gook, 204
  killer-victim, 161
  in object relations approach to
    psychotherapy, 35
  with therapist, 90, 92-94
  in traumatic neurosis, 164
  with victims, 53, 82

Imipramine, 245, 246
Interpersonal relationships
  with combat stress, 111
  as focus for therapy, 293
  identity mergers with, 111, 112
  insecurity of, in war neurosis, 108,
    111
  parental, affecting war neurosis,
    107, 108
  in posttraumatic stress disorder,
    105
  trauma affecting, 105-106
  with women, 205-206
Iproniazid, 230
Israeli wars
  battle of Latrun, 271-276
  combat neurosis from, 269-302
    delayed psychological reactions
      in, 278-279
    guilt in, 285
    masked psychological reactions
      in, 277-278
    mechanism of reactions in, 280-
      285
    symptomatology and content of
      symptoms, 285-286
    treatment of, 286-302
  cultural factors in, 285-286
  psychological and physical injury
    from, 276-277
  sociocultural context of, 270-271

James, William, 10
Janet, Pierre, 11

Kardiner, Abram, 17, 30-31, 104, 106
Kohut, H., 111-112, 118

Lebanon war, 279
Lithium carbonate, 246-247

Magnetism, 2, 5, 6, 7-8
Masculinity, 93, 94, 147-148
Masochism, 60, 75, 76
Memory disturbances
  amnesia, 1
  in combat neuroses, 27
  of fixating trauma, 142
  in general stress response, 128
  with night terrors, 104

[Memory disturbances]
  in stress response, 126, 127
  in survivor syndrome, 19
Mesmer, Franz Anton, 3, 5, 6-7
Monoamine oxidase inhibitors
  for anxiety-related states, 231
  in brain, 233
  chronic posttraumatic reactions
    and, 229-238
  for depression, 230-231
  experimental, 230
  history of, 230-233
  phenelzine sulfate, 226
  platelet, 233
  for posttraumatic stress disorder,
    226
  studies of, 232-233
Monoamine oxidase, 230
Muscle spasms, 27

Narcissism
  rage and, 202
  as support against combat reac-
    tions, 280
  in war neurosis, 35, 109, 110
    nightmares and, 112
    treatment of, 119
Narcoanalysis, 294
Neurasthenia, 16
Neuroses
  combat. See Combat neuroses
  peacetime, 18, 32
  sexual trauma in etiology of, 27-
    28
  traumatic, 15
    history of, 15-16, 106-113
    organic basis for, 16
    psychoneurotic complications
      from, 17
    symptoms of, 106, 165
  war. See War neurosis
Night terror
  characteristics of, 103-104
  sleep stages correlating to, 239
Nightmares
  anxiety of, 114, 115
  of dead bodies, 258
  disruption of self and, 112
  ego psychology of, 114-116
  group therapy for, 200

[Nightmares]
  implications of, for therapy, 119-
    120
  in masked psychological reactions,
    278
  night terror vs, 103
  oedipal conflicts and, 114
  phenelzine sulfate for, 226
  in posttraumatic stress disorder,
    224
  in REM sleep, 104, 239
  self-psychology of, 118-119
  suicidal repression via, 108
  from traumatic experiences, 1
  in traumatic neuroses, 33-34, 49,
    103-120
  vulnerability and helplessness in,
    104
Nocturnal enuresis, 239
Noise hypersensitivity, 68
Norpinephrine, 230

Object relations
  in personality development, 165
  in psychoanalytic psychotherapy,
    34-39
  in war neurosis, 110, 165
Operation Peace of Galilee, 279
Oppenheim, Herman, 16
Organic syndromes, 16

Pan-suspicious attitude, 163-164
  group therapy for, 207
  of rap group members, 176
Paralysis, 27
Paranoia, 60
  rage and, 202
  rap group members exhibiting, 176
Parenting competence of Vietnam
    veterans, 163
Patient education
  in group therapy, 175
  on transference, 95-96
Persecutory guilt, 73
Personality
  dreams in elucidation of structure
    of, 104-105
  multiple, 9
  predisposed to war neurosis, 104
  for psychotherapy, 131

[Personality]
  in somnambulism, 9
  in survivor syndrome, 19
  traumatic experiences affecting, 1
  traumatic war neurosis affecting,
    106
Pharmacologic treatment of war
    neurosis, 226, 229-248
  lithium carbonate, 246-247
  monoamine oxidase inhibitors,
    229-238
  tricyclics, 245-246
Phenelzine sulfate, 222-226
  for anxiety, 226
  for cardiac neurosis symptoms, 231
  case studies with usage of, 227-
    229, 234-238, 240-245
  clinical studies of, 232-233
  dosage for, 227
  for flashbacks, 245
  for nightmares, 226-227, 240
  sleep affected by, 245
Phenylethylamine, 230
Phobias
  rap groups for treating, 175
  in survivor syndrome, 19
  of trauma, 225
  from traumatic experiences, 1
Physical injury, 16, 276-277
Physioneuroses, 222
Posttraumatic stress disorder
  acute and chronic phases of, 223,
    224
  alcohol and drug abuse with, 161
  battle fatigue in, 126
  diagnosis of, 105
    difficulties in, 226
  group therapy for, 162
  monoamine oxidase inhibitors for,
    230, 233-234
  outcome studies of, 225-229
  stress responses and, 126
  symptoms of, 199-207
    Agent Orange anxiety, 206-207
    alienation, 201
    anxiety, 206
    authority factor, 203-204
    automatic incursive phenomena,
      200-201
    depression, 207

[Posttraumatic stress disorder]
  [symptoms of]
    gook-identification guilt, 204
    guilt of commission and omis-
      sion, 204
    guilt-about-guilt, 204-205
    impacted grief states, 203
    intimacy and relationship with
      women, 205-206
    laundered aggression, 203
    life course alteration, 207
    long-term course of, 225
    narcisstic rage, 202
    nontrusting attitude, 201-202
    pan-suspicious attitude, 207
    paranoid rage, 202
    reactive numbing of self, 199-
      200
    self-against-self aggression, 203
    self-maintenance aggression, 203
    survivor guilt, 205
    symptomatic aggression, 202-
      203
  treatment of, 224, 226
  war neurosis vs, 126
Preconscious state, 113
Projection, 57
  in fear of death, 266
  of guilt, 71-72
Psychoanalytic psychotherapy
  analytic space for, 80-81
  attitudinal change and, 40
  brief, 131-148
    barometer of anxiety in, 139-
      142
    focus of, 137-139
    masculinity and, 147-148
    outcome of, 148
    patient selection for, 131-133
    technical consideration for, 137-
      146
    termination of, 137
    work-up for, 133-136
  for character disorder, 40-41
  for combat psychopathology, 26-
    27, 40
  countertransference in, 96-99
  gauging anxiety in, 139-142
  in group therapy, 168, 188-192
  for guilt, 71-82

[Psychoanalytic psychotherapy]
  for Israeli war veterans, 291-292
  motivation in, 132
  object relations approach to, 34-39
  psychic trauma in, 27-30, 32-34
  regressed character in, chronic, 42-
    44
  regressed character in, delayed, 42
  therapeutic alliance in, 87
  therapeutic pitfalls in, 96-98
  therapist's personal history influ-
    encing, 81
  timing of, 301
  transference in, 86, 87
  for Vietnam veteran, 23-44, 131-
    148
  for World War II veterans, 30-32
Psychodynamic group therapy
  for alcohol and drug abuse, 161
  for becoming comfortable and
    aware of feelings, 207-208
  critical issues in, 156
  diversity of members in, 169
  for enhancing growth by character
    change, 208-214
  for expediency of treatment, 156
  experiential, 160
  flexible treatment plan in, 166
  group development via, 169
  homogenous group composition
    for, 168
  indications for, 156
  individual therapy concurrent with,
    157
  individuation as goal in, 168-169
  limitations of, 156
  model for, 163-214
    cognitive-emotional, 161-162
    integration in, 192
  life-cycle group development in,
    169
  linear-progressive group develop-
    ment in, 169
  linear-regressive group develop-
    ment in, 169-170
  multiple-group, 166-170
  pendular group development in,
    169
  psychoanalytically-oriented
    group in, 188-192

[Psychodynamic group therapy]
  [model for]
    rap group in, 170-188
    rap group members in, 192-198
    single-group, 169-170
  overview of, in treatment of
    veterans, 153-163
  parental figures represented in,
    172-173
  power play in, 171
  primary group cohesiveness in, 168,
    169
  rap groups in. See Rap group
  reattribution process in, 162
  secondary group cohesiveness in,
    169
  setting for, 158
  for special needs and problems of
    Vietnam veterans, 163-166
  therapeutic group interactions in,
    198-207
    on Agent Orange anxiety, 206-
      207
    on alienation, 201
    on anxiety, 206
    authority factor in, 203-204
    on automatic incursive phenom-
      ena, 200-201
    on depression, 207
    on guilt feelings, 204-205
    on impacted grief states, 203
    on intimacy and relationships
      with women, 205-206
    on laundered aggression, 203
    on life course alterations, 207
    on narcisstic rage, 202
    on nontrusting attitudes, 201-
      202
    on pan-suspicious attitude, 207
    on paranoid rage, 202
    on rage reactions, 202
    on reactive numbing of self,
      199-200
    on self-against-self aggression,
      203
    on self-maintenance aggression,
      203
    on symptomatic aggression,
      202-203
  value of, 155

Psychogenic pain, 233
Psychopathology
   combat, 26-27, 40
   of war, 33-34
Psychophysiologic aspects of war
   neurosis, 221-248
Psychosynthesis, 153
Psychotherapy
   group. *See* Psychodynamic group
      therapy
   psychoanalytic. *See* Psychoanalytic
      psychotherapy
Puysegur, 7-8

Rage
   towards authority figures, 88, 89
   group therapy for treatment of,
      202-203
   laundered aggression and, 203
   narcisstic, 202
   narcisstic injury with, 109-110
   paranoid, 202
   rap groups for treating, 175
   self-against-self aggression and, 203
   self-maintenance aggression and,
      203
   symtomatic aggression and, 202-
      203
   in war neurosis, 39
Rap group
   affinity in, 160
   catalyzing group agents in, 182
   concentric circle concept of, 173
   in dealing with posttraumatic stress
      disorder symptoms, 199-207
      Agent Orange anxiety, 206-207
      alienation, 201
      anxiety, 206
      authority factor, 203-204
      automatic incursive phenomena,
         200-201
      depression, 207
      gook-identification guilt, 204
      guilt of commission and omis-
         sion, 204
      guilt-about-guilt, 204-205
      impacted grief states, 203
      intimacy and relationship with
         women, 205-206
      laundered aggression, 203

[Rap group]
   [in dealing with posttraumatic
      stress disorder symptoms]
      life course alteration, 207
      narcisstic rage, 202
      nontrusting attitude, 201-202
      pan-suspicious attitude, 207
      paranoid rage, 202
      reactive numbing of self, 199-
         200
      self-against-self aggression, 203
      self-maintenance aggression, 203
      survivor guilt, 205
      symptomatic aggression, 202-
         203
   dependency in, 171
   description of members of, 192-
      198
   developmental crisis in, 181, 183
   for dealing with posttraumatic
      stress disorder symptoms,
      199-207
   diagnosis issues in, 176-177
   goals of, 174-175
   group-centered approach to, 184
   phallic stage of psychosexual
      development in, 186
   qualities of leader of, 177-180
   selection criteria for membership
      in, 176
   in first-phase group therapy, 170-
      180, 215
   frontal technical approach to, 160
   function of, 170
   ghost presence of leader in, 179
   group cohesion in, 171-172
   group-centered, 184
   hatching process of, 181
   historical overview of, 158
   honesty in, 178
   integration of tri-phasic, 192
   leader-centered, 184
   maturational–developmental pro-
      gression in, 173
   motivational factor in selection of
      members for, 177
   oblique technical approach to, 160
   with posttraumatic stress disorder
      members, 177
   power play in, 171

[Rap group]
  in second-phase group therapy,
    180-188, 215
  anal stage of psychosexual
    development in, 186
  for becoming comfortable and
    aware of feelings, 207-208
  ego autonomy in,
  goals of, 184-185
  leader-centered approach to, 184
  qualities of leader of, 187-188
  selection criteria for member-
    ship in, 185-187
  self-generation in, 160
  size of, 177
  therapist in, 158-160
  in thrid-phase group therapy, 188-
    192, 215-216
  characterological resistances in,
    210
  cohesion of, 191
  for enhancing growth by char-
    acter change, 208-214
  goals of, 188
  individual identity in, 209
  oral stage of psychosexual
    development concerns in, 191
  qualities of leader for, 189-192
  selection criteria for member-
    ship in, 189
  transference in, 159
  for Vietnam veteran therapy, 157-
    158
REM sleep, 240
  in awakened state, 245
  dreams in, 239
  lithium carbonate effect on, 246
  night terrors in, 104
  nightmares in, 104
  role of, 117
  tricyclic antidepressant effect on,
    246
Regression, 37-38
  character disorders, 42-44
  failure of psychologic function vs,
    104
  in fear of death, 263
  guilt and, 75, 76, 77
  id, ego, superego, in combat neuro-
    sis, 281

[Regression]
  reactive numbing of self and, 199
Relaxation as group therapy tech-
    nique, 175, 200
Repression
  postwar, 51
  of psychic trauma, 28
  in stress response, 128
Revenge in war neurosis, 111
Rolfing, 153

Scapegoats, 71
Schizophrenia
  postwar, 54
  of rap group members, 176-177
Self-esteem, 110, 111, 165
  in mechanism of combat reactions,
    282
  rap sessions for improving, 174
  in short-term psychotherapy, 302
Self-punshment, 58, 61, 65
  fear of dead and, 260, 262
  guilt and, unconscious, 71
Semler, Johann Saloman, 5
Sensitivity training, 153
Separation anxiety, 107
Serotonin, 230
Sex in neurosis etiology, 27-28
Shell shock, 15
Shock trauma, 31
Sleep
  delta, 239
  NREM, 239
  REM. See REM sleep
  stages of, 239
Sleep disturbances
  nightmares. See Nightmares
  noise-sensitive, 247
  postcombat, 50
  in survivor syndrome, 19
Smith, Helene, 10
Social adjustment, postwar,
    48
Socioeconomic class vs breakdown,
    283
Sodium amytal, 224
Somatoneuroses, 222
Somnambulism, 7-8, 239
State anxiety, 283
Strain trauma, 31

Stress
in combat psychopathology, 39, 40
conditions of event perspective on
reactions to, 154
dreams reflecting, 116
general response to, 126, 127
in posttraumatic stress disorder,
105
predisposition perspective on
reactions to, 154
process perspective on reactions to,
154
techniques for reduction of, 175
Stress response syndrome, 126, 127,
128
Suez campaign, 274
Suicide attempts, 51, 52
Superego, 18
auxiliary, in therapy, 78
father identification and, 73-74,
76, 77
in fear of death, 264, 265
guilt and, 71, 72, 73
regressed postcombat, 76, 78, 281
Superstition, 2-3
Survivor syndrome, 19, 75

Therapist
as authority figure, 89
in countertransference, 96
errors of, in therapy, 97-98, 100
identification with, 90, 92-94
personal history of, influencing
therapy, 81
as rap group leader, 158-160, 170,
177-180
reactions of, to brutality of war
crimes, 96-97
sympathy of, for Vietnam veteran,
97-98
Trait anxiety, 291
Tranquilizers, 224
Transactional analysis, 153
Transference
authority and, 87-89
definition of, 86
with ego development arrested, 159
with fear of dead, 259
in group therapy, 156
guilt and, unconscious, 72, 75

[Transference]
handling, in therapy, 90
by identification with therapist,
90, 92-94
by interpreting via extra therapy
situations, 90, 92
negative reactions, 90, 94-96
by restraint from early interpretation, 90-92
therapists reactions in, 96-99
in historical development of psychotherapy, 12
negative, 94-96
in object relations approach to psychotherapy, 38
patient education on, 95-96
in therapy for guilt, 52, 58, 79-
80
in veteran rap groups, 159
Trauma, psychic
cumulative, 1
definition of, 104
dramatic rehearsal of, 18
dreams and, 103
ego affected by, 19
problems of, in psychoanalytic
theory, 32-34
in psychoanalytic theory, 27-30
shock vs strain, 31
superego affected by, 18
tolerance for, 1
Traumatic neuroses
classical symptoms of, 164
description of, 106
historical overview of, 15-16, 106-
113
organic basis for, 16
psychoneurotic complications of,
17
Tremors, 26-27
Tricyclic antidepressants, 245-246
Trust
as criterion in psychotherapy
patient selection, 131
group therapy for improving, 201-
202
rap sessions for improving, 175
trauma affecting sense of, 105
Tryptamine, 230
Tyramine, 230

Unconscious state
    dreams as outlet for, 114
    guilt in, 47-82

Veith, Ilza, 6, 14
Veterans Outreach Program, 26
Vietnam Veterans Against the War,
    158
Vietnam war
    CIA in, 124
    casualties from, 23
    combat wounds and deaths in, 24-25
    hypocrisy of, 87
    nature and style of, 23
    political and moral support for, 85,
        165
    psychic numbing of, 53
    societal response to soldiers re-
        turning from, 85-86, 164-
        165, 254, 264
    soldiers of, statistics on, 24, 164
    special needs and problems of com-
        batant in, 163-166
    violence of, uncontrolled, 53

War neurosis
    characteristics of, 111
    combat. See Combat neuroses
    death instinct in, 108
    etiology of, 18, 108
    fatigue in, 31
    Freudian theory on, 28, 29, 108
    group therapy for. See Psycho-
        dynamic group therapy
    guilt in, 47-82
    historical overview of, 1-21, 106-
        113
        from past to World War I, 1-16
        from World War I to present,
        16-21
    insecurity in, 111
    from Israeli wars, 269-302
        symptomatology and content of
        symptoms in, 285-286
        treatment of, 286-302

[War neurosis]
    libido affecting, 108
    motor symptoms of, 126
    narcissism in, 109, 110
    from neuronal damage, 222
    nightmares as symptom of, 103-120
    object relations approach to, 35-39
    organic basis for, 15-16
    prior parental relationships to, 107
    peacetime vs, 18, 32
    pharmacologic therapy for, 221,
        229-238
        lithium carbonate, 246-247
        monoamine oxidase inhibitors,
        229-238
        tricyclics, 245-246
    posttraumatic stress disorder vs,
        126
    psychoanalytic therapy for. See
        Psychoanalytic psycho-
        therapy
    psychophysiologic aspects of, 221-
        248
    revenge in, 111
    separation-anxiety in, 36
    traumatic dreams of, 29
    treatment environment for, 166
    treatment refractoriness in, 281
    vulnerability in, 111
War of Attrition, 275, 277
War superego, 18
Wish fulfillment theory of dreams, 114
World War I
    combat psychopathology in, 26
    historical overview of war neurosis
        up to, 1-16
World War II
    combat psychopathology in, 27
    historical overview of war neurosis
        following, 16-21
    psychoanalytic theory from, 30-
        31

Yom Kippur War, 269, 274, 275, 277,
    281